Bodies of Evidence

Dedicating objects to the divine was a central component of both Greek and Roman religion. Some of the most conspicuous offerings were shaped like parts of the internal or external human body: so-called 'anatomical votives'. These archaeological artefacts capture the modern imagination, recalling vividly the physical and fragile bodies of the past whilst posing interpretative challenges in the present. This volume scrutinises this distinctive dedicatory phenomenon, bringing together for the first time a range of methodologically diverse approaches which challenge traditional assumptions and simple categorisations. The chapters presented here ask new questions about what constitutes an anatomical votive; how they were used and manipulated in cultural, cultic and curative contexts; and the complex role of anatomical votives in negotiations between humans and gods, the body and its disparate parts, divine and medical healing, ancient assemblages and modern collections and collectors. In seeking to recontextualise and reconceptualise anatomical votives this volume uniquely juxtaposes the medical with the religious; the social with the conceptual; the idea of the body in fragments with the body whole and the museum with the sanctuary, crossing the boundaries between studies of ancient religion, medicine, the body and the reception of antiquity.

Jane Draycott is Lord Kelvin Adam Smith Research Fellow in Ancient Science and Technology at the University of Glasgow. Her research focuses on health and well-being in antiquity. She has published on a wide range of subjects relating to the history and archaeology of medicine.

Emma-Jayne Graham is Senior Lecturer in Classical Studies at The Open University. Her research focuses on the archaeology of Roman Italy, with a particular interest in the treatment of the body and its representation in material culture. She has published on mortuary practices, infant health and death, sensory experience and the materiality of votive religion.

Medicine and the Body in Antiquity

Series Editor: Patricia Baker
University of Kent, UK

Series Advisory Board

Lesley A. Dean-Jones
University of Texas at Austin, USA

Rebecca Gowland
University of Durham, UK

Jessica Hughes
Open University, UK

Ralph Rosen
University of Pennsylvania, USA

Kelli Rudolph
University of Kent, UK

Medicine and the Body in Antiquity is a new series which aims to foster interdisciplinary research that broadens our understanding of past beliefs about the body and its care. The intention of the series is to use evidence drawn from diverse sources (textual, archaeological, epigraphic) in an interpretative manner to gain insights into the medical practices and beliefs of the ancient Mediterranean. The series approaches medical history from a broad thematic perspective that allows for collaboration between specialists from a wide range of disciplines outside ancient history and archaeology such as art history, religious studies, medicine, the natural sciences and music. The series will also aim to bring research on ancient medicine to the attention of scholars concerned with later periods. Ultimately this series provides a forum for scholars from a wide range of disciplines to explore ideas about the body and medicine beyond the confines of current scholarship.

Bodies of Evidence

Ancient anatomical votives
past, present and future

**Edited by
Jane Draycott**

University of Glasgow

Emma-Jayne Graham

The Open University

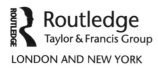
Routledge
Taylor & Francis Group

LONDON AND NEW YORK

First published 2017 by Routledge

2 Park Square, Milton Park, Abingdon, Oxfordshire OX14 4RN

52 Vanderbilt Avenue, New York, NY 10017

Routledge is an imprint of the Taylor & Francis Group, an informa business

First issued in paperback 2020

British Library Cataloguing in Publication Data
A catalogue record for this book is available from the British Library

Library of Congress Cataloging in Publication Data
Names: Draycott, Jane (Jane Louise), editor.
Title: Bodies of evidence : ancient anatomical votives past, present, and
    future / edited by Jane Draycott, University of Wales, Trinity Saint
    David and Emma-Jayne Graham, The Open University.
Description: New York : Routledge, 2016. | Includes bibliographical
    references and index.
Identifiers: LCCN 2016029146 | ISBN 9781472450807 (hardback : alk. paper)
Subjects: LCSH: Greece—Religion. .| Rome—Religion. | Votive offerings—
    Greece. | Votive offerings—Rome. | Human body—Miscellanea.
Classification: LCC BL795.V6 B63 2016 | DDC 292.3/7—dc23
LC record available at https://lccn.loc.gov/2016029146

ISBN: 978-1-4724-5080-7 (hbk)
ISBN: 978-0-367-59557-9 (pbk)

Typeset in Bembo
by Apex CoVantage, LLC

Contents

Figures

Contributors

Ellen Adams is Lecturer in Classical Art and Archaeology at King's College London. After receiving her PhD from Cambridge on Minoan Crete, she spent two years based at Athens on a Leverhulme Study Abroad Studentship, and then two years at Trinity College Dublin on an Irish Research Council for Humanities and Social Sciences (IRCHSS) Postdoctoral Fellowship. She has published a variety of articles on Minoan Crete and also researches the classical tradition in the museums of London, and how Classics may engage with Disability.

Sara Chiarini is presently Lecturer at the University of Magdeburg. After receiving her PhD from the University of Milan she lectured at the Freie University, Berlin, and at the University of Exeter. Among her awards are a research grant from the British Academy and a scholarship from the Fondation Hardt. She is the author of *L'archeologia dello Scutum Herculis* (Aracne, 2012). Her coming second book is a comprehensive study of nonsense inscriptions on Greek vase painting, and she has just started her next project on the tension between formularity and subjectivity in the Greek and Latin curse tablets.

Olivier de Cazanove is Professor of Roman archeology at the University of Paris I – Sorbonne. He is particularly interested in Roman and provincial religion and has published widely on the archaeology of ritual, especially the votive offerings of Italy and Gaul.

Jane Draycott is Lord Kelvin Adam Smith Research Fellow in Ancient Science and Technology at the University of Glasgow. After receiving her PhD from the University of Nottingham, she was 2011–2012 Rome Fellow at the British School at Rome, Associate University Teacher in the Department of Archaeology at the University of Sheffield and Lecturer in Classics at the University of Wales Trinity Saint David. She has published on the history and archaeology of ancient medicine.

Rebecca Flemming is Senior Lecturer in Ancient History in the Faculty of Classics, and Fellow of Jesus College, University of Cambridge. She has published widely on medicine and gender in the ancient world, both jointly and separately. She is co-editor of the forthcoming volume *Reproduction: A History from Antiquity to the Present Day*.

Fay Glinister is presently a Lecturer at Cardiff University. She has previously been a Research Associate at Cambridge University on the Wellcome Trust's Generation to Reproduction project, and before that was a Research Fellow at University College London as part of the Festus Lexicon Project and as a British Academy Postdoctoral Fellow. She has published articles on votive offerings, on gender and religion, and on the religious contexts of Roman colonisation, and co-edited the book *Verrius, Festus and Paul* (Institute of Classical Studies, Bulletin Supplement No. S93, 2007).

Emma-Jayne Graham is Senior Lecturer in Classical Studies at The Open University. She was Rome Fellow at the British School at Rome (2005–2006) and previously taught at the Universities of Cardiff, St. Andrews and Leicester. Her research focuses on the archaeology of Roman Italy, with a particular interest in the body and its representation in material culture. She has published on mortuary practices and the treatment of the human body in death, swaddled infant votives, sensory experience and the materiality of religion. Together with Jessica Hughes she runs the research network *The Votives Project* (www.thevotivesproject.org).

Jen Grove is an Engaged Research Fellow in the Centre for Medical History at the University of Exeter, on a Wellcome Trust–funded research project *Rethinking Sexology: The Cross-Disciplinary Invention of Sexuality: Sexual Science Beyond the Medical, 1890–1940*. She has published on the history of sexuality, focusing on the modern collection and reception of sexually related artefacts, and is the editor of a forthcoming book *Sculpture, Sexuality and History: Encounters in Literature, Culture and the Arts from the Eighteenth Century to the Present* (Palgrave, 2017, with Jana Funke). Jen was consultant on the Wellcome Collection's major exhibition 'Institute of Sexology', 2014–2015, and she works on the award-winning Sex and History project, which collaborates with museums, schools, charities and young people throughout the UK, using artefacts from the past to get people talking about sex today.

Laurent Haumesser is Chief Curator in the Department of Greek, Etruscan and Roman Antiquities at the Louvre Museum, a former student of the Ecole Normale Supérieure and a member of the French School of Rome. His research focuses on Etruscan paintings and bronzes, as well as on the history of archaeological and historical collections. He was one of the commissioners of the Italian exhibition *Gli Etruschi dall'Arno al Tevere. Le collezioni del Louvre a Cortona* in 2011 and the exhibition *Les Etrusques et la Méditerranée. La cité de Cerveteri* at the Louvre-Lens and in Rome in 2013–2014. He is one of the authors of *L'Art étrusque. 100 chefs-d'œuvre du musée du Louvre*, published in 2013.

Jessica Hughes is Lecturer in Classical Studies at The Open University. Her research focuses on the themes of objects, memory and religion, and her publications include a forthcoming monograph on anatomical votives from classical antiquity. Together with Emma-Jayne Graham she runs the research network *The Votives Project* (www.thevotivesproject.org).

Georgia Petridou is Lecturer in Ancient Greek History at the University of Liverpool and works on Classical Literature, History of Greek and Roman Religion, and Ancient Medicine in its sociopolitical context. She is the author of *Divine Epiphany in Greek Literature and Culture* (OUP, 2015) and the co-editor (with Chiara Thumiger) of *Homo Patiens. Approaches on the Patient in the Ancient World* (Brill, 2016).

Justine Potts is a doctoral research student in Ancient History at Balliol College, Oxford, and a UK Arts and Humanities Research Council award holder. A fair weather archaeologist, she has worked on various excavations in Italy, most recently on the north slope of Vesuvius, and at Aeclanum, for the Apolline Project. Her doctorate is on the confession of sin in the Roman world and her research interests include the history and archaeology of ancient religions, classical reception in Arabic and Persian literature, and the cult of Isis.

Preface

The core of this book stems from a conference entitled *Bodies of Evidence: Re-defining Approaches to the Anatomical Votive* organised by the editors and hosted by the British School at Rome in June 2012. Additional papers were commissioned on the subjects of confession stelai and footprints, in addition to two new chapters contributed by the editors (on votive hair and on personhood in Italy, respectively) as well as an afterword. Other papers were also presented in Rome by Letizia Ceccarelli (a votive deposit at Fidenae), Jessica Hughes (hybridity and rites of passage), Ergün Lafli (ear plaques from Asia Minor) and Matthias Recke (polyvisceral votives).

Modern scholarship has categorised as 'anatomical' a range of *ex-votos* which depict parts of the human body. Reliefs and models depicting arms, legs, eyes, fingers, hands, feet, uteri, genitals, internal organs and other recognisable parts of the internal and external body have attracted attention from scholars exploring religion and health alike in different disciplines. Nevertheless, the category of 'anatomical offering' remains noticeably ill defined. The Rome conference sought to bring together scholars working on anatomical offerings in their broadest sense from across a range of historical and cultural contexts in order to explore and refine understandings of this phenomenon. Key questions posed by speakers at the conference included what anatomical votives were for, what they represented to those who dedicated, encountered or made them, and what factors influenced the selection of a particular item. Presented papers were concerned with what these distinctive offerings can reveal, not only about past religious and medical contexts and practices, but also about identity, society, politics and concepts or constructions of the human body, both past and present. In particular, speakers and participants at the conference debated how we might define and interpret the 'anatomical' votive. The results of some of these discussions, along with new explorations of their consequences, are presented in this volume.

We are especially grateful to the British School at Rome for hosting the original conference, especially Christopher Smith, the director of the school, but also all of the other staff members who provided administrative and technical support on the day, not to mention vital sustenance for our bodies. Special thanks go to Peppe Pellegrino and Antonio Palmieri for generously giving up their time to

help with this. We would also like to thank all of the speakers and other participants who provided sustenance for our minds by making it a dynamic day of
discussion and debate which has culminated ultimately in the chapters presented
here. These thanks extend, of course, to those noted earlier whose work is not
included in the final publication. Thanks are due also to Jean Turfa and Jessica
Hughes for their critical and thoughtful reading of early drafts of each chapter.
We are grateful to all individuals, museums and institutions that have provided
illustrations or allowed us to publish material in their collections.

Jane Draycott and Emma-Jayne Graham

Abbreviations

CIG	*Corpus inscriptionum graecarum.* (Berlin 1828–77)
CIL	*Corpus inscriptionum latinarum.* (Berlin 1893–)
Drew-Bear	Drew-Bear, T., Thomas, C.M. and Yildizturan, M., 1999. *Phrygian votive steles.* Ankara: Turkish Republic Ministry of Culture.
IDelos	*Inscriptions de Délos,* 7 vols. (Paris 1926–72)
IEleusis	Clinton, K. ed., *Eleusis: the inscriptions on stone. Documents of the two goddesses and public documents of the Deme.* (Athens 2005–8)
IG	*Inscriptiones graecae.* (Berlin 1895–)
IGBulg	Michailov, G. ed., *Inscriptiones Graecae in Bulgaria repertae.* (Sofia 1959–66)
IGUR	Moretti, L., *Inscriptiones Graecae Urbis Romae,* 4 vols. (Rome 1968–90)
LIMC	Boardman, J. ed., *Lexicon Iconographicum Mythologiae Classicae.* (Zürich, München, Düsseldorf 1981–99)
New Documents	Hermann, P. and Malay, H., 2007. *New documents from Lydia.* Vienna: Verlag der Österreichischen Akademie der Wissenschaften.
Petzl	Petzl, G., 1994. Die Beichtinschriften Westkleinasiens. *Epigraphica Anatolica,* 22, pp. 1–143.
Researches	Malay, H., 1999. *Researches in Lydia, Mysia and Aiolis.* Vienna: Verlag der Österreichischen Akademie der Wissenschaften.
Syll.	*Syllecta Classica.* (Iowa)
TAM	*Tituli Asiae Minoris.* (Vienna)

Introduction

Debating the anatomical votive

Emma-Jayne Graham and Jane Draycott

Consider the following scenes. The first involves a visit to the Asclepieion on the south slope of the Acropolis at Athens, during the early third century BC. Upon entering the monumental temple of Asclepius we meet a number of men in the process of taking an inventory of the items arranged on the walls and in the rafters, as well as those placed directly onto the cult statue itself. Eventually, they tell us, the results of their survey are to be inscribed on a large, rectangular slab of marble, which will be set up somewhere in the vicinity of the temple (*IG* II² 1534A; Aleshire, 1989, p. 166). Following the men as they work their way around the darkened sacred space, their attention piqued by items made of precious metal, our own eyes take in the gold and silver of the cult statue against the west wall and the objects that cluster around it, those which sit on or hang from the rafters, cross-beams and ridge-beam of the roof, and others arranged in rows on the walls to right and left (Aleshire, 1991, pp. 42–3). The inventory makers make notes about models and relief images of eyes, ears, mouths, an abdomen, a silver hand, a jaw, legs and male and female bodies, sometimes recording their weight and consequent economic value (Aleshire, 1991, pp. 199–200). Although the inventory makers pay them scant attention, we can also make out objects made of less precious materials. Amongst these, clustered largely on the lower levels of the right-hand wall, are a number of stone models and reliefs depicting human body parts including breasts, genitalia and feet (van Straten, 1981, pp. 106–8; Aleshire, 1991, p. 45). The scene is reminiscent of a similar arrangement within the Asclepieion of Corinth where relief plaques featuring breasts, genitals, ears and eyes, as well as terracotta arms, hands, feet and legs moulded in the round can be seen suspended from nails or leather thongs, with others freestanding or placed against a wall (Roebuck, 1951, p. 116) (Figure I.1).

In our second scene we find ourselves wandering the winding streets of the medieval town of Arezzo, Italy. It is 1493, and our stroll brings us to a shop specialising in the sale of religious items made from wax. Upon entering we find the shop filled with objects including, according to the owner's inventory, anatomical models in the form of 'heads, eyes, teeth, chests, breasts, arms, hands, legs, feet, hearts, swaddled babies . . . in large, small and medium sizes' (Holmes, 2009, p. 161). Many of these items, says the owner, will subsequently find their way

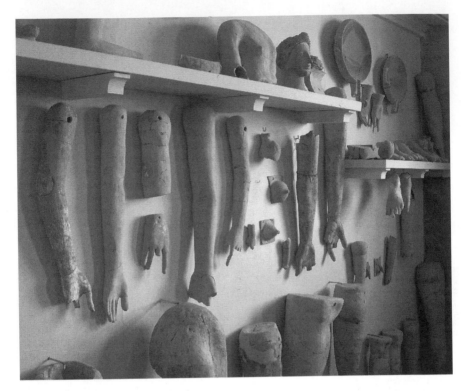

Figure I.1 Terracotta votive body parts dedicated at the Asclepieion of Corinth, shown hanging from nails and resting on shelves as they may once have been displayed in the sanctuary.

Source: Courtesy of www.HolyLandPhotos.org.

into local churches where they will be left as material testimonies to miraculous acts of healing (Thompson, 2005, pp. 214–15; Holmes, 2009, p. 163) (Figure I.2).

Finally, we are transported to the twenty-first century, to the sanctuary of Santa Quitéria das Frexeiras in northeastern Brazil where we encounter an ordinary-looking building painted sky blue with a roof of brown terracotta tiles (Terra, 2014). Inside the building the walls are covered – one might even say cluttered – with offerings: paintings, drawings, photographs, clothing, flowers, posters, crutches and, most strikingly of all, a series of wooden carvings of human figurines and body parts. Into one wall is set an arched doorway opening into the area containing the altar to the martyr. This wall is covered with near-life-sized hands, arms and legs made from heavily varnished wood (Figure I.3). Shelves lining other walls bear individualised busts, breasts and feet, some of which carry painted names, along with terracotta models re-creating scenes from the modern operating theatre.

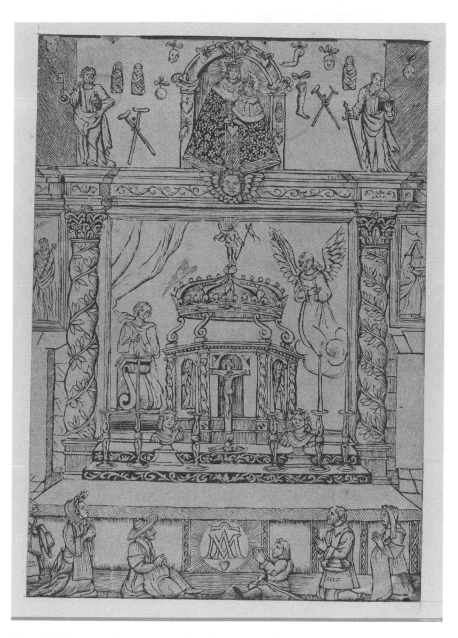

Figure I.2 Seventeenth-century woodcut showing an altar surmounted by a statue of the Virgin surrounded by votive offerings, including hearts, swaddled babies, crutches, legs and arms. In the foreground sick or troubled people are praying.

Source: Wellcome Library, London. Wellcome Library Iconographic Collection 643133i.

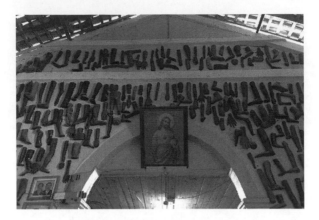

Figure I.3 Wooden anatomical votives in the shape of arms, legs, hands and feet in the sanctuary of Santa Quitéria das Frexeiras, Brazil.

Source: Image courtesy of Anna Terra.

All of the dedicated (or yet to be dedicated) objects described in these scenes are by definition the same: they are all examples of *ex-votos*. They are offerings (*donaria* or *anathema*) given as part of a ritual request for divine intervention in the human realm. Within these scenarios we can detect other broad similarities: in all three the human body is represented in complete or fragmented form, and these anatomical models appear as dedications alongside objects which take a variety of other shapes. Similarly, all of these objects are offerings dedicated (or soon to be dedicated) in a sacred setting – be that a temple, Christian church or shrine – to the inhabitants of a divine world. But, at the same time, these three scenes overflow with diversity and creativity. Most noticeably of all the materiality of each of these offerings is different, ranging from precious metals with an economic value determined by their weight to comparatively inexpensive but durable materials such as terracotta and stone, as well as items moulded or carved from malleable but ultimately perishable substances including wax and wood. The gods or sacred figures to whom these objects are (or are to be) devoted range from an ancient god of healing to a Christian martyr. As a consequence, the processes, rituals and religious knowledge produced and experienced when dedicating or encountering each of these dedicatory contexts remain substantially different. Indeed, look closely and the list of differences perhaps outweighs the similarities: some involve the written word, others do not; some will remain on view, others will be periodically cleared away – perhaps even deliberately disposed of or destroyed. Despite these fundamental differences which serve to emphasise the great variety of practice and changing tradition associated with offerings of all types, one thing unites all of the examples given earlier: all of the offerings that reference the human body can be described as 'anatomical votives'.

Getting off on the right foot: defining anatomical votives

But what *is* an anatomical votive? Despite the broad similarities noted earlier, a critical reading of the three scenarios sketched out here suggests that answering this question may be far from straightforward, especially once the historical, religious, social and cultural contexts in which these objects are (or were) used are brought into the picture. Nevertheless, at a most fundamental level an anatomical votive is defined customarily as an *ex-voto* – a gift of thanks made to a divine being – which directly references the human body usually, but not always, by means of visual representation (see, for example, Dasen, 2012). More specifically anatomical votives, both past and present, are categorised as dedicated objects which display or take the form of recognisable *parts* of the body's interior or exterior, most commonly its individual elements (or sometimes pairs of body parts in the case of eyes, ears and breasts), which are depicted as isolated, detached or fragmented from the somatic whole. They include models and relief images of limbs, eyes, ears, hands, genitals, hearts, bladders, uteri, intestines, lungs and a wide range of other parts of the body which are notable largely because they are represented as autonomous objects. It is this which marks out anatomical votives as a category of offering distinct from those which take the form of full-length standing or seated statues and figurines which represent the complete and nonfragmented human body. Traditional definitions of anatomical votives therefore focus on the intentional fragmentation or dismemberment of the human form (although see Hughes, 2008, pp. 222–3 for a compelling critique of this assumption).

It is this rather crude definition based principally on the appearance and form of a dedication which allows us to make connections between the ancient Greek, medieval and modern examples cited earlier. It also makes it possible to identify the occurrence of similar votive objects within a range of other historical and modern religious practices, including those of the ancient Egyptian, Greek and Roman cultural worlds; the many denominations of modern Christianity (such as Roman Catholicism and the Greek and Russian Orthodox churches); Islam; and Hinduism. In many respects the anatomical *ex-votos* which continue to be dedicated at modern shrines and holy places in association with almost the whole gamut of world religions are similar in nature to their ancient counterparts, at least when comparisons are based on their form alone. Look beyond this, however, and the picture becomes more complicated. Modern offerings may often (but not always) be considerably smaller and made more frequently from other materials such as thin sheets of silver or tin and even plastic, although some continue to be carved from wood or moulded from clay by hand or with the aid of a mould. What becomes clear is that even today there is no singular way to produce an anatomical votive, nor indeed has there ever been.

In ancient contexts objects identified as anatomical *ex-votos* are frequently carved or moulded in relief on stone or clay plaques, but might also be fashioned in the round using terracotta, metal, wood, wax or ivory, with or without an accompanying inscription. In the case of some stone reliefs, largely from Greek contexts, multiple different body parts might be displayed either as a group or as individual parts, and some even include images of the human dedicant and/or the divine recipient themselves (Forsén, 2004). Probably the most well-known example of the latter is the late fourth century BC stone relief found in association with the sanctuary of Amynos the hero-physician at Athens shown on the cover of this volume (National Museum of Athens, inv. 3526; see also Figure 11.6). An inscription names the dedicator as Lysimachides, son of Lysimachos from Acharnai, and the relief image depicts him holding a model of an over-life-sized leg with a pronounced (varicose?) vein, alongside two separate feet contained within a recessed panel. With the exception of those from Corinth, the best-known models in the round come from sites in Italy, where the majority of surviving examples are made not from stone but from fired clay (for an introductory overview, see Recke, 2013). However, substantial numbers of three-dimensional anatomical votives from Italy and the western part of the Roman world were also made from bronze or silver (either cast or in the form of thin sheets) and sometimes, more rarely, from gold (for instance, the pair of sheet-gold relief eyes recovered from the baths-basilica complex at Roman Wroxeter in Britain: Painter, 1971). Ancient anatomical votives can also be life sized and miniaturised, or indeed any size in between. Over-life-sized models in the round seem to have been produced rarely, although the example of Lysimachides cautions against the assumption that this was completely unknown, and the nature of the evidence may mean that such items are easily mistaken for fragments of broken statuary or temple decoration.

This volume seeks to infiltrate these cracks within definitions of 'the anatomical votive'. The intention is to move treatments of ancient votive artefacts and assemblages away from a narrow focus on typological characteristics towards a greater understanding of how these objects were used and manipulated in a range of cultural, cultic and curative contexts, both past and present, as well as the meanings and knowledge associated with and produced by their use. In order to do this individual chapters adopt diverse but compatible approaches, investigating the motivations that led to the dedication of offerings which reference directly the human body and the meanings and significance attached to these activities; the ways in which anatomical votives as objects with agency were used, viewed and engaged with and the contexts in which this occurred; the nature of the relationship between anatomical *ex-votos*, concepts of the body, religious experience, medicine and divine healing; and the anatomical votive as part of a commemorative or curated assemblage. Accordingly, the chapters in this volume recontextualise and reconceptualise these apparently familiar artefacts, broadening the traditional parameters of votive studies to include material, ideas and themes which are not regularly integrated into these analyses, including questions of reception and theoretical models derived from anthropological studies of religious materialities and body theory. They ask new questions about exactly where the boundaries circumscribing definitions of 'the anatomical votive' lie, pushing against the margins between humans and gods, the body and its disparate parts, divine and medical healing, collections and collectors. Some of the chapters evaluate dedicated objects not defined traditionally as anatomical votives, such as confession stelai, footprints and hair, as well as the unfragmented bodies of swaddled infants which sit at the fringes of existing definitions. Others look beyond traditional chronological boundaries in order to consider how anatomical *ex-votos* have continued to have meaning for later generations and in turn how these meanings have generated many of the conceptual boundaries subsequently imposed upon them. Stretching the edges of 'the anatomical votive' in this way, integrating these objects within the broader materiality of religious and medical performances, as well as considering an alternative array of contexts in which the agency of votive objects is significant for the articulation of knowledge concerning the human–divine relationship and the body, makes it possible to problematise the idea of *the* anatomical votive. It also makes it possible to consider how positioning these objects in relation to alternative theoretical and methodological frameworks, examining them from new angles, bringing fresh sources to bear on their interpretation and creating more lenses through which to view them can blur established boundaries and typologies, allowing their complex properties as multivalent objects to come into greater focus.

Getting a head: votive practice in ancient contexts

Before going much further, however, we must address briefly the issue of terminology and context against which all of these chapters are set, beginning with the term *ex-voto* and the nature of votive religion in the ancient world. Contributors to this volume focus primarily, although not exclusively, on objects, practices and contexts associated with Greek and Italic/Roman culture, but providing a catch-all definition of votive cult can prove troublesome even for regions and cultural groups known to share at least some cultural and religious connections. The terminology used to write about votive practice – indeed the term 'votive' itself – is derived largely from textual and epigraphic sources of the Roman period and later. This imposes, intentionally or unintentionally, a degree of homogeneity on a type of ritual practice and material culture that might well involve considerable discrepancies in terms of the acts, beliefs, experiences and materialities concerned. Nonetheless, the use of standardised terminology also has its benefits, making it possible write about a type of activity – and a category of object – which finds distinctive expression across space and time and to identify and explore notable points of intersection and divergence from more general sequences of activities and practices.

The term *ex-voto*, still used widely in modern contexts, derives from the Latin formulation whereby a human seeks support, assistance, protection or some other form of specific intervention by means of a direct request or petition made to a divine figure (or figures) and vows to offer something in return if that request is fulfilled (Osborne, 2004; Frateantonio, 2006; Dasen, 2012; Hahn, 2012). The term itself is associated with the second part of this process: the vow (*votum*) that an offering would be made in return for a successful petition. This could be made in relation to everything from personal well-being to the security of a public figure or the Roman imperial family, on either an ad hoc basis or as part of a recurrent periodic vow connected with public religion or stages of the life course (van Straten, 1981, pp. 88–102; Rüpke, 2007, p. 163; Derks, 2014, pp. 59–65). It was this return offering which in Latin was known as an *ex-voto*, commonly anglicised today as 'votive' (for more on the technicalities of votive terminology, see van Straten, 1981; Bodel, 2009). Sometimes this formal relationship is framed as *da ut dem* ('give so that I may give'), providing a powerful reminder of the reciprocal but formal relationship which lay at the heart of this process of negotiation (Hahn, 2012). However, as Rüpke (2007, p. 163) has pointed out, the gods need not uphold their side of the bargain and 'there were no strings attached: the outcome was open'. If this remained the case then there was also no compulsion to make a return gift, meaning, of course, that 'failed vows produce no votives; the system renders its failures invisible' (Rüpke, 2007, p. 164). Nevertheless, the frequency with which objects recovered from sanctuaries, temples, shrines and other sacred places attest to the dedication of items which appear to offer thanks for an answer received or the successful completion of a vow suggests that this process was often considered to have been completed satisfactorily.

The underpinning principles of votive activities, comprising an initial request (probably via a spoken prayer) accompanied by a vow and the promise of a thank offering, followed by a prayer of thanks and the gift itself, can therefore be established with a reasonable degree of confidence (Rives, 2007, pp. 24–5). Sometimes Greek terms are used in modern scholarship to refer to these different stages, including *euchomai* (spoken prayer), *euchē* (vow) and *anathema* (votive gift), but the terms used most commonly to write about this type of religious performance tend to be Latin. They therefore promote a rather Romano-centric formulation of a type of ritual activity that had existed in the ancient Mediterranean for millennia before these terms came into use, even if it is widely accepted that they do offer a useful way of describing the broad outline of this long-lasting tradition. It is, therefore, necessary to remember that a Greek person of the fourth century BC making their offering in thanks to Asclepius at Athens, Corinth or any other healing figure at another sacred site would not have articulated their actions using these words, even if, as epigraphic sources attest, the same recognisable process of making a thank offering was followed (for instance, the public expressions of thanks and offerings described in inscriptions at the Asclepieion of Epidaurus: *IG* IV^2 1, 121–4; Edelstein and Edelstein, 1945 and 1998; LiDonnici, 1992).

The offerings dedicated to commemorate successful vows include the anatomical votives which are the focus of this volume, but also encompassed a range of other dedications, the least ambiguous of which were accompanied by Latin inscriptions employing the revealing phrase *votum solvit libens merito* ('has fulfilled his vow willingly and with good reason') (Turfa, 2006a, p. 91; Rüpke, 2007, pp. 164–5). Offerings might vary not only in terms of their materiality – bronze, silver, gold, ceramic, terracotta and most probably wax and wood, but perhaps also fabrics, foodstuffs, liquids and animal sacrifice – but also their form (van Straten, 1981 remains a useful overview of different types of offerings across the ancient world; see also Rouse, 1902; Forsén, 1996; Turfa, 2006a). *Donaria* could be intended to be durable or ephemeral, or they might comprise objects used in daily life and subsequently surrendered to the gods. Commonly cited examples of the latter include dolls given up on the occasion of marriage and the tools of retired craftsmen (*Palatine Anthology* 4.103–4; van Straten, 1981, pp. 89–96). Alternatively they might take the form of purpose-made models, vessels or figurines (for miniature votive offerings, see Kiernan, 2009). Indeed, the range of possibilities is endless and the opportunities for individuality unlimited as petitioners chose to dedicate items that were meaningful to them, just as visitors to modern holy sites continue to do so today. A comprehensive survey of all votive practice across the length and breadth of the Greco-Roman Mediterranean and its bordering regions is inappropriate in this context, but it should not be forgotten that the anatomical votives singled out for discussion here were part of this considerably larger phenomenon of dedicated objects and a tradition which encompassed a high degree of convention but also creativity.

Challenges arise when attempting to reconstruct and explain the nuances of these shared activities, especially because so few written accounts of votive rituals survive and interpretations must rely heavily on surviving material culture. What is more, by its very nature this evidence represents only one act – and the final one at that – in a potentially protracted sequence of activities. In most instances it can be assumed that the material offerings recovered from sacred sites were dedicated at the end of the petitioning process as a gift of thanks to the deity in question and that they are, by definition, true *ex-votos*. Indeed, this behaviour is precisely what is attested in epigraphic evidence, such as that provided by the inscribed Epidauran *iamata* (tales of miracle cures) and later inscriptions from Pergamum (Edelstein and Edelstein, 1945 and 1998; Petsalis-Diomidis, 2010). It remains possible that gifts were also given in association with the prayer spoken on the occasion of the initial petition, perhaps as a means of formalising the relationship and a demonstration of appropriate respect for divine power. It is not impossible to imagine that a less durable offering might be an appropriate accompaniment to this initial request: food or a libation, something that was tangible but transient which might deteriorate or disperse before any final offering was made as a way of embodying the passing of time or the ephemeral nature of the spoken prayer, even a way of ensuring that the god did not receive more than they were due as part of the 'no strings attached' nature of the vow.

The nature of anatomical votives has prompted further speculation about the point at which offerings were made. Their potential to draw attention to an afflicted, diseased or injured part of the body and therefore to the specific request that was being made of the god – even to act as a 'visual' reminder of the anticipated outcome – has led to the suggestion that in some circumstances they were dedicated along with the initial request for divine assistance or cure (see discussion in Schultz, 2006, pp. 102–5). There is no corroborative evidence for this, and the absence of pathological indications on the majority of anatomical votives suggests that this was at least not typical (Turfa, 2004, pp. 360–61; de Cazanove, 2009). Jean Turfa (2006b) has also questioned whether it was even possible for petitioners suffering from incapacitating illness or disease to travel to the site of shrines and sanctuaries, which in many Italian cases were located in inaccessible locations or at a considerable distance from settlement centres. Not only does this seem to preclude the presence of hospitals and treatment centres – in contrast to the major healing sanctuaries of the eastern Mediterranean, including Pergamum – but she argues that it also suggests that most dedicants visited sacred sites only when they had become well enough to do so (Turfa, 2006b, p. 72 and p. 79). Observations such as this raise broader questions about the nature of ancient pilgrimage and the fact that the difficult journey undertaken to reach a sanctuary, as well as movement around it upon arrival, might form a crucial part of the supplicant's 'offering' of worship and thanks to a deity (for healing pilgrimage, see Petsalis-Diomidis, 2005; 2006; 2010; on pilgrimage more generally, see chapters in Elsner and Rutherford, 2005). Perhaps, therefore, we should conceptualise the process of making offerings as a more protracted one involving multiple dedications of differing types, both material and immaterial. Moreover, it must not be forgotten that the timing of offerings of discrete types may have been connected directly with the specific nature of the request, or indeed of the offering itself, as chapters in this volume make clear (Glinister on infant socialisation and Petridou on eyes as a testament to mysteric enlightenment).

On the one hand: studying anatomical votives

Bridging the spheres of religion, medicine, the body and reception studies, as well as very specialist coroplastic and regional-based fields, the anatomical votive sits comfortably in multiple categories. In fact they are in one sense quite well known: visually evocative examples are often used to illustrate general discussions of ancient votive practice or 'name-checked' as a particularly striking and intriguing example of the type of object that might be given to ancient gods. They are also popular features of museum cabinets, where they are connected with topics including ancient medicine and religion (see the discussion of Case 3 in the Greek and Roman Life gallery at the British Museum in the chapter by Adams).

The first academic interest in anatomical votives was expressed by the Paduan bishop and intellectual Giacomo Filippo Tomasini, who published his *De donariis ac tabellis votivis liber singularis* in 1639 (Hughes, forthcoming). In this work he discussed a range of *donaria* made to the gods of ancient Italy, including anatomical ones.[1] However, more serious interest in these objects – the scholarly importance of which was diminished for a long time in favour of more traditional forms of classical sculpture and 'high art' (see Adams, this volume) – began in the early twentieth century and has slowly gathered pace. Most notably, for the

1 We are very grateful to Jessica Hughes for bringing this early work to our attention.

Greek world, influential syntheses range from the early work of William Rouse (1902) to that of Folkert van Straten (1981) and more recently Björn Forsén (1996), supplemented by important if now somewhat dated site-specific studies, including those of the Asclepieia at Athens (Aleshire, 1989; 1991), Corinth (Roebuck, 1951; Lang, 1977) and Epidaurus (Edelstein and Edelstein, 1945 and 1998; Dillon, 1994). For Italian contexts, general surveys by Maria Fenelli (1975; 1992; 1995) and Annamaria Comella (1981) and regional studies such as that of sites in Latium by Jelle Bouma (1996) continue to be influential. These are now supplemented by the *Corpus delle stipi votive in Italia*, which is an ongoing series of site publications with a standardised series of types and categories, which have brought about the systematic publication of many assemblages excavated in the twentieth century (and earlier) which had previously lain unstudied or at least unpublished. Some newly identified sites, including those where the integrity of the assemblage is threatened by the activities of *clandestine*, have also been published recently (De Lucia Brolli and Tabolli, 2015).

Nonetheless, and especially for Italian contexts where anatomical votives were often made in series, these approaches have tended to lend themselves to the establishment of typologies and categorisations rather than analytical discourses. As a consequence, many studies still focus on the groups, patterns and connections produced by these works, as well as individual site studies and the identification of tutelary deities often at the expense of an evaluation of the wider context. Important though they are, the major surveys outlined earlier also promote a way of thinking that remains grounded in the counting of particular 'types' (examples include Potter and Wells, 1985; Fridh-Haneson, 1987; Oberhelman, 2014). Perspectives on the anatomical votive as a cross-cultural phenomenon, including its chronological nuances and the implications for changing ideas about healing, cult practice and the divine and human body, have been more rare (Linders and Nordquist, 1987; Weinryb, 2016; Hughes, forthcoming).

In all of these studies it is possible to identify a series of consistent themes which have underpinned and thus been responsible for shaping existing approaches to anatomical *ex-votos*. The impact of these is evaluated, often critically, in the context of the individual chapters of this volume, but as themes that have to date provided the driving force for studies of anatomical votives, it is necessary to pause briefly to review this background. Unsurprisingly, given the clear reference that these offerings make to the human body and its constituent parts, one of the most common contexts in which the anatomical votive is set is that of ancient medicine, health and healing cult (the literature is vast, but includes Comella, 1982–83; Potter and Wells, 1985; Girardon, 1993; Baggieri, 1999; Turfa, 2004; 2006a; 2006b; Petsalis-Diomidis, 2005; 2006; 2010; Edlund-Berry, 2006; de Cazanove, 2008; Oberhelman, 2013; Recke, 2013; Turfa and Becker, 2013; Draycott, 2014; Flemming, 2016). Indeed, this is entirely logical given that the direct connection between such offerings and the process of divine healing is often made explicit by the evidence itself (Figure I.4). Under this umbrella of healing, the cult of Asclepius has proved particularly dominant, especially for studies of the eastern Mediterranean and the Greek world, where

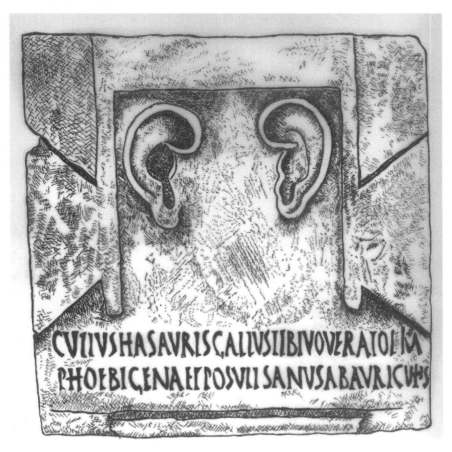

Figure I.4 Marble votive relief depicting a pair of ears accompanied by a dedicatory inscription stating that the dedication was made by Cutius Gallus in thanks for healing. Epidaurus, Roman period.

Source: Image courtesy of G. Bissas.

the association between anatomical *ex-votos* and the healing god is well attested (Lang, 1977; Rynearson, 2003; Wickkiser, 2008). The same is not true, however, for Italy, where relatively few sites can be definitively connected with the cult of Asclepius and where local deities take centre stage (Coarelli, 1986a; Renberg, 2006–7; Turfa, 2006a). Seen from this standpoint anatomical votives have been looked to as a source of evidence for particular diseases or medical conditions (for a summary for Etruscan Italy: Recke, 2013, pp. 1075–6; see also the examples of Sambon, 1895a; Stieda, 1901; Holländer, 1912, Fenelli, 1975; Ferrea and Pinna, 1986), for the healing specialisms of particular divine figures and their cults (Oberhelman, 2014) and for the extent and development of medical knowledge concerning the interior and exterior of the human body (examples include

Baggieri, 1998; 1999; Turfa, 2004; Turfa and Becker, 2013). In some instances this medical context is combined with related issues concerning human reproduction, fertility, pregnancy, birth, motherhood and infant health, especially in relation to votives which reference the uterus or genitals, as well as swaddled babies and more rare Italian examples depicting the pregnant torso (Baggieri et al., 1999; Turfa, 2004; Ammerman, 2007; de Cazanove, 2008; Graham, 2013; 2014; Derks, 2014).

Healing and medical contexts dominate scholarship on the anatomical votive, but the fact that these offerings were an integral part of religious ritual has not been overlooked. Votives that reference the human form are studied frequently as significant features of sacred sites and as part of a broader tradition of religious practice (in addition to the general studies noted earlier see Linders and Nordquist, 1987; de Cazanove, 1991; Fabbri, 2004–05; Comella and Mele, 2005; Gleba and Becker, 2009; de Grummond and Edlund-Berry, 2011). In recent years a range of other approaches have also begun to be applied to the study of these artefacts. These include body theory, sensory experience and material religion (Hughes, 2008; 2010; 2016; forthcoming; Graham, 2014; 2016; forthcoming), art and gender (Johns, 1982; Bonfante, 1986; 1989; 1997; Reilly, 1997; Schultz, 2006), 'Romanisation' and cultural interaction (de Cazanove, 2000; Glinister, 2000; 2006; 2009), as well as more restricted surveys of individual sites and geographical regions (Blagg, 1985; Comella, 2002; Melfi, 2007). Given the range of issues and contexts to which anatomical votives can be related, these disparate studies with different approaches and agendas frequently remain isolated from one another, confined by their own disciplinary, methodological or linguistic boundaries, preventing the creation of a more comprehensive and critical understanding of the anatomical votive as a broader phenomenon. Publication of assemblages excavated many years ago is often slow, as newly recovered material takes priority and new studies are hampered by the difficulties of identifying and accessing unpublished (and often simply difficult to find) material held in museum warehouses.

A body of evidence: votives in space and time

Like many other types of *donaria* which seem to have been popular at certain moments and in particular regions, the anatomical votive was not a constant feature within the votive assemblages of ancient sacred sites. As chapters in this volume demonstrate (most notably de Cazanove's investigation of chronological issues), accurate dating of the phenomenon of anatomical *ex-votos* can be notoriously circular, especially for the anepigraphic models from sites in Italy (just five rare inscribed examples: Turfa, 2004, p. 363; 2006a, pp. 101–2). Although anatomical votives appear to have reached their floruit in Greek contexts during the period covered by the fifth to third centuries BC, this estimation is based largely on the evidence from sanctuaries dedicated to Asclepius from which the most substantial evidence derives (Forsén, 2004, p. 311). This evidence takes the form of individual objects from sites including Corinth (Roebuck, 1951) and Pergamum (Radt, 1999; Petsalis-Diomidis, 2010), the famous epigraphic inventories from Athens (Aleshire, 1989; 1991) and the series of inscribed 'miracle tales' (*iamata*) from Epidaurus (Edelstein and Edelstein, 1945 and 1998; LiDonnici, 1992; Dillon, 1994). At sites in Italy anatomical dedications appear slightly later than those in Greece, beginning in the fourth century BC and peaking during the third and second centuries before declining – maybe to be replaced by votives of a different type – by or during the first century BC (Lesk, 1999; 2002; Glinister, 2006, pp. 30–31; Rüpke, 2007; although see the revised dating presented by de Cazanove, this volume). Not least amongst the new types which gained popularity in the first century BC were commemorative inscriptions that provided different opportunities for memorialising the circumstances and outcome of a vow, as well as the identity and social position of the individual concerned (Schultz, 2006, pp. 102–5).

The difficulties associated with dating a series of objects which, for the most part, are unaccompanied by inscriptions and which are often found in unstratified dumps of material cleared away from their original place of deposition to be buried in pits (sometimes referred to by modern scholars as *favisae, stipes* or *bothroi*: Glinister, 2000; Schultz, 2006, p. 97), make it difficult to draw precise conclusions about when and where the concept of dedicating body parts arose (Recke, 2013, p. 1073; de Cazanove, this volume). Regardless of specific dates, it would appear that across the Mediterranean region this tradition had peaked and largely faded by the turn of the first millennium, although evidence from Roman-period sites in the Greek East, most notably the Asclepieion at Pergamum where the Roman orator Aelius Aristides spent two years seeking relief from his bodily ailments, suggests that anatomical models and reliefs continued to be dedicated, even if in smaller quantities (Radt, 1999; Petsalis-Diomidis, 2010). Moreover, artefacts recovered from sites in Gaul attest to the continuity of this practice in other regions of the Roman Empire (Deyts, 1983; 1994; Rey-Vodoz, 1991; 2006; de Cazanove, this volume). Indeed, the fact that traces, or at least the memory of such practices, remained into late antiquity is attested by the description given by Gregory of Tours of 'barbarians' of a previous age dedicating wooden models of body parts 'touched by pain' (*Vitae patrum* VI.2 *De sancto Gallo episcopo*; cited in Hughes, forthcoming). As already observed, the descendants of these early anatomical objects are still dedicated across regions of modern Europe and further afield where largely Catholic and Orthodox faiths prevail, indicating that the compulsion to make offerings in the form of body parts has never completely disappeared even if the form, materiality and ritual context have undergone a number of changes (Cole and Zorach, 2009; Weinryb, 2016; Hughes, forthcoming). It is more difficult, not to mention inappropriate, to connect the anatomical votives of other world religions explicitly with this Mediterranean heritage.

On the other hand: new approaches

The apparent continuity or correspondence of practice implied by the ongoing dedication of offerings that are so strikingly similar to those of the ancient world and that apparently serve a similar function – that is, as part of a negotiation for divine assistance, in many cases connected with concerns about well-being, health and the inherent fragility of the human body – creates at best a sense of comfortable familiarity and at worst one of complacency about their seemingly 'obvious' and uncomplicated meanings (for instance, Capparoni, 1927). In other words, if we understand why a modern Catholic or Hindu might dedicate an anatomical *ex-voto*, then surely we can easily transfer that same understanding back into the past? Can we not use this knowledge to draw direct parallels with much older objects that were evidently articulating similar concerns? Unfortunately not. Even in ancient contexts it is evident that discrete types of anatomical votives might be associated with a range of meanings (see chapters by Draycott, Chiarini, Flemming, Graham, Petridou and Potts). What is more, this process of meaning making was one which extended also to the later stages in the biography of these dedicated objects as they became collected, curated and even created in new contexts (chapters by Haumesser, Adams, Grove and Hughes). In order to tease apart these meanings, it is necessary to acknowledge that anatomical votives could, and still can be, multivalent and that simple categorisation based on the fact that an object references the human body is not sufficient in order to really understand its significance as a material agent within religious, curative and even social activities. Appreciating this encourages new questions: Were different types of anatomical votives implicated in different types of activities or used in context-specific ways? How did the experience of dedicating an anatomical votive differ from that of making an offering in another form, perhaps a coin, a libation or an inscription? How important was the materiality of these objects and their interaction with the senses for creating religious experiences and knowledge? Not all of these questions are answered in the current volume, but the chapters presented here offer new perspectives that encourage the development of alternative questions such as these which, we hope, will move studies of anatomical votives in increasingly original and exciting directions.

Where this volume differs from existing studies, then, is that each chapter seeks to go beyond a mere catalogue of what, where and when in order to consider how these often quite varied artefacts were used, understood, experienced and were part of a broader material process of negotiation between communities composed of humans and the divine. How do they address the questions and concerns held by ancient (and some modern) people about their lives, health, bodies, fortunes and futures or about the nature of the gods, their identities and their curative powers? What is more, how do our evaluations of these questions change when we extend our perspective to include curated assemblages such as those put together by Sir Henry Wellcome? What roles do these objects, and most importantly ongoing interaction with them, have to play in the creation of bodily knowledge and understanding amongst much later generations? As a result, the chapters of this volume aim to emphasise the necessity of bringing studies of the anatomical votive into line with recent developments in related scholarship in the field of body studies within both the disciplines of archaeology and ancient medicine, as well as broader movements, including the material turn of religious studies.

There are, nonetheless, some caveats to this. Despite chapters that deal with specific types – eyes, hair, footprints, uteri, infants, open torsos, genitalia – this volume does not claim to provide a comprehensive 'head to toe' survey of ancient votive practice. Instead, the case studies included here have been selected because of the opportunities they present to debate questions about how to define, study and understand the anatomical votive phenomenon. There remain significant lacunae in the study of anatomical *ex-votos* as a whole, not just within this volume. Models of hands are one example, whereas the votive heads of Italy which take the form of relief plaques and busts (Figure I.5), as well as distinctive half-heads are another notable absence from the chapters presented here. These heads have certainly not gone unstudied and have proved crucial for providing chronological data for votive assemblages (Söderlind, 2002), as well as making a vital contribution to debates concerning the connection between votive cult and cultural interaction between Rome and the peoples of Italy (de Cazanove, 2000; Glinister, 2006; 2009). However, in many ways these objects remain – pun intended – out on a limb in terms of their integration into studies of anatomical

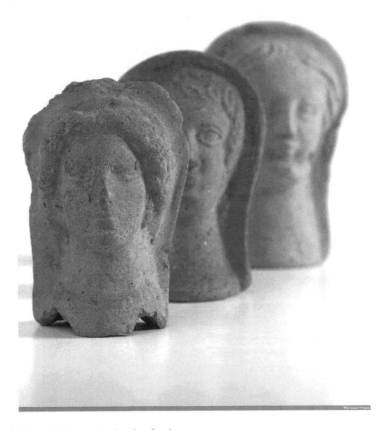

Figure I.5 Three Italian votive heads of unknown provenance.

Source: Wellcome Library, London.

votives. Their similarity to other forms of plastic art, including freestanding sculpture, the favoured topic of traditional classical archaeology, is perhaps responsible for focusing attention on the characteristics of their production and form and on questions of prototypes and artistic development rather than their meaning and significance as dedicated objects. Examples of heads were included in the discussions that took place during the original *Bodies of Evidence* conference in Rome (including the half-head finds from Fidenae discussed by Letizia Ceccarelli) and feature in the chapter by Draycott, but it is notable that none of the abstracts submitted for the conference or the papers presented focused exclusively on heads or half-heads as 'anatomical' votives. Whether this was nothing more than a coincidence, or whether it was a result of a more widely held understanding that heads should not be considered 'anatomical' in the same way as limbs, feet or uteri remains unclear (Figure I.6). Questions might be asked, then, about the extent to which ideas about fragmentation, religious knowledge and healing can be usefully applied to this abundant and well-recorded material, as well as all of the many other types not included in this volume such as legs, hands and other more uncertainly identified internal organs (such as bladders and hearts).

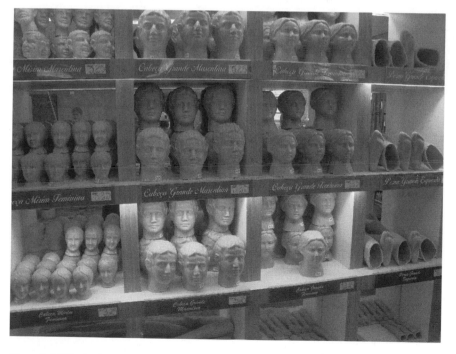

Figure I.6 Wax body parts for sale as votive offerings at the modern-day religious centre of Aparecida, Brazil. Note that heads are included alongside limbs, as they were also in ancient contexts: Are they both 'anatomical'?

Source: Wikimedia Commons. Author: Alexandrepastre.

An eye on the future

By focusing exclusively on one type of offering – although not at the expense of the wider context in which they must remain situated – this book therefore brings together for the first time a range of deliberately diverse approaches in order to challenge the simplistic categorisation applied to anatomical *ex-votos*. The volume does not attempt to situate the anatomical votive wholly in the context of either ancient religion or health/medicine, but instead exploits the interpretive potential of the intersection of these spheres, a complicated intersection that undoubtedly existed in the minds, bodies and experiences of past communities. In order to achieve this, chapters juxtapose the medical with the religious, the social with the conceptual, the idea of the body in fragments with the body whole, the museum with the sanctuary. The contributors consider a wide variety of examples, contexts and approaches but are united in their concern for exploring the complex resonance of the anatomical *ex-voto* for the people who produced, deposited or otherwise encountered them in both the distant and more recent past.

Just as the open torsos examined by Haumesser provide us with a view of the somatic interior of a terracotta body whilst their organs remain firmly contextualised within the bigger picture of its exterior, we hope that the different scales of analysis presented by this volume will make it possible to view the bigger – and indeed sometimes the smaller – picture of anatomical votives in new ways. The structure of the volume has been designed to emphasise this, moving between studies focused largely on methodological approaches and theoretical questions, those which address specific types of anatomical votive and chapters which consider how understandings of votives intersect with their later history and reception as collected objects. Nevertheless, the boundaries between these categories are deliberately fluid. Laurent Haumesser's study of 'The Open Man' demonstrates how evaluations of specific types of anatomical *ex-votos* – even in this case specific individual artefacts – must also take place with due regard to the history of an object and its own biography. Equally, Olivier de Cazanove argues that issues of chronology and methodology must remain rooted in the close analysis of specific votive types, just as Fay Glinister raises questions about what constitutes an anatomical votive by reminding us that the sum of parts can be as important as their dismemberment. From this perspective a swaddled infant votive is as anatomical as the confession stelai examined by Justine Potts, the uteri studied by Rebecca Flemming or the real and artificial hair offerings evaluated by Jane Draycott. The role of anatomical votives in the production of religious knowledge and experience for participants in ancient ritual activities also requires new theoretical standpoints which seek to offer fresh interpretative frameworks, such as those advocated by Emma-Jayne Graham, as well as detailed studies of specific types of offerings, including the different meanings attached to footprints by Sara Chiarini and eye votives by Georgia Petridou. Chapters by Laurent Haumesser, Ellen Adams and Jen Grove, on the other hand, emphasise the value of bringing together these interpretations with searching examinations of how such objects have continued to be used, collected and studied. In these instances disentangling the ancient and the modern is neither appropriate nor especially valuable, as the Afterword by Jessica Hughes concludes.

So why does the anatomical votive fascinate? The chapters collected here suggest that it is perhaps because there are so many ways in which we might understand them. They complicate our view of how the people of the past experienced not only their relationship with the divine world, but also their own bodies, as well how later generations have sought to make sense of this. Perhaps, too, it is because these objects, with their easily recognisable configuration of a human body with which we are all so familiar, provide a tangible connection with ancient people in a way that a fragment of pottery or a well-worn coin cannot. Anatomical votives capture the imagination vividly and creatively at the same time as they recall the very real, physical and fragile bodies of the past. And even if only for this they deserve our undivided attention.

1   Corpora in connection

Anatomical votives and the confession stelai of Lydia and Phrygia

Justine Potts

Introduction: transgressing boundaries

Scholars of anatomical votives have, on the whole, been far less transgressive than those whose examples of wrongdoing and punishment were written up on stelai in Roman Asia Minor. Although the subject of anatomical votives has interested generations of historians, the most exciting anatomical votives are almost never mentioned in their discussions. These, I suggest, are the confession stelai of Lydia and Phrygia published (and numbered) as a corpus by Petzl in 1994 under their traditional genre-delineation of '*Beichtinschriften*'. The distinctive nature of their inscriptions, characterised by a confession which details wrongdoing or divine punishment or both, has caused the stelai to be circumscribed by their own strangeness. In no other context of Greco-Roman epigraphy are expiatory purposes so apparent. As a result of scholarly preoccupation with the peculiar, subsequent discourse has been constrained at least as much as it has been advanced by adherence to a corpus mentality. The purpose of this chapter is to suggest how by transgressing boundaries and by viewing some confession stelai as anatomical votives, there are significant implications for both corpora of material. On the one hand, the evidence suggests that there was a hierarchy of propitiatory epigraphy available to the transgressor, highlighting a previously underacknowledged expiatory motive behind anatomical votives. On the other, this study hopes to recalibrate our understanding of the confession stelai by showing that they were not the product of an isolated and archaic religious mentality which was distinct from that held by dedicants of what might be deemed 'conventional' anatomical votives in the same region. Rather, there seems to have been a shared cultural, material and intellectual milieu among the dedicants of the two corpora. This will suggest, in turn, that the dedication of confession stelai was determined not so much by a distinct, isolated and 'un-Greco-Roman' religious inclination, but rather by structural factors such as the circumstances of illness, the nature of the punishment, the conventions of the local sanctuary, financial means and even existential exigencies. Equally, if we accept Ricl's (1995, p. 68) inference that confession was a Hittite hang-over in this region of Anatolia, the dedicants of anatomical votives may have been party to this inheritance more than is otherwise apparent. The confession stelai call into question the boundaries of the category we delineate as 'anatomical votives', demonstrating striking fluidity between two (modern) genres of epigraphic religious expression.

Incorporation

Around AD 235–236 a stele of white marble was inscribed with the narrative of a certain Theodorus. In direct speech he reveals that despite being a temple slave he had intimate assignations not only with a married woman in the temple courtyard, but also, on separate occasions, with two virgin priestesses. The gods' displeasure at this profaning of the sacred is made clear, as a divine voice in the first person informs the reader that they punished Theodorus in his eyes 'because of his wrongdoings' (Petzl 5). Reconciliation seems to have been achieved eventually, as the divine concludes that the once-blinded Theodorus has made good his mistakes by propitiating the gods and erecting a stele on the appointed day. Glaring out at the admonished reader is a representation of a pair of eyes incised on the upper-right side of the stele next to a crescent moon, which is a symbol of the god Men. On another stele, a woman called Glykia declared that she was punished by the goddess Anaitis with an infliction on her bottom. It was as a result of this punishment that she set up the stele on which was carved a relief of a leg and buttock in profile in addition to the inscription (Petzl 75). We find another transgressor in the figure of Ammias who was 'punished on her breasts because of a wrongdoing' in the second century AD, and her stele bears two round breasts which represent the afflicted area (Petzl 95). These stelai and a number of similar ones are categorised as confession inscriptions because they conform to the general framework of wrongdoing, divine punishment, statement of transgression and erection of a stele that characterises the corpus, but this chapter will demonstrate that they should also be regarded as anatomical votives: textual elaboration is no grounds for their segregation.

The corpus referred to as the confession inscriptions of Asia Minor now includes around 150 documents, all stelai with two exceptions (a tablet: Petzl 96; a statue of Men: Petzl 67), dating mainly to the second and third centuries AD, with the earliest dated to AD 57–58 (Malay, 2003). The terminology used to refer to the corpus has been the subject of long debate.[1] This chapter will continue to follow the convention of 'confession' stelai, although it is acknowledged that 'confession' is a loaded word, with Christian connotations that should not be imparted to the material. Contrary to terminological revisionists, however, it is my view that confession – by which I mean the verbalised acknowledgement of wrongdoing and culpability – should be emphasised as a central concept in our

---

1 Rostad (2002) proposed the term 'reconciliation inscriptions' and later revised this label as 'propitiation inscriptions' (Rostad, 2006) following Arnold's (2005) criticism of the former term. For Buckler (1914–16) and Chaniotis (1995) they are 'propitiatory' inscriptions and later 'expiation' inscriptions for Chaniotis (1997), as they were for Zingerle (1926). Gordon (2004) has them as 'confession-texts' (see Paz de Hoz, 2009, p. 358 n.1; also Belayche, 2008, pp. 181–2).

understanding of the inscriptions at least as much as reconciliation and propitia-tion have been. The term is not a misleading descriptor of those stelai which lack an explicit statement of the wrongdoing because a declaration of having received divine punishment was tantamount to an acknowledgment of culpability; the relative infrequency of verbs meaning 'to confess' in the corpus is no indication that the stelai in general should be regarded as any less concerned with confes-sion (*contra* Rostad, 2002, p. 151; see Chaniotis, 2009, p. 135).

The majority of the inscriptions come from the Katakekaumene in northeast-ern Lydia, around the middle-upper Hermus basin, and were set up across a num-ber of sanctuary sites to a range of gods. They have been found in the vicinities of a number of villages in Lydia and Phrygia, including Sardeis, Philadelphia, Tabala, Silandos, Thermai, Maeonia, Collyda, Tripolis, Saittai, Akmonia, Tiberiopolis, Eumeneia and Pergamum, although the precise nature and location of the origi-nating Lydian sanctuaries remain obscure (Mitchell, 1993, p. 193). A significant group of inscriptions originates from the sanctuary of Apollo Lairbenos near Motella in Phrygia. This sanctuary has been partially excavated and is expected to yield yet more additions to the corpus (Ritti et al., 2000; Akıncı Öztürk and Tanrıver, 2008; 2009; 2010). Events narrated in the confession inscriptions locate the stelai firmly in the context of divine justice familiar from other parts of the Greco-Roman world (Versnel, 1991; Parker, 1996, pp. 235–56; Chaniotis, 1997; 2004; 2009).[2] Misfortune, often in the form of a physical malady, is felt to be a punishment from the gods for a transgression. As a key step in the process of propitiation (and thus healing), the transgressor, or their relatives, would erect a stele which commonly narrated the nature of the wrongdoing, the punishment inflicted and, occasionally, a confession of their wrongdoing in direct terms (as in Petzl 100, 106, 111 and 116). However, this was not an entirely autonomous response to physical affliction: some stelai tell us that the gods commanded the transgressors 'to write up on a stele the powers of the gods' (στηλογραφειν τὰς δυνάμεις τῶν Θεῶν) (see Petzl 3, 14, 33, 35, 37, 38, 39, 47, 55 and 69).

The act of *stelographein* was not just a matter of writing up a textual account on a stele; often that text was accompanied by images either incised or carved in relief.[3] Although many of the stelai are fragmentary, images survive on roughly half of the corpus. Scholarship has tended to overlook these images and pursue a logocentric approach, attracted by the 'otherness' of the stelai's textual con-tent.[4] As strikingly different as the texts are from epigraphic religious testimonia known elsewhere in the Greco-Roman world, their images show them to be

2 Several confession stelai talk of the 'setting up of a sceptre', by which act the plaintiff who had suf-fered an injustice opened the judicial process. Petzl 60 tells us of a certain Artemidorus who set up a πιττάκιον because he was the victim of slander by Hermogenes, and so the latter was punished. Ricl (1995, pp. 67–76) highlights that curses and judicial prayers have been found not only in Greece and Asia Minor, but also in Spain, Sicily and Britain.

3 In Greek, *graphein* denotes both writing and drawing an image. There are some intact stelai which clearly never bore an image (Ricl, 1997; Hermann and Malay, 2007, hereafter *New Documents*, 84).

4 On their idiosyncrasy see Chaniotis (1995, p. 334); Belayche (2008, p. 181). Scholarship that has con-sidered images includes Gordon (2004); Belayche (2008).

typically Anatolian in appearance and in the language of their iconographical presentation. By acknowledging both text and image on the stelai, a number of inscriptions emerge which can be classified as anatomical votives, albeit accompanied by an informative amount of textual detail that is unusual for anatomical votives as conventionally conceived. It tends to be the case that anatomical votives of the Greco-Roman world, if epigraphic at all, bear a relatively short and simple inscription. Typical Greek formulae include the name of the dedicant followed by the god to whom the votive was offered, accompanied by the word εὐχή ('vow', or '*ex-voto*') in the accusative, although it could suffice to omit the verb 'to dedicate' or even to be anepigraphic altogether (such as the terracottas from the Asclepieion in Corinth: Roebuck, 1951, pp. 114–28). Occasionally the inscription might be lengthier if epithets of the gods are included, but detailed narratives of the sort found on the confession stelai are extremely unusual for anatomical votives as we know them. Textual elaboration stating a wrongdoing or the imposition of divine punishment has determined inclusion in the confession corpus. This not only brings into relief the arbitrary nature of modern genre construction, but also calls into question how distinct the intellectual world behind these two categories of inscriptions really was. A certain corpus mentality, together with logocentricity, has caused scholarship to underestimate the potential offered by considerations of epigraphic comparanda.

Although comparative observations between the corpora have been made, they have been of limited scope. Van Straten (1981, pp. 101–2, and nn. 40–8 in the appendix) highlighted a connection between anatomical votives and the confession stelai by including them in his catalogue of votive offerings representing parts of the human body. Belayche (2008, p. 182) also made the association by noting that text and image are combined in these inscriptions, just as they are in '*les types traditionnels*' – that is, votives – of the area. Chaniotis (1995, p. 325) acknowledged that 'vows and propitiatory inscriptions are closely related', and Gordon (2004, p. 181) views them as 'scarcely distinguishable'. Chaniotis (1995, p. 325) implicitly alludes to the classification of some stelai as 'anatomical' and, looking beyond the corpus to other epigraphic material for his study of illness and cures in the area, highlighted that both groups of texts could be dedicated to the same gods and could express similar religious sentiments.[5] More recently he has also stated the importance of studying the confession stelai in close connection with dedications and vows, recognising that their appellation has drawn up 'unnecessary boundaries' (Chaniotis, 2009, pp. 117–18) and has asserted that complex processes of assimilation and cultural transfer are revealed by their texts (Chaniotis, 2009, p. 143). Nevertheless, the implications for how this might affect our understanding of both genres remain unexplored.

It should be noted that not all confession stelai can be classified unproblematically as anatomical votives. For instance, Petzl 4 is a stele dedicated 'in thanksgiving' by the foster daughters of Severus, who forbade the cutting of wreaths, an act

---

5 Chaniotis (1995, p. 327) notes that, as in the case of 'anatomical votives', eyes take a prominent position, but aside from this he does not discuss anatomical votives specifically.

which resulted in the god 'inquiring after the wrongdoing' (εὐχα- / ριστουσαι (ll. 8–9); ἐ- / πεζήτησεν ὁ θεὸς (ll. 4–5)). It is not made entirely explicit that Severus was punished, although the fact that his daughters are 'giving thanks' suggests he was punished and then cured. Moreover, the scene of the relief depicts the act of the wrongdoing: one man appears to prevent another from cutting down branches from a tree. Any anatomical overtones are therefore absent from this stele. Other stelai narrate events in a rather impersonal, factual manner, lacking the names of dedicants or culprits, such as Petzl 3 which is a third-person account of a cloak thief who was punished, returned the cloak and confessed. Stelai such as these, therefore, can less reasonably be categorised as anatomical votives, at least at the level of their presentation, although the following comparison of confession stelai and anatomical votives will prompt a reconsideration of how distinct in terms of function and dedicatory context Severus's stele really was from that of a votive representing a body part. What is clear, despite sophisticated attempts to identify coherent patterns in the corpus (Gordon, 2004, pp. 177–96; Belayche, 2008), is the extent of variation in presentation among the stelai: there was no set blueprint for how to *stelographein*, and they appear to have been individually tailored.[6] Unlike Severus's stele, a substantial number are indeed explicitly anatomical in nature: the body part punished is specified in the inscription and/or represented by an accompanying image. It is this group that forms the focus of the present chapter.

The anatomical nature of inscriptions in the corpus of Anatolian confession stelai constitutes a significant point of divergence from the confession inscriptions from ancient South Arabia.[7] No inscription of the latter provenance represents an image of the body part punished, despite the fact that the punishment was sometimes considered to take the form of a physical infliction: we hear of illness and death (Arbach and Audouin, 2007, YM 23643; Agostini, 2012, Y.03.B.A.1), and one god even 'took vengeance' on a transgressor's molar teeth (Jamme, 1962, no. 702). The detachment and visual emphasis of a particular part of the body as a *locus poenis* is therefore, within the genre of confession texts, a peculiarly Anatolian phenomenon.

Comparing corpora and delineating delinquents

With a pair of breasts carved in relief above the inscription, confession stele no. 217 in Malay (1999, p. 176, hereafter *Researches*) bears an inscription that reads: 'Attikilla, who was punished on her breasts, set this up as an *ex-voto*

---

6 The greatest number of stelai dating to any one year is four (Petzl 54, 57, 67 and 78, in AD 118–119), and these display little stylistic similarity. One is an inscription without any image, one is a statue, one bears a figure of a woman accompanied by divine symbols and one bears the image of an arm. All were found in the Katakekaumene. There appears, therefore, to have been no contemporary uniformity of fashion.

7 There is as yet no collection of these inscriptions and some remain unpublished. For a recent discussion of the Minaean texts alone, see Agostini (2012).

with thanks to Thea Oline' (Ἀττικίλλα κολ- / ασθῖσα μαστο- / ὑς Θεᾷ Ὀλινη εὐχὴ- / ν ἀνέστησεν). When this stele is compared with an anatomical votive from the Katekekaumene in Diakonoff's catalogue of dedications to Artemis Anaitis (Diakonoff, 1979, no. 33), the layout and iconography of the two stelai are strikingly similar: the latter reads 'Alexandra dedicates [this] *ex-voto* to Artemis Anaitis and Men Tiamou for her breasts' (Ἀρτέμιδι Ἀναε[ίτι] / καὶ Μηνὶ Τιάμου Ἀ[λε]- / ξάνδρα ὑπὲρ τῶν / [μ]αστῶν εὐχὴν / ἀνέστησαν), and a pair of breasts carved in relief is located above the inscription. What appears to make the former regarded as a confession inscription and the latter not is the detail that Attikilla evidently considers the physical affliction regarding her breasts to be a punishment. However, the absence of this detail on the *ex-voto* does not necessarily mean that Alexandra thought about her breast problem in different terms from Attikilla. The malady may nevertheless have been conceived of as a punishment, with Alexandra not expressing it in those terms, but by means of what might be considered a 'conventional' *ex-voto* formula.

A relief carving of a leg from mid-thigh to foot in a square niche is another image common to both anatomical *ex-votos* and anatomical confession inscriptions where the leg has been the ostensible target of divine punishment. In the corpus of inscriptions to Hosios and Dikaios there is a votive stele dedicated to the gods by Hermes and Meltine for their son Philippikos (Ricl, 1991, no. 8). Above the inscription is a leg in a niche carved in relief. This is almost identical in presentation to an image of a leg in a niche on a confession stele to 'Zeus from Twin Oaks' (Malay and Sayar, 2004), as well as to a relief on the confession inscription no. 66 in Herrmann and Malay (2007) and to Petzl 83. As a result the stelai are scarcely distinguishable in appearance from one another. Yet they differ on the textual level: the *ex-voto* describes itself as a εὐχὴ for the dedicants' son, whilst the latter three bear detailed accounts of wrongdoing together with the gods' commands to *stelographein*. In each case the image makes it clear that a leg has been afflicted with an illness, although none of the texts specify this.

Should some *ex-votos*, such as *Researches* no. 215, be set up alongside anatomical confession stelai, they would not seem out of place. Above the inscription of 'Loukianos and Loukiane dedicated an *ex-voto* to Thea Meter Olline who is attentive to prayer' is a relief of a leg from mid-thigh to foot (not in a niche) which resembles closely the representation of a leg on Petzl 70 (Figure 1.1). This confession stele is emphatically anatomical in its iconography: three different body parts are represented despite no punishment being specified in the text. This is one example of a number of stelai for which the image 'fills in' the detail and does a significant amount of the narrative work (for example Petzl 70, 78, 83, 90, 99, 102 and 110; *New Documents* no. 66; Malay and Sayar, 2004). As Belayche (2008, pp. 182–3) has argued, there exist different degrees of engagement with the narrative offered by representations of the body part. Some stelai specify in both text and image the afflicted body part, and so they are mutually supportive on both the visual and textual register (Petzl 5, 16, 50, 75 and 95; *Researches* no. 217; Akıncı Öztürk and Tanrıver, 2009, no. 2). Others specify in the text the body part punished but not in the image (Petzl 45, 49, 63, 69, 84, 85, 89 and 122;

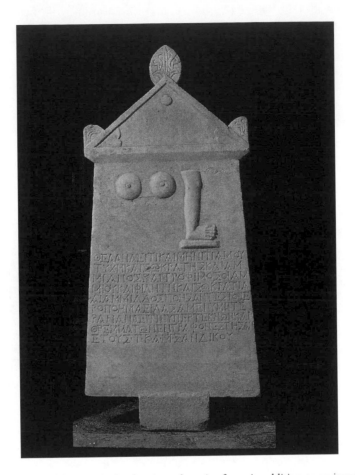

Figure 1.1 Petzl 70, depicting a leg, breasts and a pair of eyes in addition to an inscription.

Source: Image courtesy of the Rijksmuseum van Oudheden.

Petzl, 1997, no. 1; *New Documents* no. 84; Ricl, 1997 = *CIG* 4142), although in most of these cases the stele is too damaged to conclusively state that there was no accompanying image. However, the image was not there simply for narratological convenience. We should be aware that the representation of a body part was a means of reification, so that the body part itself was dedicated to the god by means of the εὐχή (*ex-voto*). Although to us images might be representation, to the dedicants of the stelai images were 'presentation' (Squire, 2009, p. 116; see also Pazzini, 1935, p. 54; Platt, 2011).[8]

8 The *Oneirocritica* of Artemidorus of Daldis is a potentially useful source for understanding the visual theology behind the confession stelai, as it dates from the second century AD and its author hails from nearby Lycia. For Artemidorus the images of the gods were synonymous with the gods themselves. He

In addition to the leg carved in relief on Petzl 70 there is a pair of breasts iconographically identical to the breasts described earlier and a pair of eyes incised in the common fashion, further demonstrating striking visual similarity with anatomical votives. However, not all anatomical votives were of the same quality as confession stelai. In *Phrygian Votive Steles* there are a number of 'mute' anatomical votives depicting legs that appear to demonstrate much rougher handiwork (Drew-Bear et al., 1999, hereafter 'Drew-Bear', nos. 40, 42–3, 46, 48, 52 and 59–66). Within the epigraphy of inland Anatolia, then, we can identify varying modes of presentation for anatomical votives: from the small 'mute' stelai of Drew-Bear's collection representing at a bare minimum the affected body part, to the more detailed and precisely carved Petzl 70 and *Researches* no. 216. The silence of the 'mute' stelai does not suggest that sentiments of punishment and reconciliation informed its dedicant any less than the dedicants of Petzl 70. It will be suggested later that there was a hierarchy of propitiatory epigraphy with which the dedicant might engage and that the nature of their dedication could be conditioned by sanctuary-specific customs.

Looking at Phrygian material alone we can see that the incised nature of some of the legs on the tablets and stelai of the Drew-Bear collection recall the incised leg adorning Petzl 102, two legs on Petzl 110 and an incised leg on confession stele no. 2 in Akıncı Öztürk and Tanrıver's (2009) publication of new finds from the sanctuary of Apollo Lairbenos. This shows regional similarity of iconographical presentation between anatomical *ex-votos* and anatomical confession stelai in Phrygia. Although the upper part of the latter representation of a leg cannot be seen because of the fragmentary nature of the stele, we know that the dedicant was punished on their buttocks thanks to the detail in the text. Similarly, had it not been for the detail in the inscription of Petzl 75, a relief of a leg in side profile from waist to foot, it might have been read as representing punishment concerning a leg rather than buttocks as the inscription indicates. These two confession stelai, thanks to their accompanying textual detail, serve to show the difficulties of interpreting the iconography of 'mute' anatomical votives.

In the representation of the other body parts, too, there is significant overlap between the confession stelai and anatomical votives. For example, *Researches* no. 216, an *ex-voto* dedicated by Loukianos and Loukiane, bears an identical inscription to no. 215 discussed earlier, but in this case male genitalia are represented above the inscription rather than a leg. We find male genitalia depicted likewise, although incised, on Petzl 110, where the image no doubt refers to the area punished rather than the crime committed (*contra* Miller, 1985, p. 62).[9]

---

says of Artemis: '[I]t makes no difference whether one see the goddess as she lives in our imagination or her statue, since, whether the Gods appear in the flesh or as statues made out of wood, they have the same significance' (*Oneirocritica* 2.35).

9 When crimes are represented, this tends to be done in a figurative narrative scene. Because two legs are represented next to the genitalia, it is more likely here that the genitals and legs were punished because of the nature of the crime (going unclean into a sacred precinct and having an intimate assignation there: Pettazzoni, 1936, p. 69). So in some sense they do allude to the crime but they acted primarily as

This function of the image to allude to the body part afflicted by the punishment can be found throughout the anatomical confession stelai. As for eyes portrayed frontally as disembodied organs, there are also strong similarities in style and presentation across the confession stelai and *ex-votos* of the area. Of all the afflicted body parts mentioned or represented in the confession corpus, eyes are by far the most numerous, and among the *ex-votos* from Phrygia they are extensive enough to have a whole section devoted to them in Drew-Bear's catalogue (Chaniotis, 1995, pp. 327–8; for eye votives see Petridou, this volume). No. 19 is a small stele which bears an incised pair of eyes with pupils above the inscription 'Asklepiades [dedicated] this vow to Zeus Alsenos' (Ἀσκληπιάδη- / ς Διὶ Ἀλσην- / [ῷ εὐχήν]). The location and presentation of these eyes parallel the eyes we find on a number of confession stelai, such as Petzl 5, 16, 50, 70 and 90.

So far we have seen how a comparison of anatomical confession stelai and anatomical *ex-votos* shows that they shared a common visual language, but it is apparent that there are similarities also in the textual language. In the Petzl corpus, for example, there are nine stelai which employ the word 'εὐχὴν' (*ex-voto*). Of these, six stelai (Petzl 122, 66, 42, 84, 90 and 91) are significant for our purpose because they self-identify as a εὐχὴ (Chaniotis, 2009, pp. 117–18). For example, Petzl 122 (ll. 2–7) reads:

Ἀφιὰς Θεοδότου / εὐχαριστῶ Μητρὶ / Λητώ, ὅτι ἐξ ἀδυνά- / των δυνατὰ πυεῖ, . . . / κὲ κολαθῖσα ἰς τὸν γλουθρὸ[?]- /ν Μητρὶ Λητὼ εὐχήν.

I, Aphias, daughter of Theodotus, give thanks to Meter Leto, as she makes the impossible possible; and [I give] to Meter Leto [this stele as an] *ex-voto*, after I had been punished on my buttocks.

In addition, the Greek verb used generally within votive inscriptions to denote dedication – ἀποδίδω – is employed widely on confession stelai (Chaniotis, 2009, p. 118). Therefore, as established earlier for Attikilla and Alexandra, the inscriptions of the confession stelai can resemble closely the dedicatory inscriptions on *ex-votos* except that we are informed additionally of someone's 'punishment'. What is especially significant, however, is that confession inscriptions which indicate in the text that someone has suffered from a physical malady do not necessarily represent a body part in the visual register. Petzl 66, which self-identifies as a εὐχὴ and linguistically resembles an *ex-voto*, bears a crescent moon as an image, not an image of an afflicted body part. It is possible that the punishment in question took the form of something difficult to represent visually such as the 'states of death' or 'madness' of which some inscriptions talk (Petzl 7, 10, 57 and 81). However, if we turn to Petzl 63 we see that it was

---

representations of the afflicted body parts. Among the Anatolian stelai there is no scene of wrongdoing that depicts intercourse, but among the 'confession' inscriptions of ancient South Arabia there is a remarkable bronze tablet from the Temple of Yġrw in Wadi Šuḏayf that shows a couple intertwined alongside the text of the confession (Sima, 1999, Appendix 1, pp. 151–2).

possible to represent something other than the afflicted body part, even when that body part could have been depicted easily. This stele tells us that Stratonike, who had delayed repayment after borrowing a *modius* of wheat, was punished on her right breast. Instead of the image showing this body part as we might now come to expect, the image portrays a crescent moon, the symbol of Men Axiottenos whom Stratonike praises in the inscription. The visual language of an anatomical votive is therefore not always employed even in stelai that we know are 'anatomical' because of the nature of their inscriptions. This point has significant ramifications for 'nonanatomical' *ex-votos*, such as those 'mute' examples that bear only the figures of people or symbols of gods, or even the aniconic *ex-votos* which tell us no more than 'X has dedicated this εὐχὴν to the god Y'. If the compiler of an anatomical confession stele should choose to employ non-anatomical visual language, it is entirely possible that contexts for other *ex-votos* are equally 'anatomical', that is involve the healing of a body part or disease even though they do not *appear* as anatomical *ex-votos*, with this aspect of them lost to scholarship because of the paucity of information contained in their inscriptions. Perhaps, therefore, the genre of the 'anatomical votive' might be stretched even further to incorporate stelai such as Drew-Bear no. 3, which bears a bust of Zeus Alsenos and reads 'Hippostrophos son of Diophantos [dedicated] this *ex-voto* (εὐχὴν) to Zeus Alsenos'. Such a conclusion is, of course, impossible to prove, but anatomical confession stelai certainly encourage us to rethink the boundaries of the anatomical votive genre in this way.

The hierarchy of propitiatory epigraphy

The fact that anatomical confession stelai are not differentiated iconographically from anatomical *ex-votos* of the same region suggests that they were different expressions of a common intellectual world. Further observations illustrate this point. First, we are told in some of the confession inscriptions that wrongdoers neglected to give thanksgiving for a vow. For example, in Petzl 45 Diogenes made a vow about cattle 'and did not fulfil it' (κὲ μὴ ἀποδούς) so his daughter was punished, in Malay and Sayar (2004) Menophila promised a votive but 'wasted time and did not fulfil it', and in Petzl 101 the wrongdoer describes himself as 'not fulfilling the vow' (μὴ ἀποδὼν τὴν εὐχήν). This demonstrates that the people who erected the confession stelai would also dedicate *ex-votos*. Two such people may be identified through a comparision of the dedicatory inscription Diakonoff no. 13 (AD 211–12) with the confession stele Petzl 70 (AD 236–7). Both of these include the names of Socrateia and Trophimos among the dedicants, and on both occasions they give a ἱεροπόημα (a sacred offering) to Thea Anaeitis and Men Tiamou. The word ἱεροπόημα is rare in the corpus, and in Petzl it is used only twice elsewhere. We might tentatively infer that these are the same people rhetoricising their piety in the same way after an interlude of 25 years. If so, the same people set up a dedicatory inscription to a deity under a particular set of circumstances and a confession stele under others. Because the confession stele, in comparison with the earlier inscription, is particularly marked by elaboration – in narrative detail, ornament, iconography and even by using patronymics – we might see the act of erecting a confession stele as a step up from merely offering a votive.

A concern for elaboration is a general feature of the corpus. It is significant that in the cases where a confession inscription is preserved well enough to show that it never bore an image the text fills up nearly all of the area of the shaft, leaving very little empty space (for example, Petzl 78 and 54). This is one aspect of their appearance that can be seen to contrast with *ex-votos*. In Diakonoff's catalogue of inscriptions dedicated to Artemis Anaeitis, no. 24 provides a good example of a lack of concern for textual detail and empty space. In the middle of the shaft an inscription bluntly reads 'Amias to Anaeitis an *ex-voto*' (Ἀμιὰς Ἀναείτιδι εὐχήν) and two horizontal laurel branches meet in the middle. The stele is 40 cm high, and at least half of the surface of its shaft is empty space. In contrast, the confession stelai tend to show a concern with proportion and good management of space. The erection of a confession stele, therefore, was a relatively effort-intensive form of religious expression.[10]

The value of taking confession stelai into consideration in discussions about anatomical *ex-votos* lies also in what the stelai can reveal about the process of votive offerings in general. We have already seen that in Malay and Sayar's (2004) confession to 'Zeus from Twin Oaks' Menophila had found herself in trouble because, having been punished, she promised to set up a πίναξ (a votive tablet) but failed to fulfil that promise. We are then told that her sister Julia joined in her prayers, and the god requested a stele from her as a result of this (presumably additional) misdemeanour. This informs us about two things: first that it is not just stelai which, despite remaining the informative witnesses of the 'confessional' mentality, were media for the religious expression of this mentality. Votive tablets (πίνακες) could be part of this intellectual world too. This shows that less elaborate epigraphy (which 'conventional' anatomical votives were) could be a product of the same religious mentality as that which informed the confession stelai. The second point offered by this example concerns the idea proposed earlier that confession stelai were somehow a step up from simple votive offerings. Menophila's default on her side of the bargain provoked the god to demand not that she fulfil her original promise of a πίναξ but that she *stelographein*. This indicates that there was a hierarchy of propitiatory epigraphy.

The same confession stele provokes the question of whether all the stelai which portray body parts do so because of the dedicant's failure to give an anatomical votive. Owing to the informative nature of the inscriptions on the stelai, we can deduce that unfulfilled vows were not always the motivating cause of the punishment and subsequent erection of an anatomical stele. Petzl 5, 16 and 110 and *New Documents* no. 66 all bear representations of body parts, but they are for crimes that are unrelated to defaulting on votive dedications. This suggests that

---

10 There are some exceptions to such intensity of effort: Petzl 105 to Hosios and Dikaios bears arguably the least competent attempt to depict figures.

the representation of body parts on the confession stelai was not an attempt to make up for what was lacking after defaulting on a promised anatomical *ex-voto*, but rather it concerns the elective employment of a visual language commonly found in contexts of divine healing.

Common contexts of production and chronological correspondence

Analysis of the images on the stelai also raises questions about the circumstances of their production. Where it is possible to tell, the image was carved before the inscription: the images on Petzl 5, 99, and 104 all demonstrate this because the text envelops the image in a way that could not be achieved if the text were carved first. This observation, together with stelai such as *New Documents* no. 66 which allude to the punished area in the image but make no mention of it in the text, raise the suspicion that they were in origin ready-made, perhaps cheaper stelai from anatomical votive workshops. However, this cannot have been the case because there seems to have been no distinction between production contexts of anatomical votives and of confession stelai. These two (to us now distinct) genres were not produced by craftsmen specialising in either one or the other. Whilst this does mean that a stele bearing an an image of a body part offered epigraphic versatility in its potential to be inscribed with either a confession text or a simple dedicatory text, we cannot say that a confession stele was ever a reappropriated anatomical votive. This indistinction in circumstances of production can be deduced from the fact that a sculptor (or perhaps workshop) can be identified at work across a number of different epigraphic genres, including an anatomical confession stele (Petzl 70) and an anatomical votive (Diakonoff no. 33). Diakonoff (1979, p. 156) has argued on the basis of lettering that a single hand can be identified in six stelai from the Anaeitis dedications and in five other inscriptions. Of these inscriptions six are dated, revealing a work span of at least 25 years. Pushing back the sculptor's dates to the beginning of the third century AD, Diakonoff finds four more inscriptions which, although there is a slight difference in epigraphic style, carry the same signature pediment and *acroteria*. One of these is Petzl 10, a confession stele to Zeus ἐγ διδύμων δρυῶν dating to AD 194–195 which extends the active period of the sculptor to 50 years, perhaps suggesting a workshop rather than one sculptor (Diakonoff, 1979, p. 157). The variety of genres of epigraphy in which we see this 'hand' at work shows that the confession stelai were not the product of craftsmen specialising in this type alone. Rather, the same sculptors who were working on grave stelai and dedication inscriptions, as well as on anatomical votives, were also working on the confession stelai.

On a confession stele ascribed to this sculptor (Petzl 70, see Figure 1.1) he has carved body parts; on another stele, this time not a confession stele but a εὐχὴ dedicated 'for healthy eyes' (ὑπὲρ ὑγείας τῶν ὀφθαλμῶν: Diakonoff no. 7), he has carved a small, barely noticeable pair of eyes off to the top right of the stele

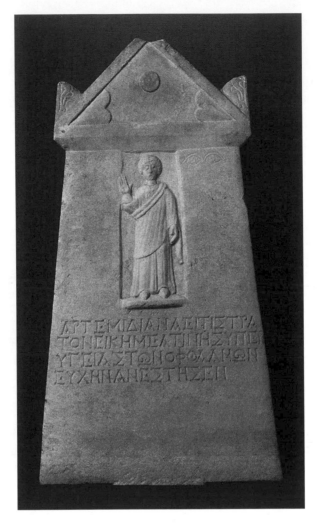

Figure 1.2 Diakonoff no. 7, in which a pair of eyes can be seen carved at the top right of the
        stele, to the side of the central figure.

Source: Image courtesy of the Rijksmuseum van Oudheden.

but, centrally and prominently, a female figure with her hand raised (Figure 1.2).
Such figures, probably shown in the act of swearing an oath, appear often in the
confession corpus (for instance, Petzl 6–7, 10–12, 20, 35, 37–38 and 97). We
might expect eyes to be depicted centrally on the *ex-voto* and the pious female
on the confession stele, but instead Petzl 70's visual register focuses solely on
body parts despite the text mentioning none, and the *ex-voto* for healthy eyes
iconographically emphasises the oath-swearing woman. This not only suggests
that correlation between 'anatomical' text and 'anatomical' image was of little

concern, as seen earlier in Stratonike's use of the symbol of Men despite her breast punishment, but it also demonstrates that no particular visual language or group of sculptors appears to have been the preserve of confession stelai alone. Equally, an otherwise blank stele bearing an image of an oath-swearing woman offered just as much epigraphic versatility as one with a body part. It also indicates that there were probably no workshops which produced ana-tomical votive stelai exclusively; no single hand can be identified on anatomical votives alone. The common milieu of anatomical votives and confession stelai is stressed yet further by studying the findspots of the seven inscriptions with reliable provenances which show that the sculptor's work was widely scattered across the Katakekaumene. Diakonoff (1979, p. 158) argues that the workshops were probably not located near to the sanctuaries, but that their products were transported there after their production. Confession stelai therefore do not appear to be the work of specialist sanctuary-resident craftsmen confined to an isolated religio-cultural context. Indeed, it appears that the dedicants themselves made no categorical distinction between a confession inscription and anatomical *ex-voto*: the *Textgattung* exists only for us, and it has been misleading.

A close relationship between the confession stelai and other votives of the region more generally can also be detected by studying change over time within the corpus. The chronological pattern of stelai that bear images cor-responds roughly to the distribution of all surviving stelai over time, with a particular peak in the first decade before and the first decade after AD 200. Whereas in general the number of stelai with surviving images in any given decade is roughly half the number of stelai dating to that time, in the two decades on either side of the year AD 200 almost three-quarters of those stelai bear images. The fact that the chronological pattern of the stelai with images roughly reflects the chronological pattern of surviving stelai in general sug-gests that the trend for images on the confession stelai did not fluctuate, but rather images were a constant part of epigraphic expression for more than two centuries. We may then compare this chronological development and the noticeable peak in numbers around AD 200 with epigraphic activity else-where in the region. The early third quarter of the second century AD saw the start of production of votive reliefs in the Upper Tembris plain and the area of Kurudere in Phrygia, and the latest votive reliefs from both areas date from the third century, around AD 240–270 (Drew-Bear et al., 1999, p. 33). Furthermore, the workshop at Kurudere achieved its greatest production in the period around AD 180–200, and the peak of the Tembris valley votive production occurred in the first few decades of the 200s (Drew-Bear et al., 1999, p. 33). This epigraphic activity in Phrygia indicates that the increase in the number of confession stelai around AD 200 is not just an accident of the archaeological record, but rather a true indication of increased production. It seems that at this time there was a certain increase in intensity of output which was common to the different epigraphic genres – confessional, ana-tomical or otherwise. This shared material milieu brings the confession stelai and anatomical *ex-votos* yet closer together as different religious expressions of a common intellectual world.

Healing wrongs

A further insight that the confession stelai provide for the context of anatomical votives concerns local medicine and conceptions of illness and healing. It is not the purpose of this chapter to reopen the dossier on this subject (see Chaniotis, 1995; Petzl, 2006), but an observation can be made. Body parts occur relatively infrequently as images, with 18 in total. This has possible ramifications for Petzl's (2006, p. 62) argument that there was medical competition between sanctuaries and secular doctors. If there was indeed fierce competition and if a primary function of the inscriptions was to *advertise* the potency of divine healing, then we might expect the majority, if not the whole corpus, to show a body part or at least foreground the healing nature of the experience in the image. This is not the case.

Scholarship highlights that behind the confession stelai lay the motive not just to atone, but to heal. It is not their resemblance to anatomical votives alone which should make us think this. Some stelai speak explicitly about healing, such as Petzl 94 in which we are told that Zenonis 'was punished and nursed back to health at the hands of Eunoia' (Ζηνωνὶς /. . . κολασθεῖσα / καὶ θαραπευθῖσα διὰ / τῆς Εὐνύας χιρὸς (ll. 2–4)), and there are a couple of stelai in which the medical context is both clear and illuminating. For example, *New Documents* no. 84 tells the story of Onesimos who was punished in his shoulder and 'was disbelieving towards the god and could not be cured by anyone, and was cured by the god' (<ἐ>κολάσ- / θη ἰς τὸν ὦμον καὶ δθσαπιστῶν τῷ θε- / ῷ καὶ ὑπὸ μηδενὸς δυνάμενος θαρα – / πευθῆναι ἐ<θ>αραπεύθην ὑπὸ τοῦ θεοῦ (ll. 11–14); Petzl, 2006, p. 60). He was then punished a second time, presumably for his disbelief in the healing powers of the god, and subsequently the god saved him again. As Chaniotis (1995, p. 332) points out, some priests had medical knowledge, as suggested by an inscription from Kula (*TAM* V.1 432) that tells of a young priest called Loukios who was a student of the doctor Tatianos. On the other hand, we should be aware of the limited nature of the information available about local illnesses and cures from evaluations of epigraphy alone. Indeed, only a certain number of afflicted body parts are mentioned: eyes, breasts, bottoms, legs, feet, knees, genitalia and arms. These cannot have been representative of all the maladies that affected the region. There are, for instance, no torsos represented, yet we cannot imagine the region was free from heart and stomach illnesses. Internal organs are absent from the corpus at both the visual and textual level, unlike in Italic/Roman corpora (van Straten, 1981, p. 101; see also chapters by Flemming and Haumesser, this volume). One inscription mentions the 'soft parts', which might well refer to an internal malady or possibly the genitals. A number of stelai mention general maladies such as being 'struck dumb', 'put in a yoke' or put in a 'state of death', where the image of the affliction is not represented, presumably because such illness are difficult to represent iconographically.[11]

11 Petzl 1 (struck dumb), 7 (death-like state), 10 (death-like state), 34 (killing of animals and daughter), 35 (destroyed), 37 (death of son and granddaughter), 54 (death), 57 (insanity), 67 (put in a yoke), 68

There seems to be no correlation between gods and illness. As Chaniotis (1995, p. 330, Table 3) concluded by looking at both the confession stelai and votives, 'practically any local deity was believed to be competent to cause any kind of health problem' (see also Forsén, 1996).[12] Female illnesses, for instance, were not the preserve of female deities. Petzl 53 concerns Stratonike who was 'punished' on her right breast. The fact that she attributes the punishment and therefore dedicates the stele to Men Axiottenos shows that considerations about the nature of the crime and the wronged deity supersede those of the type of illness in question. Stratonike had borrowed a *modius* of wheat from land sacred to Men Axiottenos, so it was he who had to be appeased. In this way the propitiatory nature of the inscriptions comes to the fore. The stelai advertised not the gods' medical competency, but rather their ability to be appeased and remove a divine affliction: sanctuary and secular healing were not equivalent alternatives. Similarly, the choice of divine addressee was not a matter of which deity could best heal, but rather whose anger needed appeasing. Despite this, the clear overlap of the concepts of 'transgression' and 'illness' demonstrated throughout the corpus challenge Chaniotis's (1995, p. 335) statement that 'the primary aim of medicine is to cure sick people, whereas the primary aim of the rites which we find in the propitiatory inscriptions is to relieve a sinner from his sin'. He uses Petzl 5, the Theodorus stele, as an example, pointing to the fact that it is 'sin' which the god is said to take away, not his affliction. But the affliction *was*, or at least was closely associated with, the state of having committed a transgression. Moreover, the fact that different ideas of pathological cause were arguably held by secular and religious healers does not mean that the primary aims of their patients were different. It is clear that the recovery and preservation of health was a primary consideration and the removal of the impurity attendant on transgression was a way to achieve it.

Ritual in relief: illuminating anatomical votives

One of the most intriguing questions concerning anatomical votives relates to the temporal context of their dedications: Were they thanksgivings for healing, or were they dedicated in the hope of a cure? Van Straten (1981, p. 103) addressed this question, finding evidence that anatomical votives could function in both of these ways. In the confession stelai, too, there is evidence that some stelai were set up in thanksgiving following the healing of the affliction and also an indication that others were set up in hope of propitiation and cure. A number

---

(death), 69 (death), 72 (death), 80 (death), 81 (insanity), 100 (became weak) and 103 (punished flocks); *New Documents* no. 51 (death). There is arguably an exception to the absence of such depictions: a marble votive relief (lot 27) sold at Bonhams, London on 24 October 2012 appears to be an entirely iconographic confession stele depicting a narrative sequence in which the transgressor ends up in a yoke, thus echoing in image the linguistic metaphor of Petzl 67.

12 Some gods appear more frequently than others such as Mater Phileis, Men Axiottenos and Artemis Anaitis, but that may be a consequence of their wider popularity (Chaniotis, 1995, p. 330).

of stelai adopt a tone of thanksgiving which is not found across the whole corpus and which show that they were set up after the afflicted body part was cured. Petzl 70, for example, was set up 'after Meter Anaitis was appeased', and the first-person account of Antonia of Petzl 43 tells us 'I confessed and set up a eulogy because I recovered my health'. Likewise, Onesimos in *New Documents* no. 84 says 'having been saved by the god, for my own part I set up this stele in praise'. In contrast, other stelai are more propitiatory in nature, although none explicitly say that they remain punished. For example, there are stelai such as Petzl 85 which convey little information other than that someone is dedicating a stele 'having been punished'. Petzl 85 simply reads 'to the goddess Phileis, Klaudia, after having been punished in her eyes [sets up a stele]' (ll. 1–4). Similarly, Akıncı Öztürk and Tanrıver no. 2, rather than being thankful in tone, is actually admonitory: '[I was punished] on my buttock. I declare that nobody should disregard [the god], because he will find my stele as a warning' (ll. 1–6). Furthermore, *New Documents* no. 83, a confession to Meter Anaitis, Meis Tiamou and Meis Ouranios from Collyda, ends with 'Tryphania, a slave of Babylonia, entered unsuitably and was punished and now confesses' (ll. 5–8). The tone of these texts suggests that such stelai aspire to the restoration of health rather than giving thanks for it. Whereas in the majority of cases where the verb ὁμολογέω or ἐξομολογέομαι appears, it is used in the past tense, there are some stelai on which the present tense 'I confess' is used, such as Petzl 100 (ὁμολογέω), 106 (ὁμολογέω), 111 (ἐξομολογοῦμε) and 116 (ἐξομολογοῦμαι). Given that the process detailed in other stelai tends to be that of punishment–confession–healing (for example, Petzl 3 and 43), this observation also indicates that such stelai were erected before, and in hope of, a cure. In this way it would be wrong to talk of *the* function of the confession stelai because it is clear that each stele was motivated by, and tailored to, individual circumstances. The functions of the confession stelai consequently match the functions of anatomical votives as identified by van Straten (1981): they could be employed in thanksgiving for the healing of an affliction after the successful granting of a vow, but they could also be part of the process of divine reconciliation to bring about healing.

Anatomical confession stelai also shed light on an ever-elusive question concerning the motivations behind anatomical votive offerings: Why would someone dedicate an anatomical votive? That they were thanksgivings for divine healing, fulfilments of promises made in prayer or requests for a cure does not illuminate the whole picture. The confession stelai, however, highlight the desire to propitiate, and even expiate, as a psychological impetus behind anatomical votives. The context for the dedication of anatomical *ex-votos* in the region was also the context of the confession inscriptions, and this chapter has argued that they were different epigraphic expressions of a common intellectual world. In appearance neither group of inscriptions is easily distinguishable from the other, with their iconography and format strikingly similar, yet they are conceptualised as different genres. Such observations call for a reconsideration of the function of anatomical votives as traditionally conceived. What if they, like the confession stelai, were offerings made in reparation for religious transgression? Their silence is, of course, inconclusive on the matter of a perceived expiatory function. However, Pazzini (1935, p. 53ff.) proposed that anatomical votives did not simply function *pro memoria* after or in search of healing, but that they in fact served as expiatory offerings. He quotes what he deems to be the first mention of an anatomical votive in literature which is illuminating in the context of this chapter because it explicitly shows an anatomical votive to function as a guilt offering. In 1 Samuel 6, when the Philistines have been punished with a plague by the God of Israel for having stolen the Ark of the Covenant, they asked 'priests and diviners':

> 'What is the guilt offering that we shall return to him?' They answered, 'Five gold tumours and five gold mice, according to the number of the lords of the Philistines; for the same plague was upon all of you and upon your lords.
> So you must make images of your tumours and images of your mice that ravage the land, and give glory to the God of Israel; perhaps he will lighten his hand on you and your gods and your land . . . '.
>
> (1 Samuel 6.4–5 NSRV)[13]

Consequently, Pazzini (1935, p. 54) understood the *ex-voto* in the ancient world to have functioned as an expiatory sacrifice, a substitution of the part of the body affected in order to transfer the 'sin' onto the object away from the actual body part. This is particularly interesting in light of confession stelai which suggest that the physical transferal of wrongdoing was in fact a concept familiar to and practised by dedicants in inland Anatolia. Petzl 6 (AD 238–239) tells of the wrongdoing being dispelled by a *triphonion* of a mole, a sparrow and a tuna fish; likewise in Petzl 5 the priest is said to take away Theodorus's first wrongdoing with a sheep, a partridge and a mole; his second with three sorts of fish; and his third with three sorts of birds (Chaniotis, 1995, p. 334). These appear to be rituals for the transmission of wrongdoing onto animals (Chaniotis, 2009, pp. 137–8). Therefore, the confession stelai call for a reconsideration of the perceived functions of anatomical votives in inland Anatolia at least and perhaps elsewhere in the Mediterranean as well. The common linguistic usage between votives of the region and confession stelai prompted Chaniotis (2009, p. 118) to reflect that 'the background of thanksgiving dedications in these regions may have been divine punishment', but the observations made in this chapter should cause us to consider this possibility yet more seriously and even beyond the confines of 'these regions'. The dedicatory context we see in the corpus – that of divine punishment, desperate hopes for cures, confession, appeasement and coercion to *stelographein* – offers a provocative lens through which to contemplate the background of the more breviloquent or even 'mute' dedications of the region, hinting at hitherto underacknowledged expiatory intent.

---

13 The word translated as 'tumours' – טְחֹרֵי – can mean 'haemorrhoids' or 'swellings'. Regardless of how it is translated, it refers to some malady of plague.

'Conventional' anatomical votives have also been silent about whether a financial transaction accompanied the dedication of a votive. Petzl 58 is unusual in that it provides information about a certain Eudoxos who paid nine obols to fulfil an oath that his wife had sworn but left unfulfilled. The inscription then suggests that he paid the sanctuary 175 *denarii* for the matter to be settled. This raises questions concerning the context of anatomical *ex-votos* in general: Were they accompanied by a financial transaction to the healer-priests or to the sanctuary? Because Eudoxos's wife had promised a votive but then not fulfilled her vow, it is significant that he fulfilled it 'by paying' nine obols as well as setting up a stele, as if he were paying off the financial obligation that came with making a vow and dedicating a εὐχή. So it is probable, especially given the close relationship between *ex-votos* and confession stelai outlined in this chapter, that at least in this part of inland Anatolia anatomical votives were accompanied by extra financial burdens. What is more, the textual and presentational elaboration characteristic of the confession stelai implies that they would have come at an even higher price than other anatomical votives, further articulating the hierarchy of propitiatory epigraphy.

Accounting for absence: why *stelographein*?

The reason why sentiments of confession and expiation might be absent from some votives yet present on others is difficult to infer. Rostad (2002, p. 163) posed the question of why sentiments present on confession stelai were absent from other votives of the area, considering whether the former were the product of 'oriental' inheritance or just peculiar expressions of ideas found in the Greco-Roman world. Whilst the aim of this chapter is not to suggest that everyone in inland Anatolia thought the same way about the gods, it is to warn against the assumption that each type of votive might be the product of a different mentality as if the dedicants of anatomical votives viewed the gods as beneficent, whereas the transgressors of the confession stelai viewed the gods as punishers. The arguments proposed in this chapter suggest that the stelai were not products of an isolated culture.

We have already seen that only certain illnesses feature as motivating causes of confession stelai, with many remarkably absent from the corpus, and that it mattered more which god required appeasement than which god could best heal the malady. These are significant observations in the context of deducing why someone would set up a confession stele rather than an anatomical votive because they indicate that the confession stelai were only erected in certain conditions: for crimes which aroused divine anger and for maladies which could be in some way connected with divine provenance. Looking at the illnesses more closely, we see that ocular illnesses account for half of those that are mentioned in the corpus, with others concerning mental illness, breasts, buttocks, legs, arms, loss of virginity and genitals (Chaniotis, 1995, p. 327; Table 1 pp. 338–9). These were either associated particularly with divine causation (such as mental illness or blindness) or denoted the part of the body responsible for the offence (as was the case for Metrodorus who broke a stele of the gods and so was punished in his arm: Petzl 78; Pettazzoni, 1936, p. 69). Even the punishments which on the surface seem to have little connection to the divine can be found to have religious resonance. For example, in Petzl 69 we hear that a sickle (δρέπανον) dropped on Sokrates's foot precipitated the attempted cancelling of the 'sceptre and the curses' (τὰς ἀράς). Although a sickle dropping on a foot might seem to be a random accident, there is evidence elsewhere in Anatolian epigraphy for religious sentiment concerning 'the curse of the sickle', based on the Septuagint's mistranslation of Zachariah 5.1–4. In the original Hebrew this passage speaks of a flying scroll (מְגִלָּה: *megillah*), which is interpreted by the prophet to be a 'curse going out over the whole land' according to which thieves and false-oath swearers will be banished. However, the Septuagint misreads 'scroll' for 'sickle' (מַגָּל: *magal*; *Septuagint*: δρέπανον), and this version is what we find in some grave curses from Asia Minor (for example, *Inscriptiones Iudaicae Orientis* II no. 175:'. . . may the sickle of the curse enter his house and leave no one alive', see van der Horst, 2014, p. 139). Given that both theft and swearing false oaths feature prominently in the corpus, this highlights also the otherwise easily overlooked religious resonance of these crimes. Assessing the corpus's collection of punishments in this way, we are left with the impression that had it been gout plaguing Sokrates's foot there would have probably been no thought to *stelographein* so elaborately but he may well have dedicated an anatomical *ex-voto*.

The other necessary condition for confession stelai was that the wrongdoing was thought to have incurred divine wrath, although it is important to note that the gods were not concerned about *any* wrongdoing, only that which directly offended them. Transgression regarding cultic purity or breaking a 'stele of the gods' leaves little ambiguity as to whether the divine was offended (Chaniotis, 2009, p. 137). If the crime was less obviously offensive or the perpetrator slow to recognise culpability, it seems the dedication of a confession stele could be precipitated by an oracular command to *stelographein* (Chaniotis, 2009, p. 131). Alternatively, the victim could curse the culprit with a *defixio* or set up a sceptre in the sanctuary, whereby victimhood was ceremonially transferred from the human plaintiff to the god so that interpersonal injustices became religious infractions, as in the case regarding Apollonius's 'lost' pig (*New Documents* no. 66) or the stolen possessions of orphans (Petzl 35; see Chaniotis, 2009, pp. 127–9). Cruel though it may seem, the gods would have been indifferent to theft from orphans had a sceptre not been set up to transfer those possessions over to the gods, making them the victims. Therefore, confession stelai were not erected for *any* illness or for *any* wrongdoing such as murder (a crime remarkably absent from the corpus), but only in specific circumstances. Thus the distinction between anatomical votives and confession stelai was not about who dedicated them and the different mentalities they possessed, but about the exigencies of the circumstance.

The existence of a hierarchy of propitiatory epigraphy also hints at why someone would *stelographein* rather than dedicate a simple anatomical *ex-voto*: confession stelai seem to have been required when particular circumstances demanded dedicants surpass ordinary epigraphic expectations. The necessary (but perhaps not sufficient) circumstances for this extra effort, as we have seen, appear to have been that both illness/punishment and wrongdoing were associated with the divine. However, we have also seen that confession stelai came with extra financial burdens which not everyone could have supported. Expiatory intent may thus have equally motivated the dedication of simpler anatomical *ex-votos*, with wealth determining the final form of epigraphic expression. It may even have depended on whether the dedicant sought a degree of anonymity (de Cazanove, 2009, p. 1). The difference, therefore, concerns not which group of dedicants was more or less fearful of the gods, but whose circumstances caused them to view their lot in terms of religious wrongdoing and divine retribution and whose financial means or capacity for self-inculpation constrained their epigraphic expression, investing nonetheless as much credence in the gods' capacity for mercy as their capacity for wrath. Those who may never have felt the necessity of dedicating a confession stele seem likely to have thought of the gods as wrathful punishers just as much as Theodorus considered Zeus and Men Axiottenos. A concern for theodicy must also account for confession stelai to some degree given their blatant advertisement of 'the powers of the gods': some self-identify as a 'witness' (μαρτύριον: Petzl 9 and 17) or a 'proof' (ἐξεμπλάριον: Petzl 106, 111–12 and 120–21). However, we should be careful not to infer from this that confession was sanctuary sponsored rather than customer driven, not least because it was in the transgressor's interest to justify and please the gods just as much as it was the priest's.

Moreover, the choice was conditioned by regional conventions and local practices. The relatively simple portrayal of a roughly incised leg seems to be a Phrygian phenomenon, and in general the Phrygian stelai seem to be of a poorer quality than their Lydian counterparts. Furthermore, it is interesting to note that in all the recent publications of finds from the sanctuary of Apollo Lairbenos in Phrygia only one nonconfessional anatomical votive has been found (Akıncı Öztürk and Tanrıver, 2009, p. 87, no. 1). Although fragmentary, this shows a breast in relief, which no doubt would have been accompanied originally by another one to the side and reads '. . . having made a vow, [dedicates this] to Apollo Lermenos'. Although the sanctuary has not been excavated systematically, it is arguably significant that in all the publications of new finds an anatomical votive has not yet been found that is not also a confession stele, except for that cited earlier. In contrast, the Phrygian votives in the Drew-Bear corpus discussed so far are dedicated to Zeus Alsenos and Zeus Petarenos, to whom no confession stele is dedicated (Drew-Bear et al., 1999, p. 17; the sanctuary has been located near Kurudere). Contrasting the abundance of 'simple' anatomical *ex-votos* there with the apparent lack of 'simple' anatomical votives at the sanctuary of Apollo Lairbenos, together with the lack of confession stelai at the former yet their abundance at the latter, adds weight to the suggestion that epigraphic expression was conditioned by local, even sanctuary-specific, practices. The worshipers at the sanctuary of Apollo Lairbenos may have been more inclined to dedicate a confession stele should they have found themselves the recipient of a divinely sent affliction, whereas those who worshipped at the sanctuary of Zeus Alsenos and Zeus Petarenos tended instead to dedicate a 'simple' *ex-voto* with little epigraphic detail. Despite these sanctuary-specific tendencies, the presence of Akıncı Öztürk and Tanrıver (2009) no. 1 at the sanctuary of Apollo Lairbenos shows that confession stelai and anatomical *ex-votos* could be, and were, dedicated at the same sanctuary. This suggests that although each sanctuary might have a customary mode of anatomical epigraphic expression, alternatives were possible. Unfortunately, the fact that the Lydian stelai have been found in mixed contexts with little known about the archaeological sites of their sanctuaries makes judgements for the Lydian material difficult to formulate. However, the same gods appear as recipients of both confession stelai and of *ex-votos* from Lydia, implying that both categories of epigraphy were dedicated at the same sanctuaries. In the Lydian context, sanctuary-specific preferences for one type of votive over the other were arguably not as influential as the simple acknowledgement of religious offence, the worshipper's financial means, the setting up of a sceptre or the command to *stelographein*. We must also consider the inscriptions' materiality in accounting for the confession stelai. The proximity of marble quarries, most notably at Dokimeion, help to explain epigraphic practice in the area: the lavishly lapidary land must have facilitated the elaboration required for the detail of confession.

Conclusions

This chapter has shown the fluidity of boundaries between the confession stelai of Asia Minor and anatomical votives of the region. Through a comparison of the two corpora we have seen significant parallels of iconography, presentation and language which highlight how the circumscription of confession stelai has hinged on the relative elaboration of their texts. With the questionable nature of the distinction thus put into focus, we are led not only to reflect on what attributes should determine the classification of votives as 'anatomical', but also to reassess our understanding of both corpora. In particular, we have seen that the 'anatomical' was not always manifested visually in the epigraphy of inland Anatolia. Due to the textual elaboration of confession stelai we know that symbols or gods could be depicted on votive stelai even when the contextual circumstances of their dedication could be just as 'anatomical' as those of votives depicting body parts. This prompts a reassessment of classificatory methodology, as votives which present neither on the visual or textual register as 'anatomical' could be equally worthy of consideration in studies of anatomical votives. Visual appearance alone has tended to dictate how scholarship determines an anatomical votive, but this analysis encourages us to consider whether it should, instead, be function or dedicatory circumstance which makes a votive 'anatomical' and even whether delineation of such a category is helpful at all. Viewing confession stelai as anatomical votives has illuminated our understanding of the function of conventional anatomical votives because the confession stelai expatiate detail about both the common religious milieu and the dedicants themselves on which most anatomical votives are otherwise silent. They confirm that votives might be dedicated in the hope of, as well as thanksgiving for, a cure and suggest that they were accompanied by extra financial burdens payable to the sanctuary.

Comparative analysis has shown that confession stelai *were* anatomical votives of a sort, albeit with supplementary textual detail, but this study has also attempted to assess the extent to which anatomical votives of the region were expiatory votives. The confession stelai underline the link between bodily affliction and punishment for wrongdoing while emphasising the role of divine healing. Although this might imply that dedicants of anatomical votives who clearly do appeal to divine healthcare also linked the malady to punishment, we cannot base our assessment on this alone. Similarity in appearance between the two corpora is not enough to suggest that dedicants of anatomical votives were similarly motivated or possessed the same religious mentality as the dedicants of confession stelai. Rather, it is the fact that the dedicants of confession stelai and anatomical votives appear to have been part of the same material and intellectual world which suggests that the corpora were different epigraphic expressions of common religious mentality. The contexts of production of the corpora were shared: the same sculptors produced inscriptions of both types, working with wide geographical reach and not confined to a particular sanctuary, and chronological comparisons further demonstrate their common contexts of production. Moreover, the people who dedicated confession stelai also dedicated votives, as well as less elaborate tokens of – as the inscriptions themselves make clear – propitiation.

The identification of a hierarchy of propitiatory epigraphy reinforces the argument that the two corpora were products of a common intellectual world and, what is more, accounts for the fundamental difference between them. For all that this chapter has stressed the similarity of confession stelai and anatomical votives, there must have been a reason why someone would employ one form of epigraphic expression over the other. It has been observed both from comparative analysis of appearance and from textual indications found in the inscriptions that confession stelai represented a step up from simple votive offerings. In the situation of Menophila and her sister Julia, where Menophila had defaulted on her promise of a propitiatory πιναξ and her sister Julia had joined in her prayers after this additional misdemeanor, it is moving to observe that Julia proceeded to *stelographein*, apparently accepting that whatever was next presented to the god would have to be even more desirable than the promised πιναξ for the initial offence. The command to *stelographein*, the setting up of a sceptre, financial means and existential exigences intensified by the natural human desire to go to the greatest lengths possible to effect salvation (particularly if a simple *ex-voto* had failed) were also important factors in determining whether a confession stele was the most appropriate response.

Analysis of the two corpora also sheds light on the dedicatory background of the confession stelai. The identification of a shared religious and intellectual milieu between the dedicants of confesison stelai and anatomical votives indicates that the stelai do not represent the vestiges of an isolated religious mentality that was distinct from that held by dedicants who expressed themselves in an apparently more 'Greco-Roman' epigraphic fashion. The specific circumstances of their dedications point to the necessity of certain structural conditions in determining whether someone would *stelographein*: the transgression had to be deemed offensive to a god and the punishment must have been conceived as a divinely inflicted penalty. This suggests that the dedicants of the two corpora cannot be polarised into those on the one hand who, associating *any* illness with their own culpability, immediately proceeded to act on a particular inclination to confess and atone for wrongdoing, and those on the other hand who dedicated anatomical votives because they did not view the gods as punishers and simply hoped for or gave thanks for divine healing. If our understanding remains that in cases where the illness was not thought to be a divine punishment an anatomical votive would be dedicated, it is interesting to note that only certain body parts are represented. This suggests that their dedication too was constrained by particular circumstances which it makes sense to interpret as the types of illness associated with divine punishment. Nevertheless, it remains probable that those seeking divine assistance for general maladies would dedicate anatomical votives, with those who had internal problems dedicating a simple votive representing a symbol or god, for instance. This chapter therefore does not argue that every anatomical *ex-voto* was dedicated by someone who felt culpable for a religious offence or punished by the god, but it does demonstrate that expiatory intent was likely behind the dedication of at least some anatomical votives in inland Anatolia. This would be particularly likely in cases where dedicants could not afford a confession stele or, in the absence of a command to *stelographein*, a more anonymous approach was the prefered first response.

There are implications here for understandings of anatomical votives elsewhere in the Greco-Roman world: If the anatomical *ex-votos* of inland Anatolia are silently expiatory, then can this judgement also be applied to the moulded body parts dedicated at, for instance, the Asclepieion at Epidaurus? This is an especially pertinent question given the fact that the only two examples of epigraphic confession from the ancient Greek world were found at this site (dating to the fourth century BC: *IG* IV² 123.67 and 91). Although their number is dwarfed by the many anatomical votives dedicated at the sanctuary, the observation is further intriguing in light of Pazzini's (1935, p. 63) argument that the healer-gods to whom anatomical *ex-votos* were dedicated, such as Asclepius, were in origin understood to be punisher-gods; it was from their function as dispensers of evil that their role as dispensers of beneficence developed. Whereas Parker (1996, p. 255) contrasts the message conveyed by the confession stelai with that of the temple record at Epidaurus (the former warning of vengeful deities, the latter praising a beneficent healer-god), the realities behind the rhetoric may have been less distinct than this suggests: epigraphy from the Asclepieion indicates that conceptions of illness as punishment and propitiation of a vengeful deity were indeed present in the background of at least some dedications there.[14] It seems, then, that not all Epidauran votives were simply thanksgivings for the cure of random illness. Furthermore, the votives of this sanctuary appear to have functioned didactically to memorialise 'the power of the god' just as confession stelai did (Dillon, 1994). It is beyond the scope of this chapter to transgress geographical boundaries, but this study does provoke the question of whether anatomical votives served expiatory functions elsewhere in the Mediterranean and whether the relative abundance of the confession stelai in inland Anatolia, representing the trumping of ordinary propitiatory dedications, was particularly facilitated there by the lapidary lavishness of the land.

Whilst the dictum that 'absence of evidence is not evidence of absence' so often marks the ancient historian's point of surrender, this chapter has shown how a better understanding of the silence might be advanced by holistic analysis of material available. The consequences of transgression do require bravery in facing them: whilst the evidence is not conclusive, it is highly suggestive. It is hoped that this initial exploration will encourage scholarship to attend to this important issue once more. As the dedicants of the confession stelai demonstrate, it is not always easy to identify where boundary lines really lie, but the confession stelai take us beyond a world of thanksgiving and prayer to a world of crimes, curses and confessions.

14 *IG* IV² 1, 121–2 details the experience of a number of dedicants: Ambrosia of Athens came to the temple and 'laughed at some of the cures as incredible and impossible' and so the god demanded that she dedicate to the temple a silver pig as a 'memorial of her ignorance' (ὑπομναμα τᾶς ἀμαθίας) before she was healed (Stele 1, no. 4; Edelstein and Edelstein, 1945 and 1998, p. 230); Hermon of Thasus was cured of blindness by Asclepius but failed to give a thank-offering so was made blind again, but when he came back the god healed him (Stele 2, no. 22; Edelstein and Edelstein, 1945 and 1998, p. 233); Cephisias accused the god of lying about his healing and so 'the god did not conceal that he was inflicting penalty for the insolence' (τὰς ὕβριος ποινὰς λαμβάνω[ν οὐκ ἔλαθε . . .) as his horse fell and crippled his foot. After he 'entreated him earnestly' (πολλὰ καθικετεύ[σαντα . . .) the god made him well (Stele 2, no. 36; Edelstein and Edelstein, 1945 and 1998, p. 236). Valerius Maximus (*Facta et dicta memorabilia* I. 1,19) calls Asclepius 'a no less effective avenger of sacrilege' ('*nec minus efficax ultor contemptae religionis*'), citing the example of Turullius who cut down the god's grove in order to build ships. When he was later executed by Caesar on the very spot where the grove had been, Asclepius 'increased the great veneration which he had always enjoyed with his worshippers'.

2 Partible humans and permeable gods

Anatomical votives and personhood in the sanctuaries of central Italy

Emma-Jayne Graham

A hilltop on the northwestern outskirts of the ancient city of Fregellae in the Liri Valley about 100 km to the southeast of Rome was the setting for an enduring series of religious activities. Evidence of the nature of the earliest cult on the site is scarce, but archaeological and epigraphic evidence indicates that it predated the refounding of what was originally a Volscian town as a Latin colony in 328 BC. The same evidence suggests that it was connected with a female divinity of water or fertility, possibly Mefitis or Feronia, both of whom were commonly worshipped in the region, as well as with Salus (Coarelli, 1986b, p. 7). During the first half of the second century BC the setting for these longstanding ritual activities underwent considerable monumentalisation, and an inscribed altar found within the built-up area reveals that by this date rituals associated with Asclepius were also taking place there (Coarelli, 1986b, p. 7). More than four thousand unstratified terracotta votive offerings were recovered from the area during excavations in the 1970s, many of which represent parts of the human body (Ferrea and Pinna, 1986). Amongst them is a clear predominance of feet, legs and heads, as well as high numbers of hands and arms and a range of other parts of the internal and external human body (Ferrea and Pinna, 1986, p. 89). Individual offerings cannot be dated with precision, but the excavators assigned the assemblage to a broad period between the fourth and third quarters of the second century BC, noting that most were probably deposited during the third and early second centuries (Ferrea and Pinna, 1986, pp. 143–4). The majority of anatomical votive objects from Fregellae consequently attest to cult activities that predate the monumentalisation of the sanctuary, an event which effectively coincided with the end of this dedicatory behaviour.

At Fregellae the stimulus for anatomical offerings was evidently not the monumental development of the sanctuary or any subsequent attraction of pilgrims that it may have given rise to. Instead, anatomical votives appeared for the first time in the context of well-established cults associated with *sanatio* (health or well-being) around the end of the fourth century BC before successively gathering pace. This phenomenon – the emergence of the so-called 'Etrusco-Latial-Campanian' votive tradition (Lesk, 2002; Glinister, 2006) – is reported at many other contemporary sanctuary sites across central Italy. From the fourth century BC onwards new and existing shrines and sanctuaries received large numbers of terracotta dedications representing the human body, both whole and more often divided into its constituent parts. At many of these sites earlier *ex-votos* attest to the presence of already long-established ritual activities, many with origins in the Iron Age (Protovillanovan and Villanovan periods; Turfa, 2006a, p. 90). The very earliest dedications at these sites reflect regional variations and encompass a range of different types of offerings, including miniature ceramic vessels and bronze or terracotta statuettes depicting divine figures (Lowe, 1978; Turfa, 2006a; Scarpellini, 2013). Particularly favoured in these early deposits were figurines of either the tutelary deity of the shrine or the god whose specific expertise or protection was sought, as well as warriors, so-called 'Tanagra' figurines and, from the end of the sixth century BC, isolated heads or busts (Nagy, 2013; Recke, 2013, p. 1068). Secure stratigraphic dating for votive assemblages is often lacking (and dating methods are notoriously circular), but from the end of the fourth century these once-common offerings were largely, although not completely, superseded by models depicting the bodies of human suppliants. Rather than focusing on the head alone, these new forms depicted humans in the act of worship or at various stages in the life course (infancy, adolescence, marriage and maternity), as well as fragmented into parts thought to reflect the area of the human body appropriate to the circumstances of the petition (Comella, 2005, p. 48; Bartoloni and Benedettini, 2011, pp. 784–5; Scarpellini, 2013).

This change in the composition of dedicatory assemblages was not restricted to major healing sanctuaries such as Fregellae. At Punta della Vipera in the vicinity of modern Civitavecchia to the northwest of Rome ceramic votive material associated with an altar dedicated to a chthonic divinity attests to the foundation of a small sanctuary in the years around 530 BC (Comella, 2001, p. 129). Also recovered from the site were three inscriptions naming the Etruscan goddess Menerva. These texts were incised onto fragments of bucchero (late sixth century BC), Faliscan ware (late fourth to early third century BC) and an amphora handle (third century BC), providing secure evidence for the duration of cult activity at the site (Comella, 2001, p. 136). The same goddess was also represented by a small number of terracotta figurines (Comella, 2001, p. 139). The site at Punta della Vipera subsequently underwent modifications during the fourth century BC before more substantial rebuilding and a 'reinvigoration' of the cult took place around the middle of the third century BC, probably in conjunction with the founding of a nearby colony and a reorganisation of the social circumstances of the local community (Comella, 2001, pp. 129–30). As at Fregellae, much of the votive material from Punta della Vipera belongs to an arc covering the late sixth to second century BC: the earliest phases (c. 530 to the early fourth century BC) are characterised by seated female figurines, with anatomical *ex-votos* belonging exclusively to the second and third periods of the site's use, that is from the late fourth century onwards (Comella, 2001, p. 138).

The changes in the nature of votive offerings observed at these sites and more widely across central Italy have been viewed as evidence for the rise of so-called 'popular' religion and greater concerns for health (Fenelli, 1975; Comella, 1981; 1996; 2005; Baggieri, 1999). However, such apparently straightforward arguments for the emergence (not to mention subsequent disappearance) of anatomical votives at Italian sacred sites remain a matter of dispute, and it seems unlikely that this phenomenon can be explained in such simple terms. More interesting and potentially enlightening questions concern what stimulated this behaviour in the first place, why the fragmented human body was adopted as a material expression of communications with the divine and what this votive behaviour suggests about the ways in which socioreligious knowledge and identities were constructed during this period. With these questions in mind this chapter investigates the anatomical votive phenomenon attested at Fregellae, Punta della Vipera and other sites of central Italy from a new perspective. It will not pursue well-trodden and unsatisfactorily resolved issues such as the meaning of individual anatomical offerings; their typological and technological development; the possible requests, diseases, conditions or experiences with which they were associated; or their connection with developing medical knowledge. Instead, the argument presented here focuses on what the dedication of an anatomical offering meant with regard to the relationship between mortal and divine persons in the ancient world. This does not mean merely what such offerings represented or symbolised. Rather, this chapter asks what the implications were of dedicating an object that took the form of a material citation of the human body and what these might reveal about how people conceptualised, performed and, most importantly, constructed their knowledge of the gods. It is argued here that an assessment of the consequences of votive activities centred on the body can provide significant new insights into the extent to which particular forms of 'social' relationship were enacted and understandings of human and divine personhood performed and produced in the context of a specific type of religious community. In turn, this makes it possible to appreciate the popularity of anatomical votives in new and unexpected ways.

Votives and personhood

The act of dedicating any votive must be understood in the context of a framework of cult practice, which like many ancient ritual activities, centred on sustaining the relationship between mortals and gods. For the ancient Italic world this is usually described with reference to Latin formulations and terminology. These set out how divine guidance or assistance could be attained by means of a contract that was articulated with a prayer or other spoken formula in the form of a vow (*votum*) that the benevolence of the god would be subsequently acknowledged with a gift (*ex-voto*) once the request had been fulfilled or following a determined period (for the formal nature of votive cult, see van Straten, 1981; Rüpke, 2007, pp. 162–5; Bodel, 2009; also the Introduction to this volume). In broad terms votives provided the tangible material reference point for the contractual relationship established between mortal and divine. This occurred most often on the occasion of a request for healing, protection or other circumstances that concerned the physical or social well-being of a person, such as transitional points in the life course and passage across the age or status boundaries of society (Pautasso, 1994, pp. 114–15; Gatti and Onorati, 1996; Glinister, 2006, pp. 11–12; Graham, 2014). Significantly, although frequently overlooked by recent studies, anatomical votives situated the body of the suppliant – both real and figurative – at the very centre of these ritual practices through the deliberate material citation of the human form. Moreover, the way in which this occurred was far from arbitrary. As Jessica Hughes (2008) has argued, these objects indicate an intentional decision to interact with the divine with reference not just to the body but also to its fragmentation. As a result, she asserts that an anatomical *ex-voto* connected with a request for healing might not only act as a metaphor for illness, but that healing itself could be perceived as 'the disassembly and subsequent remaking of the body' (Hughes, 2008, p. 232). Divine healing and other forms of divine intervention concerning the well-being of a suppliant might therefore be conceptualised as a complex embodied experience capable of exemplifying but also generating religious knowledge with reference to the materiality and inherent fragility of the body. In order to investigate the significance of such embodied experiences, this chapter situates anatomical votives in the context of recent studies of personhood. In particular it draws upon the insights derived from anthropological and archaeological analyses of relational forms of persons and the maintenance of these identities through reciprocity and forms of enchainment.

Although comprehensive discussion of the scholarly background of personhood theory is beyond the scope of this chapter (notable works include Strathern, 1988; Battaglia, 1990; Busby, 1997; LiPuma, 1998; Fowler, 2001; 2004; Jones, 2005; Kirk, 2006), it is necessary nonetheless to highlight the central principles crucial to the argument that will be developed. Theories of personhood assert that a 'person' is a contextually variable and multiauthored form of identity, something which is 'attained and maintained through relationships not only with other human beings but with things, places, animals and the spiritual features of the cosmos' (Fowler, 2004, p. 7). Indeed, according to Chris Fowler (2004, p. 7) personhood

> in its broadest definition refers to the condition or state of being a person, as it is understood in any specific context. Persons are constituted, de-constituted, maintained and altered in social practices through life and after death. This process can be described as the ongoing attainment of personhood.

In other words, personhood is a dynamically constructed form of identity that results from active participation in sociocultural practices which involve interaction with the bodies, material culture or essences of others (not necessarily restricted to humans) in particular places and at certain times. Personhood is therefore a context-specific and social form of identity, a product of the location of persons within a nexus of reciprocal relationships. These relationships might shift and change through time and across space as well as in response to changing sociocultural contexts. Specific senses of what it means to be one type of 'person' can therefore be related to distinct situations and circumstances but not necessarily to all. Together these different context-specific experiences and the senses of personhood that result from them generate the disparate components that make up one's composite identity, each coming to the fore in the appropriate context. As an example, the sense of personhood produced by a participant in an ancient votive cult might vary from that created by their participation in local politics or domestic relationships because of the different participants with whom they interacted, the varied nature of the relationships shared with them and the specific ways in which these relationships were performed and produced. From the perspective of personhood, it is the patterns of behaviour required in each of these settings and the different social relationships they involve which are responsible for producing and maintaining the part of the participant's identity that is specific to each of those circumstances and interactions. Moreover, as Fowler (2001, p. 148) observes, 'social ideals and categories of personhood are neither transcendentally "real", nor ideas simply reflected in the material world'. Instead, these types of person are created and maintained through active interaction with other human, animal, divine or inanimate persons and things: persons do not exist in passive isolation.

Central to concepts of personhood is therefore an understanding of *how* the social relationships crucial to producing these ways of understanding one's place in the world are enacted. This is commonly brought about through exchange, not only of material culture but also the parts and essences of the human body itself. Ethnographic studies suggest that persons can be described as 'dividual' or, put another way, persons are believed to be composed of the relationships, objects or substances they share and exchange with others within a community (Fowler, 2004, p. 8; Jones, 2005, pp. 194–200). Such dividuality can take two forms: partibility and permeability. The first involves the extraction of a 'part' of a person, object or animal believed to be integral to their state of being which is then transferred to another person; the second comprises the qualities or essences of one person permeating another in order to influence their respective compositions (Fowler, 2004, pp. 7–9). The two are not necessarily mutually exclusive, and the degree of partibility or permeability of a person may vary over the life course or in relation to the activities in which they participate or other elements of their identity such as age and gender. The communities of persons which result from and are sustained by dividual relationships might therefore be defined in a number of ways and might not consist exclusively of a group of humans, because it is the mutual activities in which participants engage and the essentially reciprocal relationships they share which define the community. A religious community might, for instance, be composed of human worshippers and the divine recipients of that worship, as well as the animals, objects and even the places used in the performance of cult activities.

For settings such as that examined in this chapter, objects are fundamental for understanding the negotiation and construction of personhood, in part because material culture often provides the only evidence for identifying past social interactions and exchanges. John Chapman (2000) advocates the concept of 'enchainment' for understanding how the forms of relational personhood outlined earlier might be produced through the exchange of material objects. According to Chapman (2000, p. 180) enchainment can be understood as the process whereby dividual persons maintain social relations through 'the exchange of inalienable objects', which for his study of prehistoric southeastern Europe entails the exchange of human bones, parts of fragmented ceramic vessels, figurines and other artefacts. 'Inalienable' essentially defines the items exchanged as things that cannot be given away, regifted or reused either in the same context or a different one because of their role in enchaining the participants to one another. This need not, however, preclude objects from taking on additional new meanings over time or bring an end to their dynamic and complex biographies. Chapman's (2000, p. 226) emphasis falls on the deliberate fragmentation and circulation of partial artefacts as a means of creating and maintaining meaningful bonds between persons or groups, but in other cultural contexts enchainment might be predicated on alternative forms of inalienable material culture or bodily substances which exemplify the dividuality of the person. So to what extent did ancient cult practice comprise acts of enchainment involving the transfer of inalienable elements of the respective dividual 'bodies' of both gods and mortals? What is more, how does categorising anatomical votives as objects which reference the partibility of persons within a religious community change the way in which we investigate gods, humans and the production of socioreligious knowledge and identities in central Italy between the fourth and first century BC?[1]

Pars pro toto? Anatomical votives and the dividual human

Alongside terracotta models of animals and buildings, typical Etrusco-Latial-Campanian votive assemblages include statuettes of men, women and swaddled infants; veiled and unveiled heads or busts; half-heads; open torsos, and other internal organs; numerous items often thought to be connected with 'fertility', including models of uteri, genitalia and breasts; as well as the ubiquitous isolated limbs and other body parts (in addition to chapters in this volume see Fenelli, 1975; Comella, 1981; 1996; 2005; Turfa, 1994; Lesk, 1999; 2002; Schultz, 2006). As noted earlier, models of deities continued to be dedicated, but from the fourth century BC a preponderance of offerings make reference to the body

---

1 Anatomical votives are the focus of this chapter, but other nonanthropomorphic votives might also serve as a part or an extension of the body. As Gell (1998, p. 123) observed, '[I]t does not matter, in ascribing "social agent" status, what a thing (or a person) "is" in itself; what matters is where it stands in a network of social relations'. Animal figurines might also be representative of the identity of a human suppliant as ethnographic parallels suggest: 'the elements which compose the 'Are' are person are distributed throughout the social world; they are to be found in the things which people grow, cultivate, rear and, most vitally, exchange. In other words, the qualities to be found in persons are found elsewhere in the world, in objects and plants and animals' (de Coppet, 1981; Fowler, 2004, p. 28).

of the human dedicant rather than to the divine recipient. Also significant is the fact that of the very few terracotta anatomical votives from Italy that bear inscriptions most name the dedicator rather than the deity to which it was given (Turfa, 2004, p. 363; Comella, 2005, p. 48; Fabbri, 2010, pp. 22–3; Bartoloni and Benedettini, 2011, p. 784). Many of the isolated body parts in these assemblages were probably intended to indicate medical conditions localised in that part of the human anatomy, but others may have been designed to act as an extension or representation of the whole person who made the offering. This is commonly explained with reference to the concept of *pars pro toto*, or 'a part for the whole'. Rather than making specific reference to headaches or injuries, heads or half-heads may therefore have represented a visual abbreviation of the whole being of a suppliant, derived perhaps from complex ancient notions of the head as the seat of personal identity (Glinister, 2006, p. 12; see also Onians, 1951). The swaddled form of a newborn infant might be emblematic of the moulding of their new bodies and the creation of a place for them in the socioreligious world (Graham, 2014; Glinister, this volume), whereas an open torso could serve to acknowledge that the dedicant was a complex being composed of different elements, as well as a person symbolically exposed to the intervention of the gods (Haumesser, this volume; Hughes, forthcoming). Indeed, it is probable that each individual *ex-voto* was invested with a range of highly subjective meanings, and it should be emphasised that the dedicant was not necessarily compelled to choose one of these over another. Opening one's body to the divine may have been just one of many simultaneous motives associated with the dedication of an open torso along with requests concerning very specific ailments, more general well-being or even recovery from nondivine medical intervention or surgery. Acknowledging this multivalent nature of anatomical votives as complex, meaning-laden objects is fundamental for an investigation of the connection between these artefacts and dividual personhood. It suggests that as well as being connected with requests or thanks for healing, good fortune and bodily welfare, anatomical votives could, like all 'religious' objects, serve simultaneously to exemplify and produce potentially more elusive religious knowledge related to the human body and the process of divine healing itself (Boivin, 2009, p. 274; Morgan, 2010, p. 12). Equally significant is the manner in which these objects present the very real surrender or, more accurately, the exchange of an aspect of the body and/or identity in gratitude for divine protection and care. Anatomical votives are, of course, inanimate models not actual body parts detached from a living person. However, the capacity of an anatomical votive to serve as an extension of the corporeal body (*pars pro toto*) and therefore to connote or to possess the fundamental essence or identity of a person makes it possible to interpret such objects in terms of the dividuality of the suppliant. Seen in the light of enchainment and dividual personhood, this behaviour suggests that, like the votive objects themselves, *pars pro toto* could operate in more ways than one. To examine this further, it is necessary to ask to what extent an anatomical *ex-voto* might be categorised as an inalienable material manifestation of a dividual human person.

In terms of enchainment it is important to observe that the act of ritual dedication rendered all votive offerings sacred. It was forbidden to remove gifts to the gods from the confines (*temenos*) of the sanctuary or shrine where they remained as tangible evidence of the relationship established and enacted between dedicant and deity. Nor could they be reused or appropriated for either sacred or profane purposes. In reality pressures on space meant that votive objects did not always remain on display in perpetuity, and cult officials or priests must have been responsible for clearing away any substantial accumulations in order to make way for more. Those of a particularly prestigious or expensive nature may have remained on display for longer, whereas others were removed to storage rooms or buried in pits (Turfa, 2006a, p. 91). Indeed, the contents of these pits, such as those at Fregellae and Punta della Vipera, are excavated more frequently than in situ dedications within cult rooms or temple structures, although the sanctuary at Graviscae provides a notable exception (Comella, 1978). Nonetheless, this process ensured that a votive became inalienable once it had been dedicated, regardless of whether it remained on display or not. In this sense a votive offering could only ever be used in one transaction, thereby establishing and embodying a relationship of enchainment between the human and divine participants in a vow. Other stages of the performance of votive ritual might involve similar unique transfers. Prayers or ritual formulae made on one occasion only and heard exclusively by the divine, as well as the making of the vow itself, can be regarded as the transmission of inalienable words imbued with the essence of the petitioner's identity which were heard, absorbed or even felt by the gods.[2] These words also belonged to that moment only and could not be shared with or given to anyone else, human or divine. A votive offering therefore denoted one petition or act of dedication. It also embodied the connection – the enchainment – between one person and one deity at a precise moment in time in the same way that Chapman (2000) writes of intentionally broken pieces of pottery being used to cement formal relationships between prehistoric people and communities. In the context of votive cult in Italy, this was an affiliation which also signified very precise circumstances. The suppliant would be required to make a new vow and therefore establish a new reciprocal arrangement should they decide to seek further help, guidance or healing from the same divinity. This relationship had to be constantly and repeatedly renewed in order for it to be maintained beyond the confines of a single vow, and it can be argued that this behaviour, mediated via material objects, was consequently responsible for the production of particular types of relational persons: suppliants and gods.

If deity and human were inextricably enchained by the ritualised process of prayer, vow, response and offering, then the votive offering itself must be understood not only as an element of exchange in this relationship, but also as material testimony to the dividual nature of the human *and* divine body. As sanctuaries

---

2 Relevant to this are comments by Onians (1951, pp. 66–8) about breath as the container of a person's 'intelligence' (i.e., identity) and Greek ideas about how 'thoughts are words and words are breath'.

came to be filled with objects that personified the presence of the human body, these assemblages themselves became a tangible sign that the divine had reciprocated or at least had the power to offer healing or protection in return. Put another way, worshippers had entrusted a part of themselves to the care of the god for whatever reason, and the *ex-voto* was left in the sanctuary as a material acknowledgment of that arrangement and its successful outcome. In turn, the very presence of objects attesting to these successful relationships bore witness to the fact that the god in question possessed the capacity to intervene directly in the human body through the transfer of healing or protective power to it. These objects therefore embodied the fundamental essence of divine power, and as a result this power came to be effectively personified by the assemblage of bodily fragments in that sacred place. By virtue of *pars pro toto* in its widest sense, anatomical votives therefore *were* the dividual bodies of worshippers combined with the healing powers or essence of the divine, and thus they secured a material bodily presence within the sanctuary not only for human suppliants but also for the divine. To enter a sanctuary or cult room involved a visual confrontation with the 'body' of this combined religious community arrayed before one's eyes, the very enchained dividuality of its human, divine and material members foregrounded by the reconstituted collection of heads, limbs, torsos and internal organs. Together these emphasised the human contribution to the creation, maintenance and manifestation of divine power.[3]

Anatomical votives dedicated by different people were therefore reassembled into a composite body, the fragmented nature of which existed as testimony to the relational forms of personhood which generated and sustained that religious community. Together these otherwise isolated body parts provided a single locus which embodied the bonds of dependency between the two types of person at its heart: by seeking divine assistance, humans provided the material body parts, which in turn enabled the incorporeal powers of the divine that they subsequently received to be made manifest in material form. After all, gods do not always need to be understood only in terms of the fully anthropomorphic forms commonly associated with cult statues, as Alfred Gell (1998, p. 98, original emphasis) explains: '[T]he idol form is the visual form of the god made present in the idol . . . Idols, in other words, are not depictions, not portraits, but (artefactual) *bodies*'. A deity can therefore be present within an object or objects even if the material form or appearance that it takes varies from what has come to be expected of religions such as those of ancient Italy which customarily produce recognisably anthropomorphic icons. As Michael Squire (2011, p. 167) also notes, '[S]tatues of the gods were as multistable as the deities that they embodied:

---

3 This contribution might also be reflected by the presence of models of animals or parts of animals, which also represented the community in its widest possible sense. Hughes (forthcoming) suggests that the juxtaposition of human and animal *ex-votos* may have led to the recognition of human–animal hybrids, an idea not incompatible with the notion that a person could be composed of the essences of animals and objects as well as gods and other humans.

in the same way that the gods were both assimilated to human bodies and different from them, images both materialised and impeded that divine bodily form'. Ways of representing the gods and their power might therefore vary from context to context, with the complete human body not always offering the most appropriate means by which to express shared knowledge of what divinity entails. For example, in the context of votive cult which involved relationships predicated on exchange and which emphasised the dividuality of both human and divine, an assemblage of fragmented body parts may have been eminently more evocative of how divine power was constituted and communicated than a cult statue of the deity alone. Under such circumstances ancient gods could be constructed not just in the image of their worshippers but also from their dividual bodies.

Viewed from this perspective it can also be argued that anatomical votives might play a role in the creation of a strong sense of community. Access to the most sacred areas may have been denied, but a sanctuary visitor familiar with votive cult would understand that as they performed their own prayers, vows or offerings they were surrounded by displays, storage rooms or pits containing the *ex-votos* dedicated by their family, neighbours and past members of their community. As such, the whole sanctuary offered compelling testimony to the shared actions and performances of the persons who made up the much broader religious community to which they belonged, both past and present, human and divine (for the sanctuary of Asclepius at Pergamum as a testimony to the community, see Petsalis-Diomidis, 2005; 2010). This knowledge could serve to reinforce the importance of cult activities and the need for continued enactment of the active relationship between human and divine in order to ensure ongoing stability, normality and security. Placing a votive limb or uterus amongst those belonging to friends, relatives and social leaders affirmed one's place in human society, and the cumulative effect of so many dedications maintained and confirmed the presence of the gods as very real participants in social relations and as persons in their own right.

Permeable and partible gods?

It has been argued earlier that both divine power and human identity were embodied by the material agents of votive practice, with anatomical *ex-votos* particularly well suited to this purpose. Indeed, as Nicholas Rynearson (2003, p. 7) notes for the healing cults of the Greek world, '[E]ach anatomical votive proclaims the power of the god by representing a successful narrative of healing', providing 'a direct proof of the power of the god himself'. However, although anatomical models might embody divine power by representing it in material form, they reveal much less about the underlying nature of that divine dividuality and precisely how this was understood to transfer to the bodies of human suppliants in exchange. Very few anatomical votives from Italy are accompanied by inscriptions recounting the names of dedicants, let alone the circumstances of their dedication, making it necessary to look elsewhere for parallels which might help to fill this gap. Consequently, despite being distant from the votive deposits of fourth to first century BC Italy in time and space, epigraphic testimony from sanctuaries of the Greek world as well as later ones operating under the Roman empire can be explored for clues about the possible ways in which the nature of the transfer of divine essence might be understood in Italian contexts. Such evidence is provided by the four stelae inscribed during the late fourth century BC at the sanctuary of Asclepius at Epidaurus recording approximately 70 tales of miraculous cures (*iamata*) performed by the healing specialist (*IG* IV² 1, 121–4; Edelstein and Edelstein, 1945 and 1998; LiDonnici, 1992). Similarly, during the Roman period at the Asclepieion at Pergamum in Asia Minor, pilgrims who had successfully sought and received healing often dedicated votives featuring a short narrative detailing the circumstances of their cure (Petsalis-Diomidis, 2010). Alongside this can be placed the experiences of the Roman-period orator Publius Aelius Aristides (c. AD 117–80) who spent two years at Pergamum seeking healing from Asclepius whose powers he used his writings in the *Sacred Tales* (*Hieroi Logoi*) to praise. The discussion which follows focuses largely on these three sources of evidence, but inscribed records of healing have also been recovered from Rome and other sites around the Mediterranean (Renberg, 2006–7), and the multiperiod *Palatine Anthology* records a selection of epigrams which recount similar experiences (although some may reflect poetical exercises rather than real dedications).

The inscribed *iamata* from Epidaurus offer valuable comparative evidence for the circumstances which led people to seek help from Asclepius, as well as the manner in which his divine power was transferred to their bodies in order to bring about healing. These accounts and others refer frequently to the process of incubation in which a person seeking cure or guidance would perform a series of stipulated rituals or sacrifices before sleeping in a dedicated room (*abaton*) in anticipation of receiving divine assistance in their sleep (Dillon, 1994, pp. 244–55; Cilliers and Retief, 2013; Ahearne-Kroll, 2014). The assistance they reportedly received included prescriptions for particular medicines, regimens of the body or ritual acts, which were often communicated in the context of dream visions, as well as direct healing and divine surgery in which the hero-god intervened personally in unconscious bodies. Although it is unknown whether these texts reflect the actual experiences of real pilgrims or the words of cult officials seeking to promote the powers of Asclepius, they provide a rare insight into ancient cultural scripts concerning the infiltration of the body with divine healing powers. Illustrative examples provide evidence for the various ways in which the divine might intervene directly or indirectly in the body of suppliants:

> A man came as a suppliant to the god. He was so blind that of one of his eyes he had only the eyelids left – within them was nothing, but they were entirely empty. Some of those in the Temple laughed at his silliness to think that he could recover his sight when one of his eyes had not even a trace of the ball, but only the socket. As he slept a vision appeared to him. It seemed to him that the god prepared some drug, then, opening his eyelids,

poured it into them. When day came he departed with the sight of both eyes restored.

(Stele 1, no. 9; Edelstein and Edelstein, 1945 and 1998, pp. 231–2)

A man with an abscess within his abdomen. When asleep in the Temple he saw a dream. It seemed to him that the god ordered the servants who accompanied him to grip him and hold him tightly so that he could cut open his abdomen. The man tried to get away, but they gripped him and bound him to a door knocker. Thereupon Asclepius cut his belly open, removed the abscess, and, after having stitched him up again, released him from his bonds. Whereupon he walked out sound, but the floor of the *Abaton* was covered with blood.

(Stele 2, no. 27; Edelstein and Edelstein, 1945 and 1998, p. 235)

Cleinatas of Thebes, with lice. He came with a great number of lice on his body, slept in the Temple, and sees a vision. It seems to him that the god stripped him and made him stand upright, naked, and with a broom brushed the lice from his body. When day came he left the Temple well.

(Stele 2, no. 28; Edelstein and Edelstein, 1945 and 1998, p. 236)

Cleimenes of Argus, paralysed in body. He came to the *Abaton* and slept there and saw a vision. It seemed to him that the god wound a red woollen fillet around his body and led him for a bath a short distance away from the Temple to a lake of which the water was exceedingly cold. When he behaved in a cowardly way Asclepius said he would not heal those people who were too cowardly for that, but those who came to him into his Temple, full of hope that he would do no harm to such a man, but would send him away well. When he woke up he took a bath and walked out unhurt.

(Stele 2, no. 37; Edelstein and Edelstein, 1945 and 1998, pp. 236–7)

It must be remembered that these examples and the others cited later relate to the cult of a specialist healing figure, whereas many of the sanctuaries of central Italy served more than one function and often more than one deity (the 'shades of cult' described by Comella, 1981, p. 762). At these sites it was routine for nonmedical petitions concerning the life course, fertility or other matters of personal safety and fortune to be made alongside those for healing. Nonetheless, the Epidauran *iamata* reveal that here, too, help was sought for a range of nonmedical matters, including missing persons (Stele 2, no. 24; Edelstein and Edelstein, 1945 and 1998, p. 234), sailing and business ventures (Stele 2, no. 8; LiDonnici, 1992, p. 27) and fertility (Stele 2, no. 42; Edelstein and Edelstein, 1945 and 1998, p. 237). Equally, evidence for incubation chambers within Hellenistic Italy is enigmatic (Renberg, 2006–7, pp. 128–9). Even the monumental Asclepieion at Fregellae lacks a designated sleeping structure, and scholars have tended to assume that two large porticoes were used for this purpose (Lesk, 1999, p. 68; for general difficulties associated with identifying an *abaton* structure, see

Baker, 2013, pp. 118–25). Once again, however, this absence of positive evidence need not be a barrier to using inscribed accounts from other cultural contexts to interrogate the manner in which divine power entered the body, not least because formal incubation was far from essential even in relation to the cult of Asclepius himself. Incubation could also occur by proxy (Dillon, 1994, p. 249) and as the epigraphic evidence makes clear suppliants could expect to receive visitations from deities in visions or dreams at other times and in other places (Dillon, 1994, p. 249). Nor were visions and dreams restricted to the cult of Asclepius. In a study of healing testimonies from Rome, Gil Renberg (2006–7, pp. 129–30) observed that the terminology used to refer to the receiving of advice or healing in dreams (*ex viso*) can be found in conjunction with multiple gods, including many who were unconcerned with medicine and not associated with incubation. This suggests that gods, including those consulted about nonmedical matters, might communicate with mortals through visions without the need for elaborate incubation rites or facilities. Other formulae such as *ex iusso* ('according to a command') 'cannot even be linked to dreams with any certainty since divine commands could also be imparted through a range of other divinatory media' (Renberg, 2006–7, pp. 130–1). Consequently, even deities who might regularly communicate through incubation need not always do so:

> [a]fter all . . . Asclepius, like any other divinity, could appear to individuals in dreams or visions whenever he pleased: his inclination to appear to his worshipers was by no means limited to those undergoing incubation, and his presence could be sensed by those nowhere near his healing sanctuaries.
> (Renberg, 2006–7, pp. 131–2)

The evidence for Asclepian healing therefore suggests that human bodies could receive divine intercession in multiple ways, including via direct intervention in the body and the use of divine surgery or drugs during dreams, but also by being commanded to act in certain ways or by being given divine visions. This testimony provides a means of thinking about how the transfer of divine curative power was effected in other contexts, including those of the votive cults of Italy.

Comparative information concerning the permeation of the bodies of mortals by the power or essence of the divine can also be gleaned from the writings of Aelius Aristides, who during the course of his lengthy residence at Pergamum encountered Asclepius on many occasions. His account of his time at the sanctuary provides evidence for very personal and charismatic religious experiences centred on his body, as the following two extracts illustrate:

> For it seemed as if I touched him and perceived that he himself had come, and was between sleep and waking, and wished to look up and was in anguish that he might depart too soon, and strained my ears to hear some things as in a dream, some as in a waking state; my hair stood on end, and I cried for joy, and the pride in my heart was inoffensive. And what human

being is capable of describing these things in words? If there is anyone who is initiated, he knows and understands.

(Sacred Tales 2.32–3)

What should one say of the matter of not bathing? I have not bathed for five consecutive years and some months besides, unless, of course, in winter time, he [Asclepius] ordered me to use the sea or rivers or wells. The purging of my upper intestinal tract has taken place in the same way for nearly two years and two months in succession, together with enemas and bloodlettings, as many as no one has ever counted, and at that with little nourishment and that forced.

(Sacred Tales 1.59)

Like the people whose cures were recounted in the Epidauran inscriptions Aelius Aristides's knowledge of divine power centred on his bodily experiences. In many instances he was directed to perform painstaking physical activities, to follow strict diets or purges and to embark upon demanding journeys. His various maladies were thereby eased as a consequence of the performance of what Alexia Petsalis-Diomidis (2010, p. 67) has referred to as 'trials of his body'. In the same way that anatomical votives could embody the power of the divine, Aristides's compliance with the directions of Asclepius can be interpreted as a corporeal enactment of the god's curative powers: the god healed him by manipulating his body. Votive dedications from the Asclepieion at Pergamum refer to other instances of the remote stimulation of human bodies. Aelius Theon, for example, was set a gruelling regimen: '. . . for one hundred and twenty days not drinking, and at dawn each morning eating fifteen grains of white pepper and half an onion in accordance with the order of the god . . .', whilst 'Julius Meidi[as] set this up in accordance with a command having been bled underneath his muscle' (Petsalis-Diomidis, 2010, p. 253). As Petsalis-Diomidis (2010, p. 253) also observes:

[T]hese inscriptions create narratives of the body suffering and enduring not on account of sickness (though this is implicit), but on account of the will of the god. Within the confines of the Asclepieion at least, the dedicants chose to identify themselves through narratives of divinely suffering bodies. The god's takeover of their bodies through the treatments was paralleled by their claiming part of the space of the god with their dedication.

In these instances the body of a human suppliant was altered physically through their own actions, but these actions were prompted by divine communications which compelled them to behave in certain ways. Fundamentally it was divine power which animated their bodies. In the course of such personal bodily performances, the living bodies of suppliants became the physical manifestation of the otherwise intangible healing powers of the dividual god. These divinely animated bodies embodied and incorporated the inalienable essence of divine power in the same way that an anatomical votive embodied the complementary essence of a mortal suppliant. Through this mutual exchange the two were enchained, as Petsalis-Diomidis (2010, p. 112) hints at when she suggests that 'these activities, as much as enemas, constitute a divine penetration of Aristides' body by Asclepius. Conversely Aristides had penetrated the god's space, the Pergamene Asclepieion, where most of these cures are said to take place'. A reciprocal and inalienable relationship of enchainment was established between Aelius Aristides and Asclepius: each 'penetrated', or in dividual terms 'permeated', the body of the other. Aelius Aristides evidently considered his own body to be constructed quite literally out of the essence and powers of the god, noting that whereas other pilgrims celebrate parts of the body that had been cured, in his own case it was 'not only a part of the body, but it is the whole body which he has composed and put together and given as a gift' (Aelius Aristides, *Oration* 42.7 Keil). Through the transfer of inalienable divine power to a permeable human body and the 'gifting' of the (living) physical body to the god in return, Aelius Aristides effectively became an animated votive, embodying and commemorating the gift of healing bestowed upon him, his physical being animated by divine instruction and through this mutual exchange of corporeal performance and divine healing he and Asclepius became enchained persons: suppliant and god.

Conclusions: reappraising anatomical votives

This paper has argued that in the context of votive cult the respective dividuality of both ancient gods and humans came to the fore, their relationship maintained via the mutual exchange of both material objects (*ex-votos*) and intangible divine powers (healing). Through acts of enchainment this behaviour not only sustained a religious community composed of deities, mortals and objects, but also produced and sustained knowledge concerning the nature of this human/divine relationship. As a result anatomical votives might be classified alongside other objects, ritual movements and sensory experiences as material 'instruments of knowledge' (Chidester, 2005, p. 57), responsible ultimately for allowing participants in votive cult 'to grasp the mysterious and elusive aspects of being, and enabling the transmission and comprehension of sacred knowledge' (Boivin, 2009, p. 269). For human members of this religious community the inalienable prayers and votive offerings surrendered to the gods were a *pars pro toto* extension of their bodies *and* of the essence of their self as members of that community. In turn, the dividual nature of the divine took the form of the transfer of otherwise immaterial healing essences or powers. Ethnographic parallels for this type of relationship include Marilyn Strathern's (1988) pioneering study of communities in modern Melanesia in which she highlights the different forms that dividual exchanges might take within a single community. Strathern writes of mediated exchange, or the giving of an objectified gift that cannot be passed on or returned. In an ancient context this might correspond with either a votive offering or unique bodily performance, such as those of Aelius Aristides. The return gift, however, might take an unmediated form more readily equated with divine healing: 'the power of the spiritual beings that will sustain the living' (Strathern, 1988, p. 264). From this perspective the giving of a votive offering was more than a gesture of gratitude for healing received; it was also integral to the production of religious knowledge, of religious communities and of religious identities, all of which were predicated on the enchainment of mortal and divine. In this way gods became multiauthored persons composed of the bodies, prayers and offerings of human suppliants, the basis of their divine power consequently sustained and made manifest by human action. At the same time, mortal participants in votive cult were also a product of their personal relationship with the divine, their healed bodies permeated by divine power. The performance of votive cult thus served to create, enchain and maintain both human and divine persons.

Nevertheless, the arguments presented here do not change the fact that for the majority of ancient cult participants an anatomical votive offering was almost certainly connected first and foremost with their personal bodily circumstances and the healing or protection offered by the divine. Nor do they contradict recent claims that the symbolic fragmentation and rebuilding of the body in its proper orderly form was an underlying principle of participation in healing cult (Hughes, 2008). Instead, this chapter has aimed to offer a new perspective on votive cult by underscoring how complex and multifaceted religious behaviours and knowledge might be. In order to understand these, it must be acknowledged that ritual performances such as those implicated in votive cult can have significant repercussions beyond an immediate petition or thank offering. Rather than focusing on the enigmatic beliefs that might have underpinned cult activities, seeking to identify their broader implications for the production and transmission of religious knowledge and religious communities has the potential to provide valuable insight into the more nuanced role of cult performances in the enactment and articulation of multiauthored social relationships, as well as personal or communal identities. Such an approach aligns studies of ancient votive objects with significant recent scholarship on the materiality of religion, which asserts that religious knowledge is produced via the performance of ritual acts and engagement with material objects rather than preexisting as an abstract idea requiring explanation or material expression (Boivin, 2009, p. 274; Graham, forthcoming).

Returning to the questions posed at the beginning of this chapter concerning the implications of dedicating a votive corresponding to the human body, the arguments developed earlier open the way for alternative approaches to an investigation of the emergence and popularity of anatomical *ex-votos* from the late fourth century BC. Contextualising anatomical votives within a relational framework centred on the respective dividuality of gods and humans suggests that the increased emphasis on the body within the votive assemblages of central Italy may not have been related exclusively to the growing popularity of healing cults, declining levels of health or the emergence of so-called popular religion. Reframing this question in the context of the role of the anatomical votive in generating a relationship of enchainment between human and divine and the production of distinctive religious communities makes it possible to suggest different explanations. It also focuses attention on other questions, including why the relationship between divine and mortal came to be expressed in this way at this particular moment in time. For example, it might be proposed that changes in society wrought by political developments and the expansion of the Roman state created a greater need to redefine and articulate personal and community identities, especially in a way that emphasised security, stability and protection and that stressed the reciprocal balance between the world of humans and that of the divine during a period of potentially momentous upheaval. The dedication of anatomical votives and the reinvigoration of the cult at Punta della Vipera around the same time as the reorganisation of the immediate sociopolitical landscape might be better understood in this context. The subsequent development of new political or economic hierarchies may also have generated different ways of thinking about identity which required material expression or which encouraged more people to seek ways to affirm their place in the world. The dedication of terracotta models therefore enabled a wider range of people to be seen as active contributors to the maintenance of the community as their bodies were placed alongside those of their social superiors within the sanctuary. Vel Tiples, for example, whose name was inscribed on a votive knee recovered from the Ara della Regina temple at Tarquinii, is presumed to have been a freedman (Comella, 1982, p. 226). In this context a full figurine or a votive statuette of a deity may have conflicted with the composite bodies being produced in these sacred settings leading to a greater preference for bodily fragments which stressed the direct connection between god and human rather than marking deities out as individual, isolated or distant figures. Wider changes to social conditions and ways of life wrought by the creation of new urban centres, as well as the simultaneous arrival of new healing cults such as that of Asclepius which emphasised holistic well-being in addition to divine cures, may also have brought about a greater concern for, or awareness of, personal welfare and identity as something situated in the body. Such developments may have led growing numbers of people to sanctuaries of all types and to the comforting support of a tangible bodily connection with the divine.

Not all of these hypotheses can be tested here, but acknowledging the role of anatomical votives within the production of religious communities predicated on dividuality and enchainment as this chapter has sought to do forces us to consider how any change (or combination of changes) to contemporary social, political, economic or other circumstances which produced a sense of insecurity or increased emphasis on social relationships and community may have resulted in a corresponding transformation in the nature of votive offerings. What is more, such an approach also makes it possible to reexamine the decline of the anatomical votive phenomenon in new ways: this coincided with another period of sociopolitical change at the end of the Roman Republic during which individuals and communities undoubtedly sought alternative media through which to articulate their place in the world of both mortals and gods. Anatomical votives evidently had more than one meaning and might intersect with a range of contemporary concerns and ways of perceiving the world in order to shape religious identities and produce distinctive religious experiences, which were potentially embedded within much wider processes of social interaction than narrow traditional 'religious' or 'healing' explanations have allowed. Rather than seeking single, universal causes for the rise and decline of the anatomical votive to comprehend this complex phenomenon, it is necessary to revise our understandings of the multivalent nature of both ritual practices and religious knowledge.

3 Anatomical votives (and swaddled babies)

From Republican Italy to Roman Gaul

Olivier de Cazanove

The purpose of this chapter is to link two classes of objects which are usually studied in a completely separate way: anatomical *ex-votos* (and related offerings) in Republican Italy, on the one hand and, on the other, those of Roman Gaul.[1] Despite traditional geographical separation one can see at first glance that these two classes present strong resemblances. These relate not only to each type of object, but also to the nature of their assemblage. It is thus advisable to go beyond regional specialisations and disciplinary boundaries in order to reconstruct a long history (from a '*longue durée*' perspective) of this kind of offering. Whilst being careful not to smooth out local and chronological differences entirely, we must seek a broad and comprehensive view of these votive practices in order to reach a better understanding of their evolution and to some extent their channels of diffusion.

Ex-voto practices in Gaul: developing a chronology

My starting point is a recent discovery made during archaeological excavations inside the Gallo-Roman sanctuary of Apollo Moritasgus at Alesia in 2011. This cult place lies at the eastern edge of the Auxois Mount at a place called La Croix Saint-Charles, the only point on the plateau where a permanent spring arises as a result of the local geology. The sanctuary has been excavated twice, although there were also limited explorations during the nineteenth century (de Cazanove, 2012). The first proper excavations were undertaken by Emile Espérandieu between 1909 and 1913 just before the First World War, with more recent and ongoing archaeological fieldwork beginning in May 2008 (de Cazanove et al., 2012a; de Cazanove et al., 2012b; de Cazanove, 2015b). An updated plan of the site (Figure 3.1) shows to what extent these excavations increased the area known to have been covered by the sanctuary.

---

1 The topic of this chapter was first presented at a research seminar organised by Ton Derks at Amsterdam in October 2011 and then, in a modified version, at the conference organised in Rome in June 2012 by Jane Draycott and Emma-Jayne Graham. I would like to thank all three for the invitation and discussion.

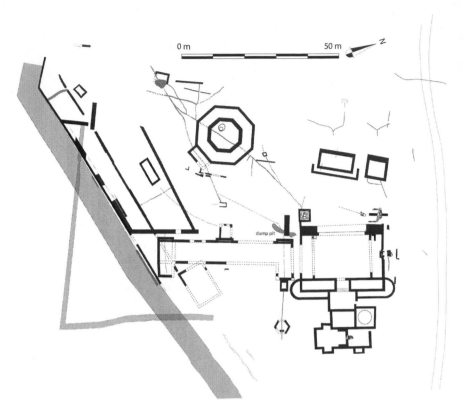

Figure 3.1 Plan of the sanctuary of Apollo Moritasgus at Alesia.

Source: O. de Cazanove.

In 2011 the opportunity arose to excavate a dump pit (Figure 3.2) located a few metres behind a large portico which from the Flavian period was used as a monumental façade for the whole sanctuary (successively, in the middle of the second century AD, the portico was rebuilt: de Cazanove, 2012). The filling of this pit can be dated precisely: it contained a *sesterce* of Lucius Verus struck in Rome between AD 163 and 168, abundant ceramic material with a *terminus post quem* in the first half of the third century and charcoal dated by AMS (accelerator mass spectrometry) to between AD 130 and 250 (with a calibrated date of AD 220). Inside the pit several pieces of limestone sculpture were found: some heads and a small bust, hands and legs, a pair of breasts on a pentagonal slab and a bird. Overall there were 22 objects, some complete but more often only fragmentary. In addition, the pit contained two fragments of limestone swaddled babies which at first sight are not easy to identify. The largest (which is headless) is recognisable thanks to the cross bands which restrain the undershirt with a broad ring

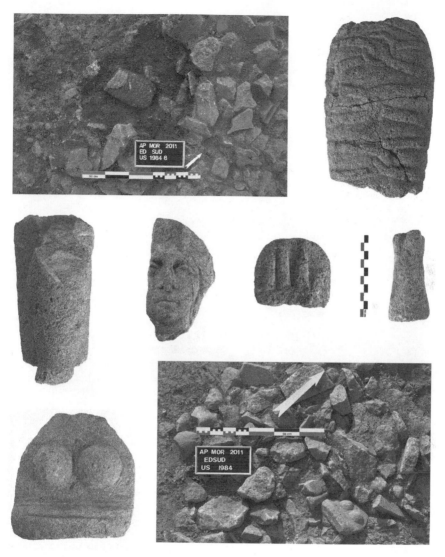

Figure 3.2 Alesia, sanctuary of Apollo Moritasgus, 2011: dump pit filled with stone offerings. Top to bottom and left to right: swaddled infant in situ, headless swaddled infant, fragmentary right leg, fragmentary female head, fragmentary left hand and fragmentary right forearm, breasts. All the objects are at the same scale.

Source: Photographs by O. de Cazanove and S. De Grandis.

placed in the middle (for the wrapping technique of infants in Gaul, see Coulon, 2004; Deyts, 2004). This kind of swaddling is very similar to that of the other swaddled infant of Alesia found by Espérandieu in 1909 and housed today in the Musée d'Archéologie Nationale at Saint-Germain-en-Laye (Espérandieu, 1910,

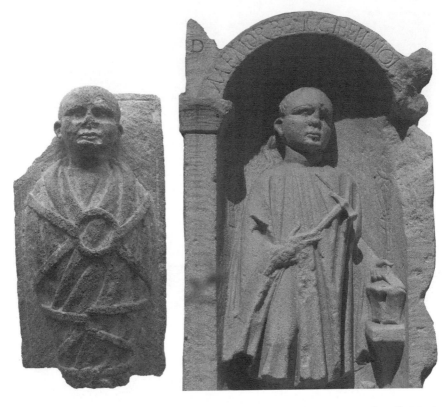

Figure 3.3 Left: Swaddled infant of Alesia found in 1909, from the sanctuary of Apollo Moritasgus, now in the Musée d'Archéologie Nationale, Saint-Germain-en-Laye; Right:
Detail of the funerary stele of Belliccus from Sens-*Agedincum* (copy).

Source: a. Photograph O. de Cazanove and S. De Grandis; b. Photograph D. Laboureix.

p. 309, n. 2387; Provost, 2009a, pp. 520–1, fig. 617; de Cazanove et al., 2012b,
pp. 116–17, fig. 21) (Figure 3.3).

Where in the sanctuary were these new discoveries from Alesia located
originally? Most probably they were placed in a small *aedicula* nearby where the
complete child in swaddling clothes was discovered in 1909. The unpublished
excavation notebook of Espérandieu indicates the findspot of this item with
precision: on the pavement slabs (which were in part reused inscriptions). In the
same pit a fragment of stucco belonging to the frieze of the *aedicula* was also
found, offering further proof that the filling materials came from this structure
(de Cazanove, 2013, pp. 10–11). The construction (or the rebuilding according to
Espérandieu) of the *aedicula* can be dated to the Trajanic period, but more probably to the reign of Hadrian or even a little later thanks to abundant numismatic
evidence. If the limestone sculptures were originally sheltered in the *aedicula*
before being discarded in a pit which was then sealed during the first half of the

third century, they are consequently datable to a period between the years AD 120 (or more likely 150) and 250.

Stylistic comparisons and epigraphy add strength to this dating. The face of the swaddled baby found in 1909 looks so strikingly similar to a male head on a funerary stele of Sens-*Agedincum* 130 km northwest of Alesia (Espérandieu, 1911, p. 12, n. 2769) that one wonders whether they come from the same workshop (Figure 3.3). This similarity helps provide a date. The stele of Sens is dedicated 'to the memory of Belliccus son of Bellator' (*CIL* 13, 2965), and although the term *memoriae* is used during the second century the formula becomes especially common at the beginning of the third century AD (Dondin-Payre and Raepsaet-Charlier, 2001, p. ix). Finally, it must be noted that two stone anatomical votives recovered from the sanctuary (but not from the *aedicula*) bear a dedication 'to the god Apollo Moritasgus' (*deo Apollini Moritasgo*: *CIL* 13, 11240 and 11241). It is generally acknowledged that the epigraphic formula *deus* + theonym seen here appears under Antoninus Pius (Dondin-Payre and Raepsaet-Charlier, 2001, p. x). All the indicators thus point to a dating of the anatomical stone offerings of the sanctuary, *inter alia* those of the *aedicula*, in the second half of the second century or at the beginning of the third century AD. This result is not unimportant. Indeed, often the dating of votive offerings is problematic because of a lack of stratigraphic context or stylistic references, especially with regard to anatomical votives. Consequently, under normal circumstances it becomes difficult to evaluate such objects in historical terms.

This precise dating offers a sharp contrast with the chronology that can be deduced for the gifts recovered from the same sanctuary which are made of bronze sheets. Inside an *ambitus* – the space between the rear wall and the terrace wall – behind the portico, some layers of dumped material were identified in 2009. These begin with the construction of the portico after AD 70 and were sealed when the portico was rebuilt around AD 130–150 (de Cazanove et al., 2012b, pp. 112–18). The abundant ceramic material from these strata once again allows for precise dating, thanks especially to the presence of forms of La Graufesenque and Central Gaul *sigillata* ware, as well as other materials. In the same strata bronze sheets with eyes were also numerous. This chronology, from the Flavian period downwards, seems to be confirmed by other sites, for instance, Mirebeau-sur-Bèze in the territory of the Lingones (Joly and Lambert, 2004). However, recently some *ex-votos* made from bronze sheet have also been found in an Augustan context associated with the sanctuary at a site known as 'La Fontaine de l'Etuvée' near Orléans (Verneau, 2014, p. 62). At least at La Croix Saint-Charles the stone *ex-votos* are later in date (see earlier).

The assemblage of stone offerings found in the dump pit behind the portico at Alesia is perfectly in accordance with the types of offerings found in nearby sanctuaries, including the large cult place dedicated to Sequana at the source of the Seine. Since the 1960s this sanctuary has been known especially for the wooden sculptures found in great quantities close to the springs (Deyts, 1983). But previous excavations also identified around 400 stone offerings in addition to more than 250 *ex-votos* made from bronze sheet (Espérandieu, 1910, pp. 314–34, nn. 2403–49; Deyts, 1994). The categories of stone offerings from this site consist of statues of men, women and children (either in the round or in relief), particularly children in swaddling clothes, male and female heads and anatomical votives, including upper and lower limbs, torsos and breasts.

In the immediate surroundings of Alesia and of the sanctuary of Sequana votive offerings made of local limestone are also widespread, found, for instance, at Sainte-Sabine (Espérandieu, 1910, pp. 148–54, nn. 2040, 2044 and 2049; Provost, 2009c, pp. 157–8; de Cazanove, 2013, p. 12), Essarois (Espérandieu, 1911, pp. 352–69, nn. 3411–39; Provost, 2009b, pp. 315–18), Le Tremblois (Provost, 2009c, pp. 406–10), La Douix (Provost, 2009b, pp. 155–7) and Massingy-les-Vitteaux (Espérandieu, 1910, pp. 310–14, nn. 2391–402; Provost, 2009b, pp. 512–13). Again these take the form of statues, including swaddled babies, heads and anatomical *ex-votos* in the shape of a limb or pelvis. It is worth noting that these stone offerings are essentially circumscribed by the ancient cities which correspond to the modern region of Burgundy, that is, the cities of the Aedui and Lingones.[2] Of course, this class of votive offering is also attested elsewhere, such as in the forest of Halatte where the usual assemblage was found: statues, children in swaddling clothes, heads, anatomical votives and animals (Durand, 2000, pp. 9–91). Moreover, the northernmost anatomical stone *ex-voto* known was discovered in the Netherlands: a male pelvis found in the Waal at Nijmegen (Espérandieu, 1925, p. 49, n. 6630). However, these few exceptions do not alter the overall framework. Elsewhere in Gaul anatomical *ex-votos* are made from bronze and primarily take the form of eyes.[3] Their distribution in any case is limited to the area north of the Massif Central, except for a few exceptions and some doubtful cases (see Fauduet, 2014, pp. 94–5; there are also specimens made from silver at Pannes near Montargis in the *civitas* of the Senones: Dondin-Payre and Cribellier, 2011; and further afield of gold at Wroxeter in England: Painter, 1971). As for wooden *ex-votos*, their conservation is exceptional, being dependent upon hygrometrical conditions and thus making it difficult to draw firm conclusions about their distribution.

A recent exhibition in Dijon provided an opportunity for the well-known wooden *ex-votos* from the Seine springs sanctuary to be reexamined, and dendrochronological analyses were carried out on 30 of them (Vernou, 2011, pp. 16–17). The results are homogeneous (Figure 3.4). The dates of tree cutting range between 30 BC and AD 30, indicating that all the dated wooden offerings from the source of the Seine sanctuary date from the Augustan and Tiberian periods. This early (but post-Caesarean) chronology is confirmed by even more recent results. At Magny-Cours (Burgundy, Nièvre Department) expansion work on the race track in 2012–2013 revealed a remarkable Gallo-Roman site

---

2 For distribution maps of babies in swaddling clothes, see de Cazanove (2008, p. 273, fig. 2); Derks (2014, p. 51, fig. 2). To these should be added an unpublished specimen (fragmentary) from Saint-Parize-le-Châtel (Burgundy, Nièvre Department).

3 Assuming that eyes on bronze sheets are anatomical *ex-votos* in the full meaning of the term, which is not completely certain. Breasts and male and female pelvises made of the same material clearly do belong to this category.

DATES ESTIMÉES D'ABATTAGE DES ARBRES UTILISÉS POUR LES *EX-VOTO*

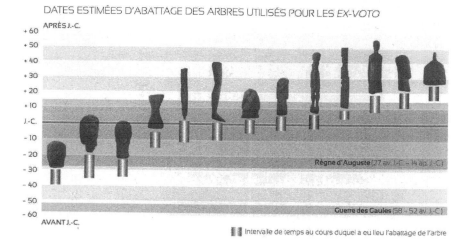

Figure 3.4 Dendrochronological dating of the wooden offerings from the sanctuary at the Springs of the Seine.

Source: From Vernou (2011).

comprising either a large sanctuary or small settlement with a complete architectural range, including temple, theatre and thermal baths (Tisserand and Nouvel, 2013). Further to the north of the site in an area of peatland pieces of wood were also found, including legs. One of them (made from oak) had been carved using material from a tree that had been felled in 26 BC (Tisserand and Nouvel, 2013). This is a very early date but one that is confirmed by the wooden *ex-votos* of Chamalières where a huge deposit can be dated to a period between the age of Augustus and the very beginning of the Flavian period (Romeuf and Dumontet, 2000). It therefore seems that wooden *ex-votos* are the oldest of all those in Roman Gaul. Nevertheless, the practice of offering wooden limbs continued during the entire period of the Roman Empire and beyond, as documented, for example, by Gregory of Tours (*Vitae patrum* VI. 2 *De sancto Gallo episcopo*).

Ex-votos between Gaul and Italy

Let us get now to the heart of the matter: the striking resemblance between the votive offerings of Roman Gaul during the imperial period and the terracotta *ex-votos* which strongly characterise, albeit several centuries earlier, the sanctuaries of Roman Italy during the mid-Republican era. The resemblance relates to each individual type of object, as well to their assemblage as a coherent group of offerings. Statues are found in great numbers in Republican Italy, *inter alia* many representations of children in swaddling clothes (Glinister, this volume), heads and anatomical *ex-votos* of all kinds: parts of the face, upper and lower limbs, genitalia and internal organs (including uteri, see Flemming, this volume) (Figure 3.5).

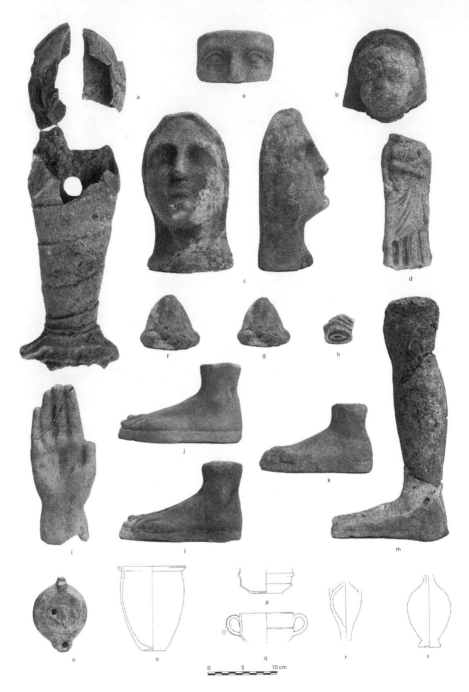

Figure 3.5 A sample of the anatomical votives and associated ceramics from the *cavernette Falische*, Museo delle Origini. a. Swaddled infant; b. Head of a swaddled infant; c. Male head; d. Standing female statuette; e. 'Mask'; f–g. Hearts (?); h. Fragment of uterus; i. Right hand; j–l. Left feet; m. Right leg; n. Disc lamp; o. Thin-walled pottery, type III Marabini Moevs; p. Thin-walled pottery, type 2/336 Curls; q. Thin-walled pottery, type 1/91 Curls; r–s. *unguentaria*.

Source: Photographs G. Imparato; drawings M. Pierobon, Centre Jean Bérard.

This striking resemblance cannot be the result of a simple coincidence. We may therefore raise a practical question: Do the anatomical votives and related offerings (including babies in swaddling clothes) of Roman Gaul derive directly from those of Roman Italy? And, if so, by which channels were these forms spread? There is certainly a chronological gap. The spread of Italian votive terracottas reaches its climax during the third century BC but soon afterwards, according to general opinion, these objects were discarded and buried in pits (Pensabene, 1979). In contrast, as demonstrated earlier, the disposal pit excavated at Alesia in 2011 was sealed during the third century AD. Nevertheless, the *ex-votos* on bronze sheets appear to be a little older than this, and the first anatomical wooden *ex-votos* have been demonstrated to be even older, some of them preceding the Christian era. Consequently, based on this evidence the gap between the two regions may not be as great as it seems at first sight.

Indeed, some Italian votive terracottas are perhaps more recent than is commonly believed, or in any case at least remained on display for a long time. Amongst other examples we might highlight the votive deposit of Porta Caere at Veii sealed around 50 BC (Torelli and Pohl, 1973), the votive deposit of Porta Nord at Vulci which contained coins that continued into the reign of Vespasian in the first century AD (Paglieri, 1960, p. 75; Pautasso, 1994, p. 91 and p. 108, n. 407) and the *caverna della stipe* in Faliscan territory with lamps and ceramics from the first and second centuries AD (Rellini, 1920; de Cazanove, 2015a). Another pertinent case concerns the excavation of Seminario Vescovile in Verona, which produced a large number of miniature anatomical *ex-votos*, especially upper and lower limbs, which were also associated with *terra sigillata* (for a preliminary report see Murgia, 2013, p. 138). These still-unpublished miniature anatomical *ex-votos* appear very close, in my opinion, to the arms and the bronze legs attested in various parts of northern Italy (Marzabotto; Arezzo, Fonte Veneziana; Monte Falterona, Lago degli Idoli; Este, sanctuary of Reitia) which are usually assigned to the Archaic period although without any conclusive evidence. Work continues on the controversial question of how to date the anatomical votives of Italy (de Cazanove, 2015a). In my opinion the chronology usually accepted for a great number of these objects is too high and requires revision. The evidence for anatomical *ex-votos* in Archaic Italy is doubtful,[4] and contrary to what is often claimed, the associated ceramics and coins show clearly that the first votive deposits which contain anatomical votives were not closed before the mid-third century BC. and in fact this often occurred much later.

Nor should such work focus only on terracotta offerings simply because they have been better preserved. There were also bronze anatomical votives and others made from precious metals including silver and gold. Evidence for such

---

4 Indeed, some bronze sheet *ex-votos* from northern Italy which are usually dated to the Archaic period (Este, and the rest of Veneto: Ghirardini, 1888, pp. 120–5; Maioli and Mastrocinque, 1992, p. 57 and pp. 115–16; Ruta Serafini, 2002, pp. 233–75 and pp. 306–10) closely resemble the eyes, breasts and phalli on bronze sheets from Roman imperial Gaul (de Cazanove, 2015a).

offerings is attested for both the Republican and imperial period, although usually the objects themselves have disappeared and only the inscription recording their dedication remains. A typical example can be found in the 'silver model' of a spleen offered to Asclepius by the imperial freedman Neochares Iulianus in the second century AD (*IGUR* 1.105; for further examples see de Cazanove, 2009, pp. 365–8). In a few fortunate cases, however, the offering survives: a bronze hemisphere interpreted as a votive breast bears an inscription dated by the publisher to the beginning of the first century AD (Iozzo, 2013, pp. 27–30, inv. 250731) but which could be a little older.[5]

The same objects also existed in miniaturised form, again made of precious metals such as gold and silver, as well as bronze. Such easily portable objects could be circulated widely. It was noted earlier that small bronze legs have been found in northern Italy and other miniature legs also exist in France, in particular in the Alps at Viuz Faverges (two miniature bronze legs associated with a *terra sigillata* bowl of Dragendorff type 36 and coins of the mid-second century AD: Canal, 1988, pp. 3–4) and Réotier (Roman, 1890, pp. 117–18). It is perhaps no coincidence that these sites are located on the road between Italy and Gaul. Small metal swaddled infants are also known in Italy (Latium, Tarentum), in Spain and in Roman Gaul, specifically at Arcis-sur-Aube in the Tricasses territory 130 km north of Alesia (Denajar, 2005, p. 233, nn. 6 and 15) (Figure 3.6). This last example was certainly produced locally and not imported, as shown by the Gallic system of swaddling with cross bands. In any case such objects, which could be carried, easily demonstrate how models could be spread.

A striking case of continuity can also be found in relation to a type of *ex-voto* with a distinctive shape: the lower part of the human body from the waist to the feet. This type is attested in central Italy (nine examples moulded in terracotta at the Latin colony of Cales: Ciaghi, 1993, pp. 185–7),[6] as well as in Roman Gaul in the Arverni territory (a wooden example at Chamalières: Romeuf and Dumontet, 2000, p.130, n. 499) (Figure 3.7a–b). The lower torso models of Cales and Chamalières are life-sized, but it might be assumed that intermediate forms existed, including those on a much smaller scale. Objects of this kind are currently unknown in central France, but some naked male bronze statuettes ending above the waist were recovered from a sanctuary excavated in the nineteenth century at Géromont near Gérouville at the border between Belgian Luxembourg and France (Grenier, 1960, pp. 821–4). The example reproduced here (Figure 3.7c) bears a dedication to the god Silvanus Sinquatis made by a certain Petronius in fulfilment of a vow *pro salute Emeriti fili(i) sui* (*CIL* 13, 3968). Perhaps we might imagine the missing link between the lower torsos of Cales and Chamalières in the shape of a similar object, although, of course, this must necessarily remain speculation. In any case, even if the means

---

5 I thank David Nonnis for this information.
6 Some more or less awkwardly made imitations of this type of anatomical offering also exist in the Samnite area at Schiavi d'Abruzzo: de Cazanove (2015a).

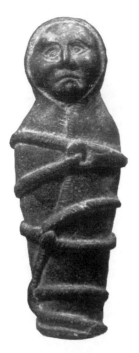

Figure 3.6 Swaddled infant from Arcis-sur-Aube, museum of Troyes (inv. 4602).

Source: Troyes, Musée des Beaux-Arts et d'Archéologie, photo by J.-M. Protte.

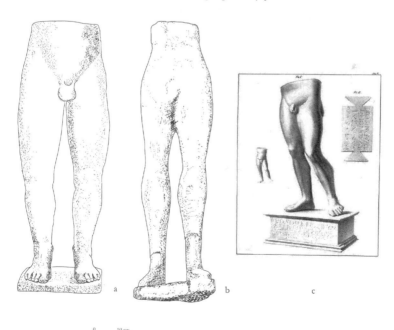

Figure 3.7 Lower torsos. a. Cales; b. Chamalières; c. Géromont.

Source: Drawings a. and b. by the author; c. after Namur (1848), figs.1 and 2, Pl. V.

of diffusion were different, the *ex-votos* of Chamalières and Géromont provide clear examples of the adoption of new types of offerings with Italian origins.[7]

The existence of close parallels between the limestone anatomical votives of Roman Gaul and the marble anatomical votives of Greece is also significant, especially given a substantial degree of contemporaneity between the two groups. The great majority of Greek stone anatomical *ex-votos* date from the Roman imperial period, with only a few from the Classical and Hellenistic periods (see van Straten, 1981; Forsén, 1996). A marble relief from Epidaurus, for instance, with a pair of ears (the ears of the man once cured, not those of the divinity, as the written text makes clear) even has a Latin dedication made by a certain Cutius with the *cognomen* Gallus, although this is probably only a coincidence (*CIL* 3, 7266: *Cutius has auris Gallus tibi voverat olim / Phoebigena et posuit sanus ab auriculis*) (Figure I.4). The shapes of some Greek and Gallo–Roman votives are very similar and might be suggestive of a direct connection, given that their exact equivalents are unknown in Italy. On the other hand, however, some assemblages which are frequent in Italy and Gaul are not found in Greece, most notably the assemblage of anatomical votives and swaddled infants (although the terracotta baby from the sanctuary of Artemis Mounychia now in the Piraeus museum offers an exception: inv. E 86; Dasen, 2013, p. 69). In brief, I believe that the Gallo–Roman, Italian and Greek series, and even Phrygian or Cypriot examples, despite local differences and also different materials, demonstrate the widespread popularity of these dedications of human parts across the various cultural areas belonging to the Roman empire, with such votive gifts and practices being themselves inherited directly from the Greek Classical period and in particular from the offerings deposited in therapeutic and health-related sanctuaries.[8] The anatomical votives of Roman Gaul made out of wood, bronze sheets or stone are only a particular case of a more general and widely diffused phenomenon. They are not a distinctive Gallic expression which made its appearance spontaneously and independently in Gaul as has sometimes been claimed. Although it is difficult to reconstruct in detail the precise channels and the intermediaries that brought about this diffusion, the general trend is clear.

Conclusion

In conclusion I would like emphasise two points. First, according to the currently available data anatomical *ex-votos* and related offerings found in Gaul all date from the Roman period, including the wooden examples which begin

---

7 Another possibility would be the importation to Gaul of terracotta anatomical *ex-votos* which were similar to those of Italy. Mentions are made, for instance, of terracotta eyes in French museums or as objects coming from excavations in France (Paris, Carnavalet Museum; Troyes, Bourg-en-Bresse, Chassey-les-Montbozon, Balmes-les-Fontaines: see de Cohën and Bailly, 1994). But in at least several cases these must be Italian objects from modern collections which were erroneously assigned to French sites.

8 I leave aside the problem of the earlier existence of anatomical votives (Georgoulaki, 1997) which does not concern us here.

in the years 40–30 BC. In contrast, the cult places of the Gallic period (that is, the enclosures of the La Tène period) demonstrate ritual traces of activity which are completely different: animal bones (Méniel, 1997; 2006), wine amphoras (Poux, 2004) and folded weapons (Brunaux, 2006; for the metal deposits see Bataille, 2008; there is also evidence for a phase of transition after the Caesarean conquest: Rey-Vodoz, 1991; 1994; 2006). Consequently anatomical votives are related to the new religious practices and the reorganisation of the sanctuaries which took place *after* the Roman conquest. In other words, they are typical votive gifts of the Roman period and the early phases of so-called 'Romanisation'. Such a term must, of course, be used with caution, but as has been pointed out recently, the concept partly maintains its utility and its operational value (Le Roux, 2004; for the situation in Roman Gaul after the conquest: Reddé, 2011, pp. 9–14).[9] Consequently, it can be argued that the situation in Italy in the third century BC, during which Rome was expanding its territory and political influence, and the situation in Gaul between Augustus and Vespasian can be compared even at a distance of several centuries. The appearance of anatomical *ex-votos* in both regions is therefore a strong indicator of 'Romanisation' and cultural change. With regard to Hellenistic Italy the doubts expressed on this matter rest on inaccurate dating of the anatomical *ex-votos*, which at least in a huge majority are unlikely to be earlier than Roman expansion (de Cazanove, 2015a).

Second, how should the immense popularity across the Roman world of this kind of practice and type of offering be explained? The vogue of the anatomical votive in Roman Gaul is not directly related to the worship of Asclepius, or even to healing cults in general. In Italy and in the western provinces the cult of Asclepius enjoys a certain popularity, but its sanctuaries do not reach nearly the same level of fame as they did in Greece and in the eastern part of the Greco-Roman world. More generally it can be argued that the importance of healing sanctuaries in Gaul was for a long time overestimated on the basis of a brief remark by Caesar (*Gallic War* VI, 17) and also on the evidence for allegedly curative water basins and for thermal complexes (as noted by Scheid, 1991). However, the sanctuary at La Croix Saint-Charles in Alesia, for example, was neither specifically nor exclusively a healing sanctuary. It was certainly a spring sanctuary dedicated to Apollo with a thermal complex, but this thermal bath demonstrates no specifically curative features. The sanctuary was in fact a versatile and polyvalent place of cult able to satisfy varied religious requests, *inter alia* requests for health, as demonstrated by the votives and the dedications recovered from the site. In the same way, at the sanctuary of Sequana at the source of the Seine one could subscribe and fulfil various types of vows, as indicated by at least one example of a *votum pro salute* (*CIL* 13, 2862: *Aug(usto) sac(rum) /*

---

9 With regard to Republican Italy a recent international congress – *L'Italia centrale e la creazione di una koiné culturale? I percorsi della 'romanizzazione'* (October 2014) – represents an attempt to provide an update on this complex issue.

d(e)ae Seq(uanae) / Fl(avius) Flav(i)n(us) / pro sal(ute) / Fl(avi) Luna(ris) / nep(otis) sui / ex voto / v(otum) s(olvit) l(ibens) m(erito)). This reflects a general vow for the safeguarding (*salus*) of the individual and his physical integrity but also his social being, his worldly goods and so forth.[10] Nonetheless, beside this kind of global request, which to some extent might be referred to as a 'general votive insurance', vows established on the occurrence of disease or accident, as well as anatomical *ex-votos* provide an additional level of precision. Representing only a part of the body was therefore clearly a statement, without risk of ambiguity, about which was the injured part for which the cure was requested by a vow, with the vow granted thereafter since the *ex-voto* was actually offered in the sanctuary. At the same time both medical and religious, this aligns well with the constant require-ment of enunciative precision which was the core of Roman piety and ritualism, but which also reflects the progress of knowledge on the human body.

10 Note that this general vow means different things in different contexts. For instance, in the inscrip-tion of Géromont (*CIL* 13, 3968) the vow *pro salute* relates specifically to health, as indicated by the nature of the anatomical votive.

4 Hair today, gone tomorrow

The use of real, false and artificial hair as votive offerings

Jane Draycott

Introduction

For the last three thousand years the anatomical *ex-voto* – whether made from terracotta, stone, metal or wood; whether in the form of eyes, ears, arms, hands, fingers, legs, feet, toes, internal organs, genitals or other recognisable parts of the internal and external body – has performed a continuous, albeit not entirely understood, role in both ritual and healing practice. But precisely what should be included in this category of artefact? Should we perhaps include votive offerings consisting of actual parts of the human body rather than just terracotta, stone, metal or wood facsimiles? For obvious reasons there are few parts of the human body that it would be possible to utilise in this way: namely hair, nails (both finger and toe) and teeth. These are the only parts of the human body that not only either fall out or fall off of their own accord but also can be removed without causing serious long-term harm or compromising the overall integrity of the human body and its ability to function. Although there is ample ancient literary, documentary and archaeological evidence for the votive offering of hair cut straight from the dedicant's head, there is somewhat less evidence for the votive offering of nails and teeth, so it is this first type of votive offering consisting of an actual part of the body that will be the focus of this chapter. However, 'real' hair was not the only type of hair that was dedicated as an *ex-voto* in ancient Greek and Roman sanctuaries, temples and shrines. 'False' hair – that is human hair that was used to create wigs and hairpieces – was also dedicated, as was 'artificial' hair – that is objects fashioned from substances such as terracotta, stone, metal, wood or textile that represent an isolated section of the hairstyle itself such as a scalp or a braid. In addition to these, supplicants dedicated *ex-voto* heads and half-heads in which the head and facial hair was frequently a prominent and thus perhaps significant feature.

How to explain the existence of this wide range of *ex-votos*? This chapter will survey the many different types of hair *ex-votos* that were offered in the ancient world, examining the use of real hair, false hair, artificial hair, head and half-head *ex-votos* with a view to establishing how these very different objects were used and whether they were used in the same ways and for the same reasons.

Hair and health

The most common interpretation of anatomical *ex-votos* is that they were offered to gods and goddesses associated with certain aspects of healing, such as Asclepius and Hygieia, at sanctuaries, temples and shrines associated with healing cult practice (see, for example, Lang, 1977; Comella, 1982–83; Aleshire, 1989; 1991; Girardon, 1993; Turfa, 1994; and the Introduction to this volume). To what extent does this interpretation accord with what is known of the dedication of hair *ex-votos*?

In his 1969 article 'Social Hair', Christopher Hallpike set out what he considered to be the 'special' characteristics of hair (Hallpike, 1969, p. 269). First, it grows constantly; second, it can be cut painlessly; third, it grows in such great quantities that it is impossible to count individual hairs; fourth, head hair is apparent on infants of both sexes at birth; fifth, genital/anal hair appears in both sexes at puberty; sixth, males develop facial and body hair even after puberty; seventh, hair on different parts of the body is of different textures; eighth, hair turns white and/or falls out in old age; and ninth, hair is a prominent feature of animals. Bearing these nine characteristics and their implications in mind, Hallpike considered that it would be surprising if all of hair's ritual and symbolic characteristics could be reduced to a single origin. Certainly in antiquity hair was utilised in a range of different religious rituals that were by no means all associated with health and healing. Hair was both grown long and cut short in the service of gods, goddesses, heroes and heroines – perhaps the most famous example, both in antiquity and today, of a votive hair offering is the Lock of Berenike (Callimachus, *Aetia* 110.7; Catullus, *Carmina* 66.9–12; Hyginus, *Poeticon astronomicon* 2.24). Whether hair remained on the head ('growing hair for the god') or was cut away from it, it took the form of an *ex-voto*. These processes of growing the hair, styling the hair, cutting the hair or shaving the head could be undertaken not only to mark different stages of life such as birth, the end of childhood and/or beginning of puberty, citizenship, marriage and/or the birth of a child, but also specific occasions such as surviving a shipwreck (for the circumstances under which hair would be dedicated see Burkert, 1987, p. 70; Rouse, 1902, pp. 240–9; these circumstances are also discussed in Levine, 1995, pp. 85–7; Leitao, 2003, pp. 112–18). Additionally, there are accounts of gods, goddesses, heroes and heroines interacting with individuals and their hair, often with lasting effects, which may have resulted in especially charged votive offerings subsequently being dedicated. Heraieus of Mytilene, for example, had a testimonial inscribed upon a stele at the Temple of Asclepius at Epidaurus:

> He had no hair on his head, but an abundant growth on his chin. He was ashamed because he was laughed at by others. He slept in the Temple. The god, by anointing his head with some drugs, made him grow hair.
>
> (*IG* IV 1.121; Stele 1, no. 19, Edelstein and Edelstein, 1945 and 1998, p. 233)

Similarly, the emperor Nero's ancestor Lucius Domitius reportedly gained the *cognomen* Ahenobarbus, subsequently borne by him and all of his descendants, at the Battle of Lake Regillus in 496 BC after having his cheeks stroked by the Dioscuri, an act that turned his beard from black to bronze (Suetonius, *Nero* 1; Plutarch, *Aemilius Paulus* 25.4). 'Ahenobarbus', taken from *aheneus* 'bronze' and *barbus* 'beard', perhaps also adds an extra layer of significance to Nero's dedication of his first beard shavings – the *depositio barbae* – to the Capitoline gods (Suetonius, *Nero* 12).

Hair was offered to a variety of gods, goddesses and other mythological figures throughout the ancient world. Herodotus's *Histories*, dating from the late fifth century BC, recounts practices that the author himself had observed being undertaken in Egypt:

> Townsfolk in each place, when they pay their vows, pray to the god to whom the animal is dedicated, shaving all or one half or one third of their children's heads, and weighing the hair in a balance against a sum of silver; then the weight in silver of the hair is given to the female guardian of the creatures, who buys fish with it and feeds them.
>
> (Herodotus, *Histories* 2.65.4)[1]

Diodorus Siculus's *Historical Library*, written several centuries later in the mid-first century BC, reported that this practice was ongoing, and he specifically connected it with the health of the children in question:

> The Egyptians make vows to certain gods on behalf of their children who have been delivered from an illness, in which case they shave off their hair and weigh it against silver or gold, and then give the money to the attendants of the animals mentioned.
>
> (Diodorus Siculus, *Historical Library* 1.83.2)

Either this practice or a similar one perhaps accounts for two mummy portraits in which young children are depicted with almost entirely shaved heads (Ikram, 2003). In the first (Figure 4.1), which is thought to date to around AD 150–200, a young boy sports an entirely shaved head except for a side-lock of youth (or 'Horus lock') on the right side of his head and two tufts of hair above his forehead. In the second (Figure 4.2), which is thought to date to around AD 230–250, a young boy has a traditional hairstyle starting farther

---

1 On the hair offerings consisting of locks of hair rolled up in clay made to the Egyptian gods during the Pharaonic period, see Tassie (1996). A study into the contents of Egyptian clay balls is currently being undertaken at the University of Manchester's KNH Centre for Egyptology by Dr Natalie McCreesh.

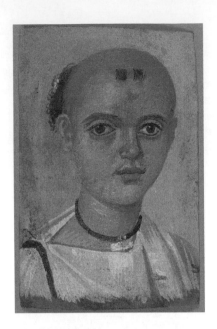

Figure 4.1 Mummy portrait, J. P. Getty Museum inv. 78.AP.262.

Source: Digital image courtesy of the Getty's Open Content Program.

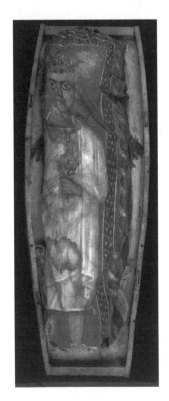

Figure 4.2 Mummy portrait, British Museum inv. 6715.

Source: Image courtesy of the Trustees of the British Museum.

back on his scalp, but the front of his head is shaved except for four tufts of hair above his forehead.

Salima Ikram (2003, p. 89) has argued that this practice of shaving part of the head is indicative of an offering having been made in an attempt to improve the health or even save the life of the child. Similar practices are also undertaken in present-day Egypt (Tassie, 1996; Blackman, 2000[1927], pp. 84–7 and p. 290). However, in both cases represented by the mummy portraits this action seems to have taken place to no avail. Although the first portrait has subsequently been separated from the mummified remains, the second has not. Analysis of the skeleton indicates that the portrait was accurate, and the deceased was aged between seven and ten years old when he died. Perhaps the hair that was shaved off was weighed and the equivalent value in gold or silver dedicated to a god or goddess as recounted by Herodotus and Diodorus Siculus.

According to Pausanias's *Description of Greece*, written in the late second century AD, Alexanor, the son of Machaon and thus the grandson of Asclepius, built a sanctuary dedicated to the latter at Titane in Sicyonia (the site is currently being explored and excavated by the Belgian School at Athens, but for interim results see Lolos, 2005; Nuttens et al., 2007). As was common in Asclepieia the sanctuary contained not only a cult statue of Asclepius, but also a number of others that depicted figures particularly associated with the god to whom suppliants could likewise make votive or sacrificial offerings:

> Of the image [of Asclepius] can be seen only the face, hands, and feet, for it has about it a tunic of white wool and a cloak. There is a similar image of Hygieia; this, too, one cannot see easily because it is so surrounded with the locks of women, who cut them off and offer them to the goddess, and with strips of Babylonian raiment. With whichever of these a votary here is willing to propitiate heaven, the same instructions have been given to him, to worship this image which they are pleased to call Health. There are images also of Alexanor and of Euamerion; to the former they give offerings as to a hero after the setting of the sun; to Euamerion, as being a god, they give burnt sacrifices.
>
> (Pausanias, *Description of Greece* 2.11.6–7)[2]

In this particular case it would appear that locks of hair were only offered to Asclepius and Hygieia, with the offerings being subsequently displayed upon the statue of Hygieia and with alternative offerings being made to the other gods. A series of inscriptions dating to the third century AD that have been recovered from the sanctuary of Asclepius at Paphos indicate that similar activities were

---

2 On the family of Asclepius, see Stafford (2005, pp. 127–34). Although it was common for cult statues of Asclepius to be accompanied by cult statues of various members of his family such as Hygieia and Telesphorus, other statue types were sometimes dedicated too, such as one of Apollonius Mys, the emperor Augustus's personal physician, in the Temple of Asclepius on Tiber Island at Rome: Suetonius, *Augustus* 59.

being undertaken there a century later. Two inscriptions record the offering of a boy's 'childhood hair' (τὴν παιδικὴν τρίχα and τὴν παίδιον τρίχα, respectively) to the god and goddess by his mother, and a third records the offering of a youth's 'ephebic hair' (τρίχα τὴν ἐφηβίην) by his father (*IG* XII 5.173.3; XII 5.173.5; XII 5.173.5). There is therefore ancient literary and documentary evidence for hair *ex-votos* having been offered specifically to deities for the purpose of ensuring good health or rectifying poor health.

Hair and religious ritual in the ancient world

Healing sanctuaries encouraged devotees to act publicly, both through making vows and through fulfilling them with sacrificial or votive offerings in a manner that was both visible and audible, thus ensuring that these activities were not only something to be performed, but also something to be seen to be performed.[3] The incorporation of such offerings into religious rituals was a product of ancient beliefs regarding the importance of reciprocity (that by making an offering to the gods they will give something in return, or that if the gods give something the recipient must make an offering to them in return) and quality (that the finer or more elaborate the offering, the more effective the prayers accompanying it will be), but these also enabled public demonstrations of piety, status and wealth (van Straten, 1981, pp. 63–77). The acquisition of a suitable offering, whether it was specially commissioned or simply chosen from an available selection, was a performance in itself, with the supplicant performing for both a human audience (consisting of the craftsman responsible for producing the votives at the very least but perhaps also the sanctuary personnel and other worshippers) and a divine one. The presentation of the *ex-voto* within the sanctuary was a second performance made not only for the benefit of the supplicant, but also for the benefit of those around them, again both human and divine. If the *ex-voto* had been made in advance and this supplication proved successful, this would necessitate a return to the sanctuary. Once there a third performance would take place during which a second *ex-voto* – a thank offering – would be presented. Consequently, the visual dynamics within the microcosm of a sanctuary were crucial: the ritual viewing of the cult image and the dedications that had been left there were part of the process by which an individual worshipped, and the display of such *ex-votos* provided evidence of divine manifestation and demonstrated the deity's efficacy and was thus central to maintaining the deity's prestige and ensuring future worship (Petsalis-Diomidis, 2005, pp. 187–8). In a very real sense the sanctuary was a theatre, their interiors the stage upon which the supplicants performed for their human and divine audiences and then,

---

3 It is worth noting that in antiquity medical practitioners such as physicians, surgeons and dentists frequently not only consulted with but also treated their patients in front of an audience consisting of the family and friends of the patient, the patient's slaves, the practitioner's slaves, apprentices or colleagues or even interested onlookers. For discussion of this see Draycott (2014). For discussion of this with specific reference to Galen's demonstrations of dissection and vivisection, see von Staden (1995).

once they had finished, the *ex-votos* they left behind would serve as a constant reminder of those performances.

The dedication of hair to gods, goddesses and other mythological figures occurred not only as part of certain specific ceremonies marking significant events such as initiations, marriages and funerals, but also on a more ad hoc basis as a thank offering for something such as recovery from an illness or escape from disaster. How exactly were these dedications made? What did the process of dedicating a hair *ex-voto* involve? It would appear that for offerings of real human hair the hair was grown, worn and then cut in public. As was noted earlier, in the sanctuary of Asclepius at Titane women hung locks of their hair upon the cult statue of Hygieia (Pausanias, *Description of Greece* 2.11.6). This was perhaps due to a belief in the power of proximity – that the closer the *ex-voto* was placed to the cult statue, the more immediate and/or effective the divine intervention would be – but it also ensured that the dedications were highly visible to those entering the sanctuary and approaching the cult statue. In the sanctuary of Zeus at Panamara in Caria hair was either – if dedicated by the wealthy – enclosed in a small stone coffer in the form of a stele and set up in the precinct with an inscription placed upon it, or – if dedicated by those with fewer financial resources – placed in a hole in the wall or hung upon the wall with a small label placed upon it (*I. Str.* 428, 434, 449 and 1263). In the case of the former, although the hair itself was no longer visible, the stele and inscription certainly were, and in the case of the latter the hair remained visible in conjunction with a label that named the dedicant. In Hieropolis in Syria hair was placed within a sacred vase, so although the hair was not itself visible, the sacred vase that contained it was (Lucian, *On the Syrian Goddess* 60). On Delos when boys and girls cut their hair in honour of the Nymphs of Hyperborea the boys wound their hair in wisps of a certain type of grass growing nearby and the girls wound theirs around their spindles, and both types of offerings were placed upon the nymphs' tomb, thus both remained visible to those who might come after them (Callimachus, *Hymn to Delos* 4.292; Pausanias, *Description of Greece* 1.43.4).

The unique nature of hair combined with its tenacity and durability ensured that the connection established between the deity and the dedicant would continue for as long as the hair was present in the sanctuary (see Pointon, 1999 for the afterlife of hair). Antipater of Thessalonica writes of an offering made to the god Phoebus Apollo by a young man named Lycon:

> Having shaved the down that flowered in its season under his temples, [he dedicated] his cheeks' messengers of manhood, a first offering, and prayed that he might so shave gray hairs from his whitened temples. Grant him these, and even as you made him earlier, so make him hereafter, with the snows of old age upon him.
>
> (*Palatine Anthology* 6.198)[4]

---

4 See also *Palatine Anthology* 6.242 in which Crinagoras asks Zeus and Artemis to protect his brother Euclides from the growth of his first beard to his first grey hair.

Indeed, it is entirely possible that such a connection could last for the entirety of the dedicant's life, with supplicants redeeming the vows they made as youngsters by offering the white hair of their old age (*Palatine Anthology* 6.193).

Yet it is clear that in addition to dedicating *ex-votos* consisting of real human hair freshly grown, styled and cut from their own heads, supplicants dedicated *ex-votos* consisting of false and artificial hair. Because hair *ex-votos* are (almost) alone amongst the entire range of anatomical *ex-votos* in representing a body part that it was possible to dedicate without requiring a facsimile, why were the latter utilised at all? A simple answer may lie in the fact that offerings of false and/or artificial hair *ex-votos* were perhaps made by those who lacked sufficient hair of their own to make an acceptable offering. Two possible examples of this practice are represented by unfortunately unprovenanced *ex-votos* that are housed in the Wellcome Collection (Figure 4.3). These mould-made terracotta *ex-votos* were painted in different colours (white on the left and black on the right), thus introducing an element of choice – perhaps even personalisation – into the process of selecting an *ex-voto*.

However, there are also examples of real and artificial hair *ex-votos* being used together with inscriptions that commemorate the offering of a lock of hair and also depict a representation of the said lock alongside the text, such as an inscription from Thessalian Thebes dating to the late Hellenistic or early imperial period which commemorates the offerings made to Poseidon by two brothers,

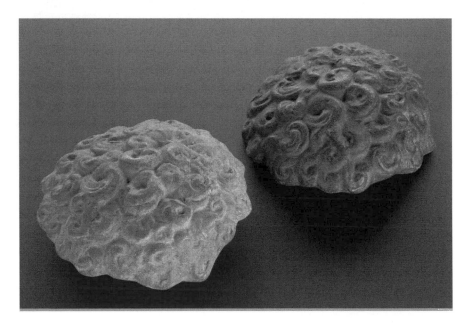

Figure 4.3 Terracotta *ex-votos*, Wellcome Museum inv. A114891 and inv. A634932.

Source: Wellcome Library, London.

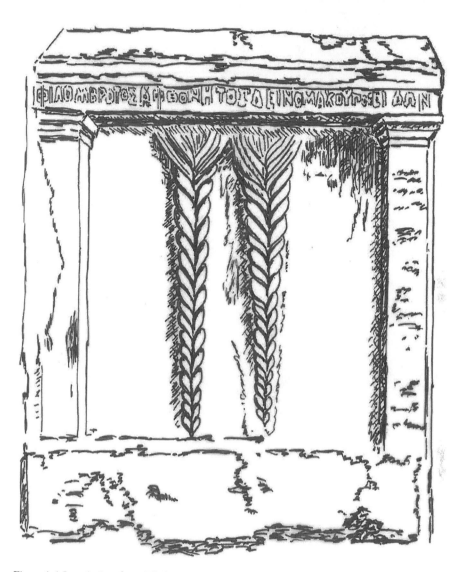

Figure 4.4 Inscription from Thebes, *IG* IX 2.146.

Source: Image courtesy of G. Bissas.

Philombrotos and Aphthonetos (*IG* IX 2.146) (see Figure 4.4). Another example can be found in the form of a terracotta braid from the Asclepieion in Corinth (Lang, 1977, p. 29, pl. 29) (Figure 4.5).

Thus it is possible that *ex-votos* consisting of real hair were destroyed periodically or whenever the cult statue or sanctuary space was cleaned, both as a way of dealing with the accumulation of tens, if not hundreds, or even thousands of

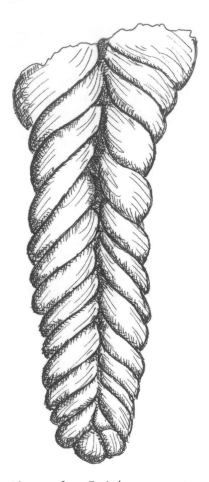

Figure 4.5 Terracotta braid *ex-voto* from Corinth.

Source: Image courtesy of G. Bissas, after Lang (1977, p. 29, pl. 29).

offerings over time and as a means of preventing the powerful hair from falling into the hands of evildoers who would pervert the *ex-voto* for their own nefarious purposes, usually as part of love spells (for examples see Euripides, *Hippolytus* 507–18; Apuleius, *Metamorphoses* 3.16; Lucian, *Dialogues of the Courtesans* 288–9; *Papyrus Michigan* 16.757).

Hair and the human body

The human body was the locus of much ritual activity in the ancient world, and thus it would not be surprising to see advantage being taken of the ready availability of hair, nails and teeth in both religious and magical practice (Hallpike,

1969, p. 257). Certainly, as discussed earlier, human hair was regularly utilised in all manner of religious rituals, and as early as 1886 George Wilken suggested that the ritual cutting of hair (or 'hair sacrifice') served as a substitute for human sacrifice on a *pars pro toto* basis. He argued that hair was considered appropriate for the purpose because the head is the seat of the soul (see also Hallpike, 1969, p. 149). The evidence for fingernails and toenails having been used in similar ways is less certain. One notable exception is found in the case of the Roman *flamen Dialis* whose hair *and* nails could only be cut by a freeman using bronze utensils, with the trimmings of both subsequently disposed of by being buried underneath a fruitful tree (Aulus Gellius, *Attic Nights* 10.15). Once removed, teeth seem to have simply been discarded as attested, for example, by the milk and adult teeth found in the drain of a bathhouse at the legionary fortress at Caerleon in Wales (Fagan, 1999, p. 87) and almost one hundred human teeth discovered in a drain below what is assumed to have been a dentist's shop near the Temple of Castor and Pollux in the Forum Romanum (Ginge et al., 1989; Becker and Turfa, 2017). However, hair, nails and teeth all seem to have been utilised in ancient magical rituals, with both Greek and Roman witches believed to harvest ingredients for their spells from the bodies of both the living and the dead. In Apuleius's *Metamorphoses* the witch Pamphile sends her accomplice Photis to retrieve the object of her affection's hair cuttings from the floor of a barber's shop:

> At the moment [Pamphile] is passionately in love with a very attractive lad from Boeotia, and she is feverishly employing all the resources and mechanisms of her craft against him . . . Yesterday on her way back from the baths, she caught sight of him by chance sitting in the barber's. She told me to steal some of his hair secretly. It lay on the ground where it had fallen after being cut off. But the barber found me as I was carefully and stealthily gathering it up and, because we are in any case notorious throughout the town for our evil techniques, he grabbed hold of me and shouted at me meanly: 'You are the lowest of the low! Is there no end to your constant theft of choice young men's hair? If you do not now put an end to this criminal activity, nothing shall stop me hauling you before the magistrates!' He matched his actions to his words. He stuck his hand down my dress and felt around, and angrily pulled out from between my breasts the locks I had already managed to hide there.
>
> (Apuleius, *Metamorphoses* 3.16)

Other ancient witches go further still, harvesting body parts from smouldering funerary pyres and digging up freshly buried corpses in graveyards (see, for example, Horace, *Epodes* 5; Lucan, *Civil War* 6.434–587). Witches were particularly associated with Thessaly (Phillips, 2002), and it is therefore interesting that the inscription and relief dedicated to Poseidon by Philombrotos and Aphthonetos (Figure 4.4) was set up in Thessaly. Additionally, in Lucan's *Civil War*, the witch Erictho not only gathers her ingredients from the dead, '[gnawing] at the pale nails of the dried-out hand', but also hovers over the living during their final moments, '[cutting] the lock from the dying adolescent' (Lucan, *Civil War* 6.507).

It is clear from a variety of sources that hair was considered to be an important component of the human body as a whole. Philippus of Thessalonica wrote an epigram describing the scattered remains of a man washed up on a beach, and hair (or rather, the body's lack of hair) features prominently as an indication of how wrong this is: 'Here lies the head, hair-stripped and tooth-bereft, there the hand's five fingers and the flesh-forsaken ribs, apart are the feet deprived of sinews and the limbs' disjointed frame. This man in many parts was once a whole' (*Palatine Anthology* 7.383). However, although hair was certainly important, possession of it was not on its own enough. Whether male or female, an individual's head of hair was expected to be healthy and attractive, so it is hardly surprising that barbers and hairdressers seem to have proliferated (Nicolson, 1891; Bartman, 2001; Olson, 2008). However, barbers and hairdressers were not the only professionals responsible for maintaining their clients' hair. Physicians circulated numerous remedies claiming not just to encourage hair growth, increase hair thickness and darken or dye hair, but also to treat more debilitating conditions such as hair loss or dandruff (on hair loss: Celsus, *On Medicine* 6.4; Pliny the Elder, *Natural History* 28.164; Galen, 12.403–5 K; Aëtius, *Sixteen Books on Medicine* 6.65; Paul of Aegina, *Medical Compendium in Seven Books* 3.1.1–2; on encouraging hair growth: Galen, 13.432–4 K; on dandruff: Galen, 12.492–3 K; on dying hair: Paul of Aegina, *Medical Compendium in Seven Books* 3.2.1). For those for whom these remedies failed to work, the one remaining option was to try to hide the affliction. Julius Caesar reportedly first tried combing his remaining hair forward before resorting to wearing his laurel crown to cover his bald spot, whereas the emperor Otho wore a wig (Suetonius, *Julius Caesar* 45.2; *Otho* 12).

As a man or a woman aged both the colour and texture of their hair would change naturally. However, the process by which hair would turn first grey and then eventually white or, worse still, thin before being lost entirely was associated not only with ageing but also with decline and then death. Philodemus of Gadara, writing of the courtesan Charito, observes that although she is 60 years old 'the long train of her black hair is unchanged' and this is in stark contrast to his depiction of himself at the age of 37, 'already . . . white hairs besprinkle me, announcers of discretion's years' (Charito: *Palatine Anthology* 5.13; Philodemus himself: *Palatine Anthology* 11.41; 5.112). This process is not easy to hide either, as Antiphilus observes that 'though you may smooth the ragged skin of your channelled cheeks and put coal-black on your useless eyes and dye your white hair black and hang around your temples curly fine crisped ringlets, all that is useless' (*Palatine Anthology* 11.66; jokes are frequently made at the expense of older women attempting to look young by authors such as Ovid and Martial).

Molly Levine elaborated upon Wilken's theory regarding 'hair sacrifice' and proposed that in antiquity hair could stand for the whole person as a metonym, observing that the Latin word *capillus* ('hair') is itself a diminutive of *caput* ('head'), so the word literally means 'little head' (Levine, 1995, p. 85). Thus

Petronius has Eumolpus sing a song that equates the loss of hair with the loss of life: 'You see in your hair's death a token of mortality' (Petronius, *Satyricon* 109). His inspiration for this is that his companions Encolpius and Giton have been forced to shave their heads and faces in an attempt to disguise themselves as slaves. This loss of head and facial hair is humiliating, serving to diminish them in not only their own eyes, but also the eyes of others and necessitating drastic steps being taken to restore them to their former glory:

> One of Tryphaena's maids took Giton below and decked him out in a curly wig belonging to her mistress. She even produced false eyebrows from a little box, and, tracing the curves where his eyebrows had been, repaired the damage to his features. All of his beauty was restored. Tryphaena recognised her own Giton, burst into tears, and gave him his first really sincere kiss since encountering him again. I was happy that the boy had returned to his original glory, but I had myself to think about. I kept hiding my face, because I knew that I was mutilated to no ordinary extent. Not even Lichas saw fit to speak to me. But the same maid noticed my embarrassment and took me aside to adorn me with a wig no less splendid. In fact, I was even more handsome than before, because my new hair was bright blond.
>
> (Petronius, *Satyricon* 110)

Giton and Encolpius's loss of hair is described as 'damage' and 'mutilation'. The use of artificial hair and eyebrows to restore them to their former glory (and even improve upon it in Encolpius's case) involves not only repairing what had been damaged and mutilated and reassembling what had been fragmented, but also replacing what had been lost and essentially creating something new in the process (on the relationship between parts of the body and the whole body, see Hughes, 2008; Rebay-Salisbury et al., 2010). The fact that the hairpieces belong to a woman does not seem to matter, at least to Encolpius and Giton, although Petronius's readers may have thought differently, as men who were deemed to be effeminate were subjected to severe criticism by their peers.

It is clear that an intact body was important, if not fundamental. Any deviation from the norm was viewed with suspicion, with physical imperfections being considered sufficient cause to disqualify someone from holding a priesthood or even result in their being excluded from one already held if they suffered injury during their tenure (Plutarch, *Roman Questions* 73). However, body parts that were lost could be replaced with prostheses, with one notable example of this coming in the form of Marcus Sergius Silus's right hand lost in his second military campaign during the Second Punic War (218–201 BC) (Pliny the Elder, *Natural History* 7.28.104–5). It was replaced with an iron one that he used to hold his shield and he continued to fight using his left hand to wield his sword. The use of prostheses can be seen as dovetailing with these concepts of repair, reassembly, replacement and the creation of something new (on prostheses in the ancient world, see Bliquez, 1996).

Although individuals born with a disfigurement or disability could be subject to assumptions that they were being punished for their (or their ancestors')
transgressions, those who acquired one during life through some sort of heroic
activity could use it to their advantage (on disfigurement and disability as punishment in the ancient world, see Vlahogiannis, 1998; 2005; on using a wound
to one's advantage, see Leigh, 1995). One notable example concerned the right
hand of Gaius Mucius, lost in a failed attempt to assassinate Lars Porsena, the
king of Clusium, in 508 BC, after which Gaius Mucius was known as Scae-
vola, 'the left-handed man' (Livy, *On the Foundation of the City* 2.12.1–13.5).
In circumstances such as these where a missing body part and its subsequent
replacement became overlaid with meanings and associations, it is possible that
the prosthesis in question might be dedicated as a votive offering in its turn
and might perhaps on occasion be intended to serve as an anatomical *ex-voto*
itself. An example is found in *Papyrus Gissen* 20 (Hermopolis, AD 117–18),
which details how a shrine is to be maintained by a manufacturer of artificial
limbs, ὁ κωλοπλάστης (*kōloplastēs*), which could have served a dual purpose as
anatomical votive offerings (Draycott, 2014). Is there evidence of 'false' or even
'artificial' hair being used in this way? The poet Myrinus writes an epigram in
which he presents Statyllius (who he refers to dismissively as 'the effeminate')
dedicating 'his borrowed curls, nard-greasy' along with items of clothing and
footwear to the god Priapus shortly before his death, presumably as a means of
easing his passing (*Palatine Anthology* 6.254). Thus it is possible that wigs and
hairpieces were dedicated as *ex-votos* in sanctuaries, as in addition to dedicating locks of their own hair people dedicated items involved in hairdressing
such as headdresses, hair nets and hair pins. Several epigrams from the *Palatine
Anthology* imagine such scenarios: upon becoming an adult woman Timarete
dedicates her dolls, ball, tambourine and child's headdress, and upon achieving a legal marriage, Alcibië (the name perhaps chosen to evoke the famous
courtesan) dedicates her hair net to the goddess Hera, and Philaenis dedicates
a purple hair net, 'protector of much-braided hair', to the goddess Aphrodite
(*Palatine Anthology* 6.280; 6.133; 6.207). Certainly, wigs and hairpieces were
deposited in tombs and graves as grave goods in the ancient world. A number
of hairpieces dating from the Predynastic Period through the Late Period
have been recovered from ancient sites in Egypt, including extensions, braids,
wigs and their storage boxes (Fletcher, 2002; 2005). There are somewhat fewer
examples dating from the Greco-Roman period, including several hairpieces
from Les Martres-de-Veyre in France (Audollent, 1923) and from Rainham
Creek in Britain (Allason-Jones, 2005, p. 133). A wig made from hair moss
has been recovered from the Roman fort at Vindolanda, and a similar object has
been recovered from Newstead, both in Britain (Allason-Jones, 2005, p. 132).
The use of such items as grave goods indicates that they were considered
necessary in the afterlife, perhaps a continuing means of repairing and
reassembling their owner's damaged and mutilated body in a similar way to
extremity prostheses.

The importance of hair in the ancient world

In antiquity the appearance of an individual's hair transmitted many complex and intertwined messages about him or her to the world at large, informing observers of their sex and/or gender, age, ethnicity, marital status and even profession (Levine, 1995, p. 80). Although the specifics varied according to territory, men and women were generally subject to different sets of expectations with regard to how they dealt with their hair. Thus the men of Classical Athens were expected to cut their hair short (and men who did not, such as Alcibiades, were regarded with suspicion), whereas the men of Classical Sparta not only grew their hair long, but also maintained and styled it, and Spartan women cut their hair upon marriage and subsequently kept it short (Athenian and Spartan men: Plutarch, *Lycurgus* 22.1; Herodotus, *Histories* 7.208–09; Spartan women: Plutarch, *Lycurgus* 15.3). Roman men were likewise expected to keep their hair short and were subject to criticism if they did not, whereas women were considered sexually unattractive if their hair was cut short (Apuleius, *Metamorphoses* 2.8). Hair played an important part in the ageing process and the accompanying markers, with boys cutting their hair or shaving their faces for the first time to mark their transition to manhood and girls wearing their hair long and loose until marriage or the birth of their first child, at which point they began to tie it back and cover it up with veils (adolescent Athenian boys cutting their hair: Pausanias, *Description of Greece* 1.37.3; adolescent Spartan boys growing their hair long: Plutarch, *Lycurgus* 22.1; boys shaving their facial hair for the first time (*depositio barbae*): *Palatine Anthology* 6.242; Petronius, *Satyricon* 29; Juvenal, *Satires* 8.166; Suetonius, *Caligula* 10; *Nero* 12; Cassius Dio, *Roman History* 48.34.3; girls with free-flowing hair as the mark of a virgin: Ovid, *Metamorphoses* 2.413; girls changing their hair upon first childbirth: *Palatine Anthology* 6.201). Hair was also used as a way to differentiate between 'civilised' Greeks and Romans and 'barbaric' 'others', such as Britons, who, according to Julius Caesar and Propertius, plastered their hair, beards and moustaches with woad (Julius Caesar, *Gallic War* 5.14; Propertius, *Elegies* 2.18.23–32) and Africans, with the latter accordingly subjected to criticism that not even members of foreign royal families were exempt from (see Cicero's criticism of King Juba of Numidia's hair and beard: Cicero, *On the Agrarian Law* 2.59; see Aldhouse-Green, 2004a, pp. 315–18; 2004b, pp. 334–45 on the Roman (mis)use of hair as a means of denigrating defeated 'barbarian' foes). It was also possible to identify an individual's profession by their haircut or style. Greek priests wore their hair long, and Egyptian priests and priestesses shaved their heads and bodies (Herodotus, *Histories* 2.36), and Roman Vestal Virgins cut their hair short and arranged it in the traditional *seni crines* hairstyle consisting of six braids covered with a *reticulum luteum* and *flammeum* (Festus, *Glossaria Latina* 454.23 L). The wife of the *flamen Dialis*, the *flaminica*, wore her hair in the archaic *tutulus* hairstyle (in which the hair was piled up on top of the head in a cone-shaped bun with locks brought forward onto the crown of the head and tied with *vittae*) and was forbidden from combing it in the months of

March and June (Ovid, *Fasti* 3.393–8; 6.226–34). Individuals in mourning were marked out because of the state of their hair, with both Greek and Roman men and women growing their hair and neglecting to style it (Aeschylus, *Suppliant Women* 6–7; Herodotus, *Histories* 2.36).

Discussion of ancient hairstyling and styles is highly pertinent to the study of anatomical votives, as one of the most common components of votive deposits is the head or half-head, whether male or female, adult or child (Steingräber, 1980; Söderlind, 2005). The prevailing interpretation of these head and half-head *ex-votos* is that they are *pars pro toto* representations and that because they are all rendered on the same scale and in the same style as anatomical *ex-votos* they must represent mortals rather than deities (Turfa, 1994; 2006a). This would seem to account not only for the stylistic differences between them, but also indicates an attempt to personalise them through the selection of particular colours of paint for the purpose of decoration or even deliberate alterations and mutilations to the face or head itself (Aldhouse-Green, 1999, discusses votive heads from Fontes Sequanae, which have been adapted to show particular pathologies). This begs the question: Were these heads and half-heads perhaps deliberately selected and then offered by people who intended them to serve as substitutes for themselves (Bartoloni and Benedettini, 2011, pp. 786–7)? This in turn raises the related question of whether the hairstyles featured on full-length figurines should be viewed likewise. Is it possible to relate with any level of confidence the hairstyle worn by a head of half-head *ex-voto* to the hairstyle of the supplicant who offered it?

Were votive heads and half-heads specially selected in order to represent the specific individual who dedicated them? Male votive heads from Etruria are generally depicted bareheaded (*capite aperto*), whereas those from Rome and Latium are generally depicted with *velum* (*capite velato*), perhaps a reflection of differing religious practices in these different regions (Söderlind, 2005, p. 359; this issue is explored more thoroughly and critically in Glinister, 2009). Female votive heads are considerably more varied due to the variety of hairstyles and hair coverings that could be worn by Greek and Roman girls and women depending on their stage of life (La Follette, 1994; Sebesta, 1994; Bartman, 2001). Thus a votive head of a young freeborn girl would depict her with her hair braided and tied with a *vitta* (Nonius Marcellus, *De compendiosa doctrina* 236 M). One of a bride or Vestal Virgin would depict her with her hair arranged in the traditional *seni crines* hairstyle (Figure 4.6) (Festus, *Glossaria Latinae* 454.23 L; Propertius, *Elegies* 4.3.15; 4.11.33; on the *seni crines* as a bridal hairstyle, see Torelli, 1984, pp. 33–7). Jean Turfa has suggested that this terracotta half-head *ex-voto* should be identified as a bride based on this specific hairstyle (Turfa, 2005, pp. 245–6, n. 272).

However, some stages of life are represented much less frequently and some not at all, perhaps due to the comparatively small numbers who successfully achieved them. Thus in theory an *ex-voto* depicting a matron might be expected to show her with her hair dressed with *vittae* and covered with a *palla* (Plautus, *The Braggart Soldier* 790–93), whereas one of a *mater familias* or the *flaminica Dialis*

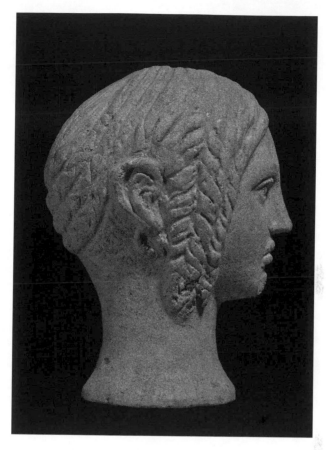

Figure 4.6 Terracotta half-head *ex-voto* from Caere, British Museum inv. 1955, 0914.1.

Source: Image courtesy of the Trustees of the British Museum.

might show her with her hair arranged in a *tutulus* (Varro, *On the Latin Language* 7.44), and one of a widow might show her having exchanged her *palla* for a *ricinium*. However, it is also possible that *ex-votos* such as these might be dedicated not as representations of the girls and women who were presenting them, but as representations of the people that they wished to become: a girl wanting to marry and become a bride or a matron wanting to become the *mater familias*. It is also possible that a head or half-head *ex-voto* might be an attempt to capture a supplicant precisely as they were in that particular moment, such as in the case of a stone head from Fontes Sequanae that depicts a woman with a fringed napkin draped over the crown of her head, this cloth having been interpreted as a cloth impregnated with sacred water from the sanctuary's spring (Aldhouse-Green, 1999, p. 71, pl. 32).

Conclusion

Real, false and artificial hair *ex-votos* all served important purposes with regard to ritual and healing practices surrounding the ancient body, as well as how it was viewed and experienced both by its owner and by those around him or her. However, these purposes were not necessarily the same. Based on the wealth of literary, documentary and archaeological evidence for the dedication of hair *ex-votos*, it would appear that real hair was the norm and was to a certain extent privileged over both false and artificial hair as it enabled and facilitated a deeper – and perhaps even lifelong – connection with the deity. Real hair *ex-votos* were dedicated for a variety of reasons such as birth, puberty, citizenship, marriage and so forth, whereas false hair *ex-votos* seem to have been dedicated at the point at which they were no longer considered necessary, such as at the end of a man's or woman's working or sexual life, assuming they were not going to be utilised as a grave good. Artificial hair *ex-votos*, on the other hand, seem to have served as replacements for real (and perhaps on occasion even false) hair *ex-votos*, offering both durability and security. With regard to the dedication of head and half-head *ex-votos*, it would appear that hair played a crucial role in the head or half-head's ability to represent the supplicant successfully, both as they were under normal circumstances, and even in one particular moment, and how they wished to be in the future.

5 Demeter as an ophthalmologist?

Eye votives and the cult of Demeter and Kore[1]

Georgia Petridou

This chapter looks at eye-shaped votives and in particular eye-shaped votives found not in sanctuaries of deities who were traditionally thought of as presiding over illness and healing, but in sanctuaries dedicated to Demeter and Kore (see Forsén, 1996, pp. 133–59).[2] These eye-shaped *ex-votos* resemble the anatomical votives we find in healing temples in terms of typology but present different interpretative challenges and possibilities, as they presuppose different models of spectatorship and visuality (Bryson, 1988, p. 91).[3] How are we to interpret them? Are Demeter and Kore conceived here as healing deities who specialise in ophthalmological diseases, or are we to think of eye votives as powerful testaments to the centrality and intensity of ocularcentric processes that informed

1 This chapter has benefited from discussions in Rome, Berlin, Reading and Erfurt. I would like to thank Jane Draycott and Emma-Jayne Graham for organising the conference where the original chapter was presented. I am grateful to Philip van der Eijk, the director of the research programme 'Medicine of the Mind – Philosophy of the Body – Discourses of Health and Disease in the Ancient World' (a programme funded by the Alexander von Humboldt Stiftung), for reading a draft of this chapter and his help with the bibliographical references. This chapter resulted from research that was partly conducted under the auspices of the aforementioned research programme and partly in the context of the 'Lived Ancient Religion (LAR). Questioning "Cults" and "Polis Religion"' project, an ERC-funded programme at the Max Weber Kolleg, University of Erfurt. I am indebted to Rubina Raja, Lara Weiss and Jörg Rüpke, the director of the LAR programme, for reading and commenting on an earlier draft. Special thanks are to be given to Dimitar Iliev and Nikolay Sharankov (University of Sofia) for providing details of the whereabouts of the Plovdiv relief, as well as with the reproduction of Figure 5.3. A shorter version of this chapter with a different methodological focus appears in *Religion in the Roman Empire* (2016).
2 Forsén (1996, pp. 142–4) mentions health-related dedications made in honour of Demeter and Kore but considers them as two goddesses who preside primarily over womanhood and childbirth ('Geburts-und Frauengottheiten' in the original). This is not a helpful distinction as Chaniotis in his *BMCR* review (98.2.10) also argues. In Forsén's view the deities that are considered paradigmatic healing deities ('Heil-gottheiten') and consequently the ones who receive the majority of the anatomical votives are Asclepius, Heros Iatros, Amphiaraos, Amynos, Apollo, Athena, Hercules and Zeus in the cultic manifestations of Alexikakos, Soter, Hypsistos, Hypatos and so on. On popular Greek and Roman healing deities and their shrines, see Petridou (2016). Vikela (2006) offers an informative discussion of healing deities and their sanctuaries in Attica, but goes too far in using anatomical votive offerings to distinguish between 'genuine' and 'not genuine' healing deities. In this view Demeter may have received such dedications, but her sanctuary cannot be called a proper healing sanctuary, and Demeter herself is not a *true* healing deity.
3 'Cultural specific visuality' and 'culturally inflected visual practices' have displaced the notion of 'vision' in an array of different scientific disciplines.

the worshipper's experiences? Are the eyes depicted the eyes of the votaries, and, if so, are they depictions of healthy or diseased eyes? Or are they to be thought of as mementos of the devotees' visual encounters with the divine in the course of an initiatory ritual? These and other related issues are raised here, and tentative answers are offered on the basis of other visual and literary evidence on the relationship of Demeter to health in general and ophthalmological disease in particular. The present chapter is aimed as an individual offering in the wider methodological debate of the volume which focuses precisely on redefining the very notion of an anatomical votive. As such its author joins forces with the editors in providing a more flexible working definition of these objects and, above all, their situational sacred dimension (see Smith, 1987, p. 104; see also the Introduction to this volume).

More specifically this study looks at these eye-shaped anatomical votives not as passive but as agentic objects. My analysis draws on Gell's (1998) influential anthropological theory of the art object which focuses on the relational problem of matter and agency. Gell's theory supposes four interactive categories: artist, index (material object), prototype (source of the form for the object) and recipient. Each of these categories is further defined by their status as agent (active) or patient (acted upon) in their social relations, with further interdependencies, reversals and cascading relations (Gell, 1998, p. 29). What is particularly helpful in Gell's analysis is that it raises awareness of the dual roles these artefacts play within their particular social networks – that is, they are simultaneously agent and patient – and the emphasis it lays on the interpretative difficulties these objects raise:

> It is important to understand, though, that "patients" in agent/patient interactions are not entirely passive; they may resist. The concept of agency implies the overcoming of resistance, difficulty, inertia, etc. Art objects are characteristically "difficult". They are difficult to make, difficult to "think", difficult to transact.
>
> (Gell, 1998, p. 23)

This chapter examines eye-shaped anatomical votives found in the sanctuaries of Demeter and Kore as exceptionally 'difficult' art objects. On the one hand, they defy our established and simplistic definition of what an anatomical votive is, and on the other hand, they challenge our modern juxtaposition of physical and mysteric vision versus physical and mysteric blindness. I use the term 'mysteric' in the same sense Sourvinou-Inwood (2003) does: to denote 'something deriving of or belonging to the Mysteria' in an attempt to avoid the misleading and anachronistic term 'mystery'.

Ophthalmological illness and eye-shaped votives

The student of archaeology, the history of art, the history of religion and, of course, the history of medicine is familiar with artefacts such as those depicted in Figure 5.1. These depict *ex-votos* in the shape of external body parts (ears,

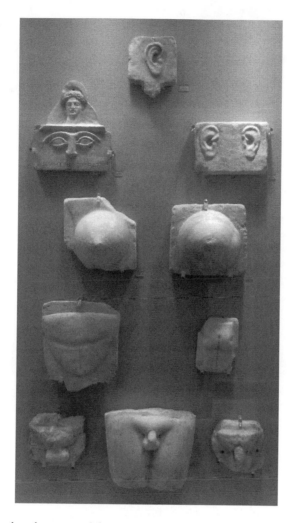

Figure 5.1 The glass showcase exhibiting (upper-left corner) the Eukrates relief (NM inv.
5256) in the National Archaeological Museum, Athens.

Source: Image courtesy of Alamy Ltd.

eyes, genitals, breasts and so on) which can be comfortably accommodated under
the rubric 'anatomical votive offering'.[4] Forsén (1996, p. 1) gives an informative

4 Representations of internal organs are very rare in Greek healing sanctuaries. For example, only a heart
(καρδία) and a bladder ([κ]ύστις) are mentioned in the inventories from the Athenian Asclepieion. On
the contrary, internal organs feature mainly in Roman and Etruscan sanctuaries (van Straten, 1981,
pp. 111–12; Hughes, forthcoming; chapters by Flemming and Haumesser, this volume).

account of the anatomical votives of the Greek-speaking world and defines them as follows:

> Anatomical votives (also known as body-part votives, anatomical *ex-votos*, or votive limbs) are representations of human bodily parts that were consecrated to deities with healing powers, as a request for healing or as a reward for the healing of the depicted bodily part.
>
> (my translation)

In short, anatomical votives could function either as requests for a cure or as thanksgiving offerings.

Forsén is not alone in emphasising the fragmentary character of these bodily parts. Other scholars, such as Hughes (2008; forthcoming), Petsalis-Diomidis (2010) and Dasen (2012, p. 402), have paid particular attention to the fragmentary character of these objects which via the act of dedication became the property of the entreated healing deity and their sanctuary. Thus, the patient's bodily parts became the *loci* of the divine conduct and healing, and these anatomical votive offerings became in turn the material evidence, if not for the act of healing itself, then certainly for the worshippers' steadfast expectation of it. It was pain and disease that fragmented the human body, and it was up to the divine healers to restore the human body to its health and its completeness, as the following extract from an oration that was dedicated to Asclepius and written by one of the most conspicuous patients of the second century AD, Publius Aelius Aristides Theodoros, shows:

> ἀλλὰ καὶ μέλη τοῦ σώματος αἰτιῶνταί τινες, καὶ ἄνδρες λέγω καὶ γυναῖκες, προνοίᾳ τοῦ θεοῦ γενέσθαι σφίσι, τῶν παρὰ τῆς φύσεως διαφθαρέντων. καὶ καταλέγουσιν ἄλλος ἄλλο τι, οἱ μὲν ἀπὸ στόματος οὑτωσὶ φράζοντες, οἱ δὲ ἐν τοῖς ἀναθήμασιν ἐξηγούμενοι. ἡμῖν τοίνυν οὐχὶ μέρος τοῦ σώματος, ἀλλ' ἅπαν τὸ σῶμα συνθείς τε καὶ συμπήξας αὐτὸς ἔδωκε δωρεάν, ὥσπερ Προμηθεὺς τἀρχαῖα λέγεται συμπλάσαι τὸν ἄνθρωπον.

> But some, I mean both men and women, even attribute to the providence of the god the existence of parts of their body, when their natural bodily parts have been destroyed; others list other things, some in oral accounts, some in declarations of their votive offerings. For us it is not only a part of the body, but it is the whole body which he has composed and put together and given as a gift, just as Prometheus of old is said to have fashioned man.
>
> (Aelius Aristides, *Oration* 42.7 Keil)[5]

Given their indispensability in connecting the body of the worshipper with the divine healer and their vital role in the very act of consecration of the diseased

---

5 The translation by C.A. Behr is slightly modified. Unless otherwise stated, translations are my own.

body part, it is difficult to approach these objects as patient (acted upon) rather than agent (active). These anatomical votives were the ones who did most of the talking in the ancient healing sanctuaries, at least in the eyes of their synchronic perceivers, the Greek and Roman pilgrims who visited them. Notice that in the passage quoted earlier Aristides compares these artefacts with the oral and written accounts of miraculous healings (including *therapeiai* and *iamata*), which were also telling of divine providence and the divine taking an interest in the innermost bodily cavities of the human sufferers (on the diseased part as being at the same time the locus of miraculous healing and therefore a sign of divine favouritism, see Petsalis-Diomidis, 2010, pp. 257–62). Such anatomical *ex-votos* are the embodiment of either the sufferers' prayers prior to their therapy or of their post-eventum homages (see Graham, this volume for anatomical votives as a material means for orchestrating mortal-immortal interaction). In either case, they are aimed at both the healing gods and the pilgrims of their sanctuaries. They speak volumes about the intensity of human suffering and the need for divine medical intervention. In this sense the votive eyes discovered all over the healing temples of the Greco-Roman world speak as loud, if not louder, than the written records of oral accounts of divine therapy.

The two questions that follow naturally are: How common were vision problems and eye-related afflictions in the Greco-Roman world and what can these eye-shaped votives reveal about their dedicants and their respective illnesses? Given the limited nature of the sources (literary, epigraphic and material culture alike), answering these questions is not an easy task. The lengthy so-called 'confession stelai' from Lydia and Phrygia, with their extensive accounts of religious transgression and the transgressor, are perhaps an exception to this rule (see Potts, this volume). Moreover, eyes are the most commonly portrayed organ in the inscriptions from Phrygia. However, some tentative answers can be given. In particular, to judge from the multiple references to ophthalmological illnesses and treatments in the ancient medical authors and the plethora of ophthalmological instruments and eye-shaped dedications excavated from the ancient healing sanctuaries, ophthalmological problems like glaucoma, trachoma, conjunctivitis and benign and malignant growths on the cornea and the eyelid must have been a constant concern amongst the communities all over the Greco-Roman world (on eye-related illnesses in antiquity, see Hirschberg, 1982; Nutton, 2013; for ophthalmological illness in the Hippocratic Corpus, see Lascaratos and Marketos, 1997; Villard, 2005; Craik, 2006; 2009, pp. 113–15; LoPresti, 2008, pp. 381–409).[6] Indeed, it is not uncommon to find these objects included in modern ophthalmological handbooks and journals as illustrations of vision-related medical problems in antiquity, quite often featuring in futile exercises in retrospective diagnosis (Chaviara-Karahaliou, 1990; for illustrative examples of the dangers of retrospective diagnosis, see Meyer-Steineg, 1912; Frohmann, 1956; van Straten,

6 I am grateful to Roberto LoPresti (Humboldt University) for his useful suggestions regarding problems related to vision and sensory perception in the Hippocratic Corpus.

1981, pp. 149–51). Jaeger (1988, p. 10) has argued that it is in fact quite rare that any pathological condition is shown on these votives.

Answering questions about the existence of healing sanctuaries that specialised in the treatment of eye diseases and conditions is riddled with analogous difficulties. Some excavations in certain healing temples have yielded richer findings than others, but judgements made from the number of the eye votives found in deposits and pronouncements that a certain temple specialised in ophthalmological illness is a difficult and often dangerous enterprise. To take the two famous temples of Asclepius in Athens and Corinth as an example, given that eye votives were the most frequently mentioned anatomical votive in the inventory from the Asclepieion of Athens (*IG* II² 1532–37 and 1539), it is surprising how few of those eye-shaped votive replicas were excavated in the Corinthian Asclepieion (Roebuck, 1951, pp. 120–21; also Lang, 1977; van Straten, 1981, pp. 109–10). Some scholars, such as Roebuck (1951, pp. 114–15) and more recently Oberhelman (2014, p. 52), have understood this surplus of one kind of anatomical votive in one sanctuary and not in another as the material evidence of different sanctuaries specialising in different kinds of illnesses. In this view eye-related illnesses were the 'specialisation' of the Athenian Asclepieion and not that of Corinth. The perishable or extremely precious material of some of these eye-shaped *ex-votos* is surely a much more important factor affecting the higher frequency with which terracotta, stone or metal eye *ex-votos* appear in the excavations (Jaeger, 1988, p. 11). By contrast, eye votives made of silver or gold occur far more commonly in epigraphic records. Indeed, van Straten's (1981, p. 150) strong reaction to Roebuck's theory of the 'specialisations' of healing sanctuaries still holds:

> However, we should bear in mind that these conclusions are only valid, if we assume that the known votive offerings from these sanctuaries form a representative collection. I doubt whether that is true. The striking predominance of eyes in Athens is incontestable, but their scarcity at Corinth is another matter. After all, out of the more than 150 Athenian dedications, only three really remain. All the other eyes were gold and silver votives that do not survive, but of which we happen to have an epigraphic record because the Athenians were rather given to inscribing all sorts of decrees and inventories on stone. For all we know, the Asklepieia of Corinth and Epidauros may have been just as rich in gold and silver *týpoi*, which, like the Athenian ones, have left no tangible trace, and, unlike the Athenian ones, no epigraphic record either. That gold and silver votives indeed occurred there may perhaps be inferred from the gilded marble relief found at Epidauros and the gilded terracottas from Corinth.

Eye-shaped votives and the Eukrates relief

But what about the votive relief depicted in the upper-left corner of Figure 5.1? Is this an anatomical votive? It depicts a pair of eyes with the nose and eyebrows and is accompanied by the following inscription: Δήμητρι Εὐκράτης, 'Eukrates (dedicates) to Demeter' (*LIMC* 4. 861, Demeter no. 161).[7] This striking artefact was excavated around 1800 in the area surrounding the Eleusinian Telestērion close to the middle round tower of the southern *peribolos*, and it has been dated to the fourth century BC (for a plan of the sanctuary and the city of Eleusis, see Mylonas, 1961, fig. 32). The modern viewer is struck immediately by its beauty and its resemblance to the anatomical *ex-votos*. Indeed, judging by the way the artefact is currently exhibited in the National Archaeological Museum in Athens – at the top corner of a glass showcase surrounded by several other votive offerings depicting body parts from the Athenian Asclepieion, the Amyneion and the sanctuaries of Zeus Hypsistos in Athens and Aphrodite in Daphne – the modern spectator is encouraged to conceptualise the Eukrates relief as a 'typical' anatomical votive. However, one's attention is quickly directed to the image of a radiant female head (one would assume the head of a goddess, presumably that of Demeter or Kore) with red rays radiating from the head, the hair and the neck, which is attached to the top of the plaque.[8] The Eukrates relief is unique in having preserved much of the paint on its surface of white marble: the red paint on the right eye, the lips and the eyes of the goddess is clearly visible, and her hair is painted in a red-brown colour. The flat area that surrounds the nose and the eyes in the lower part of the relief must also have been painted in a bright red-brown colour.

There are two distinct levels of action in the marble relief from Eleusis: a) the rectangular plaque with the pair of eyes, eyebrows and nose, which is already familiar from other eye-shaped votives; and b) the head of the light-emanating goddess on the top. The viewer is faced with a riddle concerning how the two levels are related to each other. Does the upper face image on the rectangular plaque represent Eukrates's visual experiences in the Telestērion? Does this vision of a light-emanating Demeter or Kore allude to what Eukrates saw in the Telestērion, perhaps in the course of his initiation? After all, light seems to be an integral element of Demeter's divine epiphany as described in the *Homeric Hymn to Demeter* (278–80). Or was this vision of Demeter imbued in light the very first sight Eukrates had after his blindness was cured? Or is the relief a thanksgiving offering to commemorate successful treatment of Eukrates's eye disease, hence the similarities with the other anatomical *ex-votos*? In order to answer these questions, it is important to note here, following Clinton (1993, p. 90), that these rays of light do not originate from anything the goddess is wearing (her clothes or jewellery) but come directly out of the divine body very much in the manner that is described in the *Homeric Hymn to Demeter*. The main source

---

7 Dimensions: H. 0.192 m, W. 0.17 m, Th. 0.18 m. The inscription of the relief was published as *IG* II² 4639 and more recently by Clinton (2007) as *I. Eleusis* 105 (pl. 47) with more bibliography. See also van Straten (1981, pp. 121–2, no. 13.1, fig. 56); Clinton (1993, p. 86 and p. 90); Steinhart (1995, pp. 34–8, pl. 9); Forsén (1996, pp. 143–4); Vikela (2006, pp. 46–7) and Petridou (2013).

8 The Gallo-Roman deity Apollo Vindonnus was also represented as radiating from the head: Green (1992, p. 32). I thank the anonymous referee for this addition.

of the vibrant glow (expressed artistically by both the painted rays and the use of vibrant colour) is the head and the neck of the goddess, not her accessories.

However, the real problem is how to reconcile Demeter the goddess of rural and human fertility with the explicit references to vision in general and eyesight in particular in this relief. As hinted at earlier, it is possible that the relief commemorated Eukrates's physical ability to see, perhaps after a miracle cure performed by Demeter. This cure may have taken place in the course of his initiation in the Mysteria of the two goddesses, or it might equally have been independent of it. The fluidity, however, between the notions of physical and ritual blindness in the context of mystery cults in general and that of the Mysteria of Eleusis in particular, prevents us from determining with any certainty whether the dedicant was indeed blind or visually impaired before his encounter with the goddess (Petridou, 2013). The relief may have been commissioned simply to celebrate Eukrates's new and illuminated mystic vision in the course of his initiation. In other words, it is not at all clear whether we are dealing with physical sight or vision versus physical blindness or ritual sight/vision as opposed to ritual blindness or, indeed, whether we are dealing with both. Consequently, a further difficulty arises in determining with any certainty whether the Eukrates relief can be classified as an anatomical relief or a memento of his mysteric initiation. In an attempt to postulate what role this artefact played in Eukrates's life and whether it could be interpreted as a thanksgiving offering for his cure from physical blindness or other visual impairment, the following two sections assess the literary and material evidence that speak of Demeter and Kore's iatric activity in general and their correlation to eyesight and ophthalmological disease in particular.

Demeter and ophthalmological illness: the literary evidence

In the following passage from his seventh book Pausanias describes the ὑδρομαντεῖον ('water-based oracle') of Patras. In this special type of divination by water (*hydromanteion*) we are told that people did not seek to cure their friends and relatives; instead, they sought a prediction, in other words a prognosis, regarding the outcome of the disease. Will their loved ones recover (or at least remain alive) or will they die?

τοῦ δὲ ἄλσους ἱερὸν ἔχεται Δήμητρος· αὕτη μὲν καὶ ἡ παῖς ἑστᾶσι, τὸ δὲ ἄγαλμα τῆς Γῆς ἐστι καθήμενον. πρὸ δὲ τοῦ ἱεροῦ τῆς Δήμητρός ἐστι πηγή· ταύτης τὰ μὲν πρὸς τοῦ ναοῦ λίθων ἀνέστηκεν αἱμασιά, κατὰ δὲ τὸ ἐκτὸς κάθοδος ἐς αὐτὴν πεποίηται. μαντεῖον δὲ ἐνταῦθά ἐστιν ἀψευδές, οὐ μὲν ἐπὶ παντί γε πράγματι, ἀλλὰ ἐπὶ τῶν καμνόντων. κάτοπτρον καλῳδίῳ τῶν λεπτῶν δήσαντες καθιᾶσι, σταθμώμενοι μὴ πρόσω καθικέσθαι τῆς πηγῆς, ἀλλ᾽ ὅσον ἐπιψαῦσαι τοῦ ὕδατος τῷ κύκλῳ τοῦ κατόπτρου. τὸ δὲ ἐντεῦθεν εὐξάμενοι τῇ θεῷ καὶ θυμιάσαντες ἐς τὸ κάτοπτρον βλέπουσι· τὸ δέ σφισι τὸν νοσοῦντα ἤτοι ζῶντα ἢ καὶ τεθνεῶτα ἐπιδείκνυσι.

Demeter's sanctuary is situated in the grove; she and her daughter are standing up, but the statue of Earth is sitting down. There is a spring in front of Demeter's sanctuary with a dry stone wall on the temple side and a way down to the spring on the outer side. There is an infallible oracle here, not for all purposes but for the sick. They tie a mirror onto some thin kind of cord, and balance it so as not to dip it into the spring, but let the surface of the mirror just touch lightly on the water. Then they pray to the goddess and burn incense and *look into the mirror*, and it *shows them* the sick man either alive or dead.

(Pausanias, Description of Greece 7.21.11–12, my emphasis)

It seems that in the *hydromanteion* of Patras the diagnosis of the illness and its treatment are beside the point. The prognosis, that is how the illness will progress and its outcome, is all that matters. More importantly, the prognosis is transmitted via easily perceivable and unquestionable visual data: the patient's friends or relatives need only *look into* the mirror (which is suspended over the water surface) to *see* whether their family member or friend will live or die. This is yet another instance of eyes and images speaking louder than words. The passage quoted here is telling, not only for the centrality of ocularcentric processes in the cult of Demeter and Kore in general, but also of the close correlation of viewing and healing in the specific *hydromanteion*. Further allusions to Demeter's therapeutic role are to be found in Artemidorus's *Oneirocritica* (2.39.10–24) where we read that Demeter, Kore and Iacchos 'raise the sick from their beds and save them' (καὶ τοὺς νοσοῦντας ἀνιστᾶσι καὶ σῴζουσι). Furthermore, in the *Orphic Hymn to Demeter* (lines 19–20) it is said that Demeter is the deity that brings health along with wealth, peace and sociopolitical stability (εἰρήνην κατάγουσα καὶ εὐνομίην ἐρατεινὴν καὶ πλοῦτον πολύολβον, ὁμοῦ δ᾽ ὑγίειαν ἄννασαν). In some cases Demeter and Kore were also connected with natural hot springs which were invested with healing qualities. This was, for instance, the case with Demeter *Thermasia* ('of the body-heat') and her sanctuary in Hermione (Pausanias, *Description of Greece* 2.34.6 and 12). Finally, a rather tenuous link to Demeter as a healing deity who specialises in ophthalmic illness might also be found in Hesychius's lemma '*Epōpis*', which may or may not be a reference to Demeter's links with ophthalmology in Sikyon, depending on whether we accept the reading Ἐπωπίς from ἐπωπάω, meaning 'to observe, watch', or we read ἐπωτίς, which is related to her cult epithet as ἐπιθαλασσία.[9]

Perhaps the strongest literary link between the cult of Demeter and Kore and ophthalmological health or disease is to be found in the following epigram (*Palatine Anthology* 9.298) attributed to Antiphilus:

σκίπων με πρὸς νηὸν ἀνήγαγεν ὄντα βέβηλον
οὐ μοῦνον τελετῆς, ἀλλὰ καὶ ἠελίου·

---

9 Hesych. s.v. <Ἐπωπίς>: Δημήτηρ παρὰ Σικυωνίοις. [καὶ <Ἐπωτίς>]; ἐπωπάω: 'to observe, watch'; ἐπωτίδες: 'beams projecting like ears on each side of a ship's bows, whence the anchors were let down, cat-heads'.

μύστην δ' ἀμφοτέρων με Θεαὶ θέσαν· οἶδα δ' ἐκείνῃ
νυκτὶ καὶ ὀφθαλμῶν νύκτα καθηράμενος·
ἀσκίπων δ' εἰς ἄστυ κατέστιχον ὄργια Δηοῦς   5
κηρύσσων γλώσσης ὄμμασι τρανότερον.

My staff led me to the temple, uninitiated as I was,
In both the secret ceremony and the light of the sun.
The goddesses initiated me in both, and that very night I truly knew
Having been purified from the darkness of my eyes.
Without my staff I walked down to the city proclaiming the sacred rites
Of Demeter more vividly with my eyes rather than my tongue.

On the night of the narrator's initiation into the mysteries of the two goddesses
(most likely a reference to the Mysteries of Eleusis), he left behind both the
actual darkness of his blindness and the metaphorical darkness of his ignorance
of the Mysteries; the same night the initiate welcomed both the light of the sun
and the light of knowledge. Note here the conspicuous position of the verb οἶδα
in line 3, which oscillates between the semantic fields of 'vision' and 'knowledge'.
The cultural metaphor of purification is utilised here in a twofold way: initiation into the mysteries of Demeter and Kore offered the initiate not only purity
from the actual darkness of his blindness, but also cleanness from his intellectual
and ritual darkness. In this context mystic enlightenment coincided with and
perhaps even facilitated the acquisition of his physical vision. This image of
purified vision could be read as a rhetorical trope, referring not simply to the
new enhanced visual capacity, the new and clear vistas offered by an initiation
presided over by the two goddesses themselves, but also to the process of purify-
ing the initiates' visuality from the secular side, or 'the screen of signs from the
ordinary life', to put it in Elsner's words (2007, p. 25).

Nonetheless, the most interesting feature in this epigram is that the narrator
remains confident that he can proclaim the sacred rites of the goddess better with
his eyes than with his tongue! That 'seeing comes before words' is certainly correct (Berger, 1972, p. 1). But what this example demonstrates is an intentionally
ambiguous reference to both the religious prohibitions regarding the secret ceremony (the *theōros* is not allowed to speak about what he saw) and the difficulties
of putting the unique visual experience of the secret segment of the mysteries
into words: the author of the epigram makes a self-conscious and self-referential
comment on the limitations of the linguistic dynamic as opposed to the visual
dynamic of the spectacles he saw. ἄρρητα could refer to both the things or the
experiences that one should not speak about and the things or experiences that
were impossible to speak about. A third possible interpretation of this cryptic
statement could be that on his return to the city the speaker's newly found
physical vision would act as the most reliable testimony to his newly acquired,
permanently illuminated vision through his participation in the mysteries. In
this way his cured blindness (if indeed this is a case of physical and not ritual
illness) would be perceived as the most obvious confirmation of the goddesses'
powers and the efficacy of their mysteries.

The connection between the Antiphilus epigram and the Eukrates relief is an easy one to make: they both appear to pose much the same questions, and they both paint the image of cured physical blindness as being the structural counterpart of cured intellectual and ritual blindness. Physical ability to see, and illuminated mystic vision in the course of an initiation into the Mysteries of Demeter may also be closely connected in the Eukrates relief and in the Antiphilus epigram, but our quest to find more concrete or, at least, less ambiguous links between the cult of Demeter and Kore and ophthalmological health and illness cannot be concluded before we survey briefly the available iconographical evidence.

Demeter and ophthalmological illness: the material evidence

As noted earlier, Demeter and Kore were traditionally venerated as deities presiding over female fertility, and as such they were often the recipients of anatomical votives depicting female genitalia and breasts (Forsén, 1996, pp. 133–59). However, this brief survey is concerned with material evidence that supports the idea that the cult of Demeter and Kore was in fact closely linked with vision and vision-related illness. Votive dedications that attest to this connection come from the sanctuary of Demeter at Pergamum where a series of votive eyes made of terracotta were found (Figure 5.2) (for the sanctuary itself, see Bohtz, 1981;

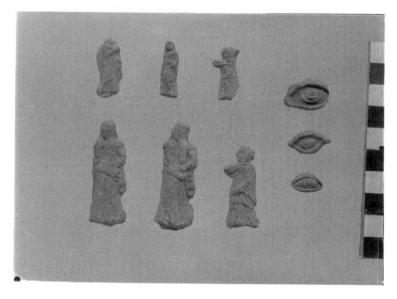

Figure 5.2 Terracotta eyes and female votaries from the sanctuary of Demeter in Pergamum now in Bergama Museum (inv. nos. 414, 415 and 416, respectively).

Source: Image courtesy of the Deutsches Archäologisches Institut.

Thomas, 1998; Agelidis, 2011). These artefacts were discovered along with other terracotta votives depicting female dedicants wearing a chiton. Deubner (quoted in Töpperwein, 1976, pp. 139–40 and p. 241) interpreted these eidola as representations of the goddess Demeter. No inscriptions accompany these votives, which makes an attempt to speculate about their original ritual role and function problematic. They are all roughly dated to the third century BC, primarily because that is the approximate dating of the figurines found nearby. Figurine b, in particular, was found together with eye-shaped votives c, d and e. According to Töpperwein (1976, p. 139) these figurines with a range of dimensions are essentially of the same type – albeit from different sized moulds – and depict female votaries, although the resemblance of some of the larger figurines to Demeter herself, as depicted on the Pergamene marble fragment from the same sanctuary, is also underlined.

Similarly, excavations in the small sanctuary of Demeter that was discovered next to the east wall of the city at the site of ancient Mesēmvria in Thrace have yielded a good number of eye-shaped τύποι (votive *repoussé* reliefs) made of bronze, gold and silver (a detailed catalogue of these objects can be found in Βαβρίτσας, 1973, pp. 77–81, pl. 93–5; see also van Straten, 1981, p. 127). These *typoi* were also found along with votives depicting worshippers raising their right hands in adoration. A number of these ἔγκμακτοι or κατάμακτοι τύποι are also mentioned in the inventories of the sanctuary of Demeter and Kore in Delos (Bruneau, 1970; Forsén, 1996, p. 143; also van Straten, 1981, p. 134, nos. 221–2 with more bibliography). Some of these *typoi* are said to have been made of gold (ὀφθαλμὸς χρυσοῦς), and some were said to have been mounted on wooden plaques (ὀφθαλμοὶ ἐπὶ σανιδίου). Needless to say, the main reason these *typoi* mentioned in the inscriptions from Delos are now lost to us is precisely because of their precious material. Some of these *typoi* have suspension holes and were perhaps meant to decorate the walls or other architectural features of the sanctuary and bear witness to the immense therapeutic capacity of the presiding deity (for the visual dynamic of votive offerings in sanctuaries, see Petsalis-Diomidis, 2005, pp. 187–8; Mylonopoulos, 2006, p. 87). Alternatively, we may imagine them suspended from the cult statue or the images of the deity, very much in the manner of the modern *repoussé* dedications found in Catholic churches, such as those dedicated to Santa Lucia (a deity presiding over ophthalmological health and illness: Cassell, 1991), as well as in modern Greek Orthodox churches like those of Agia Paraskevē.[10] A suspension hole is

10 I thank Matteo Martelli (Humboldt University) for information on the cult of Santa Lucia. On 26 July the miraculous icon (θαυματουργός) of the Hagia Paraskevē, who is thought of as presiding over vision and vision-related illnesses in the Greek Orthodox Church, is paraded throughout the streets in many cities and villages of the Greek mainland (for example, in Chalkis) and islands (for example, in Spetses). These icons are often heavily decorated with eye-shaped dedications, votive jewellery and whole-body schematic reproductions (*typoi*) of the dedicants, and they are in the majority made of precious metals. Regardless of their shape and value, these *ex-votos* are referred to in modern Greek as *tamata*, 'dedications'.

also situated in the centre of the upper level (just above the goddess's head) of the Eukrates relief, an indication that it was meant to remain in the temple and commemorate for eternity the extraordinary visual experiences of its dedicant for both the eyes of the goddesses presiding in the sanctuary and the eyes of the other *theōroi*.

The advantage of having an epigraphic record for these dedications (regardless of the extreme brevity of the entries) is that in addition to providing evidence of their existence, we occasionally gain a rare insight into the ways these *typoi* were exhibited in their original setting. From epigraphic records found in the temple of Asclepius in Athens, we also find that dedications of *typoi* representing diseased body parts were often accompanied by dedications of the full-body images of the dedicators: ἀνδρὸς καὶ γυναικὸς καὶ ὀφθαλμοὶ ἕτεροι χρυσοῖ (*IG* II² 1534, 74), τύπος ἀνδρὸς καὶ γυναικὸς καὶ πρόσωπον (*IG* II² 1534, 77) and τύπος γυναικὸς καὶ ὀφ[θαλμοί or ός] *IG* II² 1534, 74) (van Straten, 1981, p. 112). But how is this habit of duplicate dedications to be interpreted? This may well be a way of localising the fragmented diseased body part and simultaneously contextualising it within the desirable reassembled – and now free from pain – body of the dedicant, which subsequently becomes wholly consecrated to the deity. Alternatively, this kind of visual representation may be read as an indication of awareness of one's own mortality – a feeling that, as van Straten (1990) remarks, must have been intensified by looking at the plethora of similar *ex-votos* on display. Then again the whole-body image of the dedicant may allude to the desire for harmonic coexistence of all body parts, the kind of corporeal harmony that can only be achieved with the god's help, as seen earlier and demonstrated by the comment of Aristides (*Oration* 48.28 Keil) that:

> After this it is impossible to imagine our condition, and into what kind of harmony the God again brought us. For we engaged in all this, almost as if in an initiation ritual, since there was good hope together with fear.
>
> (τὸ δὴ μετὰ τοῦτο ἔξεστιν εἰκάζειν ὅπως διεκείμεθα, καὶ ὁποίαν τινὰ ἁρμονίαν πάλιν ἡμᾶς ἡρμόσατο ὁ θεός. σχεδὸν γὰρ ὥσπερ ἐν τελετῇ περὶ πάντα ταῦτα διήγομεν, παρεστώσης ἅμα τῷ φόβῳ τῆς ἀγαθῆς ἐλπίδος.)

More significantly this kind of doubly phrased dedication, which depicts not only the worshipper's disjointed body part but also contextualises it within their entire post-treatment body, provides a serious challenge to our notion of what should be classified as an anatomical votive. To add further to these conceptual challenges and to return to the original quest for material evidence that attests to Demeter and Kore's connection with therapy from physical blindness and visual impairment, I will now turn to a striking artefact from ancient Philippopolis (Figure 5.3).

The third-century relief from ancient Philippopolis (modern Plovdiv, Bulgaria) may well be both the most fascinating and unambiguous material reference to Demeter's ocularcentric activities and thus the more vocal and agentic of

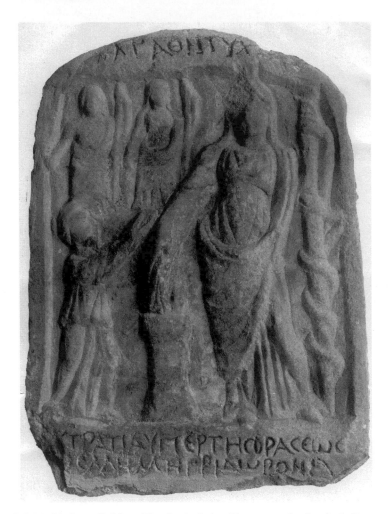

Figure 5.3 Marble bas-relief from Plovdiv depicting Demeter and a female dedicant named [S]tratia. Dimensions: 0.30 m × 0.23 m. Currently held at the Collegio Carlo Alberto, Moncalieri near Turin.

Source: Image courtesy of the Order of the Clerics Regular of St Paul (Barnabites).

all the eye-shaped votives discussed here.[11] The relief depicts a standing Demeter holding in one hand a sceptre with a coiling snake – which brings to mind immediately the snake on Asclepius's staff – and perhaps ears of corn in the other, which seem to touch the fire on the altar. Alternatively, what the goddess

---

11 I am particularly grateful to Nikolay Sharankov of the University of Sofia for kindly helping me to locate the relief. On the circumstances of its discovery, see the first edition of the inscription by Τσουκαλᾶς (1851, p. 35).

holds in her right hand may not be ears of corn, but the flames that flare up from the fire of the altar. On the left stands a female worshipper (one assumes the dedicant herself) who may be represented as blind or visually impaired, although the badly preserved relief does not allow this to be determined with any certainty. The much smaller female figure extends her hands in adoration towards the goddess, and her diseased eyes are also turned towards her in an attempt to meet Demeter's healing gaze. This sort of representational strategy whereby the worshipper is depicted in full body but with an unmistakable focus on her visual impairment or blindness is comparable to the doubly phrased dedications from the Athenian Asclepieion discussed earlier. Moreover, if indeed the Pergamene figurines found together with the eye-shaped votives depict Demeter, one may be tempted to read them as an abbreviation of the representational trope found in the Plovdiv relief. The visually impaired or blind dedicants have put themselves in plain view of the goddess and hope to meet her therapeutic gaze. But this is perhaps an overstatement given the difficulty in determining whether these figurines represent worshipers or the goddesses themselves.

The two figures on the upper-left corner of the Plovdiv relief have variously been identified as Demeter and Iacchos, Zeus and Hera or Kore and Plouton (Bruzza, 1861). Perhaps a safer identification would be to simply name them as *theos* and *thea*, the divine couple who must have played a protagonist role in the sacred rites performed in the sanctuary and whose names may have been part of the *arrhēta* of the ceremonies. The inscription (*IGBulg* III 1, 932; see also *Syll.*² 774; *Syll.*³ 1141), which visually frames the image of the blind suppliant, reads:

Αγαθῇ Τύχῃ
[Image of dedicant and Demeter]
Σ]τρατία ὑπὲρ τῆς ὁράσεως
θεᾷ Δήμητρι δῶρον

Agathē Tychē (Good Fortune).
[S]tratia dedicated this as a gift
to Demeter for the sake of her sight/vision.

The similarities between the Eukrates relief and that dedicated by [S]tratia are numerous. Both votives are inscribed (the inscription in the Eukrates relief could even be read as an abbreviated version of the latter), and they are both meant to be gifts for Demeter (note the dative *Dēmētri* in both inscriptions). They both speak of vision-related miracles performed by the goddess. They both show images of Demeter imbued in light: in the Eukrates relief the source of light is the divine body itself; in the [S]tratia relief the light comes primarily from the flames of the altar. However, the question of whether both *ex-votos* hint at miraculous healings of blind or visually impaired patients remains open because, once again, we may be faced with the thorny issue of fluidity between ritual blindness and vision versus physical blindness and vision unless, of course, we think that the prepositional phrase ὑπὲρ τῆς ὁράσεως in the Stratia dedication tilts the scales towards physical vision/sight or the lack thereof.[12]

Demeter was a rather prominent deity in ancient Philippopolis to judge from her frequent representations on the city coinage (Varbanov III 1347 var). In all likelihood her mysteria were modelled on the rites of Eleusis, and therefore it is possible that her role as a πυρφόρος θεά was also emphasised in Philippopolis. She is, after all, depicted as a torch bearer on the civic coinage. This would explain the representation of Demeter touching the flames of the fire on the relief from Plovdiv. The Eleusinian πῦρ ('light or fire') was so famous in the ancient world that it could often be taken to refer metonymically to the secret rites of Eleusis (for example, Aristides, *Oration* 22.11). Furthermore, the iconographical trope of Demeter and Kore as torch bearers is an extremely common one. One way to approach this rather modern and perhaps even overstated dilemma of physical vision or blindness versus ritual or mental vision or blindness is to consider that in ancient Philippopolis, like in Eleusis, Demeter was not ordinarily a healing deity and yet occasionally the blazing *pyr* (encountered by the participants at some climactic point in the secret rites) had the power to heal physical blindness in conjunction with the neophyte's ritual blindness (Clinton, 2005–8, p. 110; see also Clinton, 2004; 2007).

Conclusion

To pull the threads together, this chapter has argued that in order to determine the nature of the allusions to eyesight and vision in the marble relief from the vicinity of the Eleusinian Telestērion (Figure 5.1), we must reconsider the modern and anachronistic opposition between healing and sacred sight/vision in the context of the cult of Demeter and Kore and, indeed, reconsider the very definition of anatomical votives in the same context. The relief from Eleusis in particular challenges its viewers and forces them to reconsider the relationship between sacred and healing vision at Eleusis by alluding to cures of blind or visually impaired dedicants. The main question posed by this chapter is therefore whether the sacred πῦρ (light or fire) of Eleusis actually cured some blind and/ or visually impaired initiates, or whether these references to curing the initiates' eyesight should be understood as metaphorical allusions to the permanently illuminated vistas provided by the *myēsis* in one of the ancient world's most popular and time-resistant mystery cults. Notwithstanding the healing properties of the sacred light/fire in Eleusis in the context of the *mystēria,* what I have argued here is that such a dilemma should not be overstated in view of the conceptual fluidity between physical vision and/or blindness and mysteric vision and/or blindness.

---

12 ὅρᾱσις may denote 'seeing, the act of sight' as in Aristotle, *Nicomachean Ethics* 1174a14 or 'the ἐνέργεια or act from ὄψις (the sense or faculty)' as in Aristotle, *de Anima* 426a13, 'a vision' as in *Acts of the Apostles* 2.17 or when used in plural 'the eyes' as in the syntactical structure τὰς τοὺς ὀφθαλμοὺς ἐκκόπτειν (Diodorus Siculus 2.6; Dionysius of Halicarnassus 8.45; Plutarch, *Moralia* 2.88d).

More importantly, the cult of Asclepius and the cult of Demeter and Kore were closely linked in Attica for various, not least political, reasons (Benedum, 1986; Wickkiser, 2008, pp. 87–9). Indeed, Rubensohn (1895, p. 365) concludes that the spatial proximity between the Eleusinion and the Athenian Asclepieion resulted in a partial and mutually beneficial exchange of identity for the two deities (on the close correlation of the sanctuaries of Demeter and Kore and Asclepius in Attica, see Petridou, 2014).

Although Demeter and Kore's iatric activity was not as prominent as, for example, that of Asclepius Sōtēr or Zeus Hypsistos, both the literary and material evidence suggest that in certain mysteric contexts the two goddesses, and Demeter in particular, were thought of as regulating eyesight. The question remains open as to whether the remainder of the eye-shaped votives surveyed here (those discovered in the Delian Thesmophorion and the temples of Demeter in Mesēmvria-Zōnē and in Pergamum) point to a closer link between ophthalmological illness and the cult of Demeter and Kore. These eye-shaped objects could have been dedicated to request a cure or as thanksgiving offerings for an ophthalmological cure implemented by Demeter and/or Kore. Alternatively, they could have been dedicated as mementos of the intense visual experiences their dedicants may have had as part of their participation in mysteric rites performed in honour of the two goddesses. Thus, they can be thought of as concrete attestations to the fluid conceptual barriers between physical and ritual vision and/or blindness. The fact that these objects were discovered in the sanctuaries of deities who are not traditionally thought of in terms of healing does not preclude the possibility that they commemorated healing processes. On the other hand, the fact that their immediate context of discovery was the temples of deities who presided over mystery cults cannot provide unassailable evidence for their intended use or what these votives were meant to say to their viewers. Without knowledge of their immediate situational context, little can be determined with certainty about their meaning, which was also situational and not static. The possibility that these objects were intentionally made to reflect this ambiguity – that is to say they were made to oscillate between anatomical votives and mementos of the dedicants' participation in the goddesses' secret rites – cannot be excluded either. Whichever interpretation one adopts, these eye votives speak loud and clear about the centrality and the intensity of the ocularcentric processes that informed the dedicants' experience in the sanctuaries of Demeter and Kore.

6 Wombs for the gods[1]

Rebecca Flemming

This chapter focuses on the rich array of votive wombs that survive from Hellenistic, or Republican, central Italy. These offerings to the divine in the shape of the human uterus form a significant and quite distinctive grouping within the wider set of votive body parts found in the ancient Mediterranean world (for general discussion see van Straten, 1981; Turfa, 2006a; Hughes, 2008; and the Introduction to this volume). The vast majority of ancient anatomical *ex-votos* represent sections of the somatic exterior: hands, feet, breasts, genitals, ears, eyes and heads, but the early tradition in central Italy also includes internal organs, with the womb the most prevalent of this latter group. This prevalence, moreover, leads to some impressive numbers, and impressive spread, overall. The uterus received serious and sustained votive attention in early Italy, a phenomenon which demands a similar level of modern scholarly attention.

The scope and scale of the phenomenon is easily sketched out. The general population of surviving Italian anatomical *ex-votos* consists of tens of thousands of predominantly terracotta objects (surveys in Fenelli, 1975; Comella, 1981; Turfa, 2004; Recke, 2013). Many lack provenance (even publication), but when their origins can be traced they are in sanctuaries concentrated within southern Etruria, Latium and northern Campania, together with their neighbouring territories, and which enjoy a certain kind of votive flourish between the fourth and first centuries BC. This is the time when terracotta dominates and the period to which the anatomical and other items in this material are consistently contextually linked, although they cannot be dated. Around 150 votive deposits in central Italy contain offerings in the form of body parts, and hundreds (if not thousands) of votive wombs have been identified at around 80 of these locations (see Turfa, 2006b, p. 63 for the overall numbers so far) (Figure 6.1). So wombs are found in over half these collections: sometimes in very large numbers, more often making a moderate

1 My thanks to the organisers of and participants in the Rome conference and to the anonymous readers for all their comments and suggestions; and my thanks also to Fay Glinister for her help in various respects. My research into votive wombs and collaboration with Fay have been undertaken within the framework of the Cambridge University 'Generation to Reproduction' Project supported by a strategic award from the Wellcome Trust (Grant no. WT 088708).

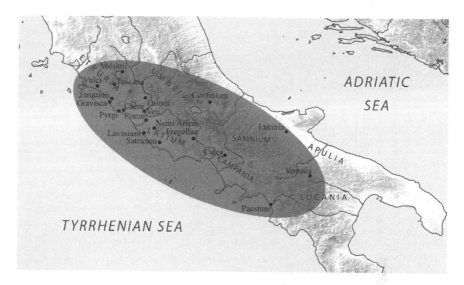

Figure 6.1 Map of Central Italy illustrating the rough distribution of votive wombs.

Source: Ancient World Mapping Centre, adapted by Alessandro Launaro and Rachel Aucott.

contribution to the overall ensemble.[2] They constitute, therefore, a substantial and widespread fraction of the whole population of surviving Italian anatomical *ex-votos* – indeed of the whole votive enterprise in the Republican period.

Despite their numerousness, distribution and distinctiveness these objects have not yet received the analytical attention they deserve (Charlier, 2000 is the only dedicated treatment thus far). Their study still poses serious practical challenges, though more detailed publication of relevant sites and their finds, including quite extensive votive typologies, have been accumulating over recent decades and as mentioned earlier a few general surveys of the material have followed. Still, further, more focused scrutiny is required as part of the kind of overall project undertaken in this volume. This chapter, for reasons of space, will be necessarily partial in its scope and argument, but the main aim is to try to advance the broader discussion about how these artefacts should be read in this particular case.[3] What are the forces at work in shaping these objects, in determining the

2 It is reported, for example, that around six thousand votive uteri and swaddled infants were found at the Italic Temple in Paestum (Greco, 1988, p. 79) but no publication has yet followed. Numbers are more often in the tens or hundreds.

3 Space means that I cannot address various general questions about the production and (presumed) retailing of these objects, about the gender and status of suppliants or about the organisation of the relevant sanctuaries, which gods are involved and so forth. These matters are all covered in a separate paper (Flemming, 2016) and in Recke (2013) as well as elsewhere in the bibliography cited and in other chapters of this volume.

somatic representations to be offered to the gods? What kind of conceptualisation of the human body and of divine action are conjoined and materialised in these items and in what social and ritual frame? The discussion will start with an exploration of those settings, providing a more substantial outline of the population of votive uteri in their religious framework by way of general introduction. Then some more somatic contextualisation will be offered, attempting to locate these artefacts in terms of wider contemporary views of the body and its parts, before bringing these two approaches together in conclusion.

A rough map: objects in a religious landscape

The more explicit evidence tends to be later and focused on Rome or on Roman practice, but the general view is that the key patterns of understanding and action which produced and distributed the surviving votive deposits both go back a long way and were shared across Italy, indeed, across much of the Mediterranean world more widely (Turfa, 2006a). The basic sequence is that a human suppliant approaches a god, optimally in a particularly sacred space, with a request, a prayer for help, together with a commitment that if assistance is provided and the desired outcome achieved the suppliant will dedicate a specific offering to the provident deity in thanks and praise (outlined in Rüpke, 2007, pp. 154–63 and more flexibly in Scheid, 2003, pp. 99–101). In later Roman contexts this commitment takes the form of a specific vow, which is where the weight of the transaction seems to fall; hence the terminology of the 'votive' or '*ex-voto*' from '*votum*', that is 'vow' in Latin (see especially Derks, 1998, pp. 215–39; 2014, pp. 59–65; also de Cazanove, 2008). Whether earlier practice followed exactly the same model, and how formalistically, across central Italy is less certain: inscription is rare and minimal, emphasising the gift to the deity embodied in the object itself (most early inscribed votives are discussed in Turfa, 2006a). Still, the basic contours of the exchange are clear, though the details may vary: a request for divine support is made and something is offered in return.

The dedicated object is then a public commemoration of divine favour. It is a material celebration of the power and beneficence of the god, a visible marker of human – a particular human's – success in dealing with divinity and of gratitude for the deity's response. Votives are displayed in the relevant temple or sanctuary, placed on and around altars, leant against or perhaps fixed to walls, covering all available surfaces, hanging from beams and fittings.[4] They remain after the dedicant has departed and greet each new suppliant, engaging all visitors to the sacred site, keeping the link with the divine open after the event and maintaining an enlarged community of the favoured, one which clearly invites

---

4 A few sites have yielded votives still in situ, for example, Lavinium (see Castagnoli et al., 1975), but the objects themselves are clearly designed for display in various ways. They have bases and pedestals (a prominent feature of many of the wombs discussed here) or holes for hanging (for example, a votive breast from Graviscae: Comella, 1978, Tav. XXX fig. 154).

further enlargement, more iterations (for the individual and communal work of votives, see Petsalis–Diomidis, 2010, pp. 238–75). Address to divinity is encouraged, empowered even, in such a setting, just as the sanctuary itself, the cult, also takes strength and substance from its accumulations of objects and materials: items with meanings in the interlocking worlds of the human and divine as they are focalised in these places.

Many such ancient offerings, probably most of these dedicated items, have long vanished, but plenty remain in a diverse range of shapes, styles and sizes and a more restricted set of materials (Figure 6.2). From the early fourth century BC terracotta increasingly dominates the central Italian scene; its durability as well as a low intrinsic value and nonreusability all count in its archaeological favour (Turfa, 2006a; it is often assumed that wax and perhaps wood offerings are now lost: Scheid, 2003, p. 100), but metal and ceramic *ex-votos* also persist in reasonable numbers through this period, and terracotta will eventually make way for stone and marble as votive trends shift again in the first century BC (Schultz, 2006, pp. 100–2; Flemming, 2016; forthcoming). The different sorts of things offered and their formal variety show that many kinds of gifts – perhaps all gifts – were pleasing to the gods. There are, however, two themes relating to the transaction with the divine itself that are most visible across the votive deposits from their most prolific periods – that is from the fourth to the first centuries BC – themes

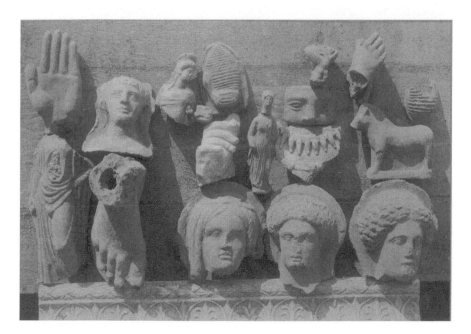

Figure 6.2 Photograph of a selection of votives and other items from Lord Savile's original glass-plate negatives of the excavations at Nemi in 1885.

Source: Nottingham City Museums and Galleries.

arising from the form and content of the human–god interaction, respectively. The first theme evokes and commemorates the ritual practice itself through the myriad *ex-votos* which represent deities, suppliants and religious personnel. In the second are placed the human body parts, animals and fruits, as well as other items which are interpreted as referring to the specific help requested: healing, fitness or function, healthy and fecund flocks, an abundant harvest or whatever it might be. There are, of course, various ways in which these two groups overlap: objects can refer to both form and content simultaneously; animals might represent sacrificial victims, for instance, as well as livestock (Flemming, 2016).

In this context the votive wombs are usually interpreted as concerned with fertility and reproduction, with uterine diseases and female health more generally. Some scholars have argued for more specific meanings for these items as a whole or in part, suggesting that pregnancy, delivery or a particular pathology is represented by some, or indeed most, of these votives (Charlier, 2000; Turfa, 2004, pp. 227–8; 2006a, p. 104; 2006b, p. 76). The implication, or assertion, is that they would have been offered after prayers for conception, birth or healing had been answered. This issue will be discussed in more detail later, but for now it seems safer to keep the full range of possibilities open (for the general move away from pathological readings of votives, see Recke, 2013, pp. 1074–7). A focused indeterminacy is one of the strengths of votive practice and of the objects it produces, including the uteri. Divinity has been successfully engaged with this part of a woman's body – a part bound up with generation and female health, as the two are bound up with each other – but the precise terms of that engagement are not recorded by the offering. Occasional inscriptions, as mentioned, name the dedicant and/or divine dedicatee but do little more than that (Turfa, 2004, p. 363 notes just five anatomical votives with inscriptions of this most minimal kind). The carrying capacity of the object as mediator and marker of that encounter remains, therefore, as encompassing as the object itself allows.

This last point serves to put the spotlight on the appearance of the *ex-votos* themselves, above and beyond their basic organic shape. The objects have to do all the work as material representations, and it is on their characteristics as such that this discussion will now focus. In so doing it must be acknowledged that the general challenge of writing about visual artefacts is exacerbated in this case by the formal diversity of the votive wombs. External body parts have a much more standard – although certainly not uniform – look to them, clearly influenced by Hellenistic sculptural styles, but not the uteri where there is real typological divergence as well as more moderate variations on the different themes evident. Nor is this simply an interior/exterior distinction since terracotta hearts are more standardised in appearance, though the approach to polyvisceral presentation – votive arrangement of multiple internal organs – is more stylistically diverse (Haumesser, this volume). There are, however, some key features which are shared across this range of uterine forms which will also be emphasised in this discussion, as well as a certain geographical division between Etruria and Latium or perhaps between southern Etruria and everywhere else.

A set of large, well-published and proximate deposits of votive wombs excavated in southern Etruria can be used to illustrate the basic point about diversity. Almost three hundred terracotta uteri were discovered concentrated in certain locations within the sanctuary of Graviscae, the port city associated with the larger polity of Tarquinii: the predominant group within a wider array of votive items more generally, including a range of other anatomical terracottas (wombs: Comella, 1978, pp. 67–81, pp. 89–95, Tav. I and XXXI–VI). Annamaria Comella has identified 63 main types within this group. Some shapes and styles do dominate, with variations on the 'almond shaped' (*a mandorla*), 'furrowed' (*scanalature*), 'pear-shaped' (*a pera*) and 'egg-shaped' (*ovoide*) models providing multiple examples which combine to make up around two-thirds of the assemblage. Still, the differences between, and to some extent within, these forms are striking: differences in respect to the overall shape of the main body of the womb, its decoration and structure – which include not just 'furrows' but also overlaid bands, cords, even 'straps', as well as buttons, crests and other protuberances – to the configuration of its mouth and neck, to size, and presentational style, that is the mode of display. Most are around 15 cm in length and 7 to 8 cm wide but can be almost 5 cm larger or smaller.

Presentation is given organisational priority in the publication of a similarly sized votive assemblage from the vicinity of the neighbouring Etruscan city of Vulci. The rich terracotta finds from the extramural sanctuary of Fontanile di Legnisina are again dominated by a collection of about three hundred uteri also accompanied by a range of figures and statues, a scattering of other body parts and assorted other items (Ricciardi, 1988–89, pp. 137–210, with the wombs at pp. 171–89). Laura Ricciardi distinguishes 48 types of votive uterus which she divides into three larger categories according to their mode of display. First are those presented 'in the round': standing upright themselves or more often supported on a base or an elaborate pedestal (Category I has 20 types generally represented by one to three examples each: Ricciardi, 1988–89, pp. 172–9). Second come those in which a ventral/dorsal view of about half the organ is moulded in high-relief on a flat base which then provides a border to the piece (Category II has 27 types with greater numbers of examples and more internal variation: Ricciardi, 1988–89, pp. 180–9). The third class consists of a handful of uterine plaques in bas relief (Category III has five examples of a single type: Ricciardi, 1988–89, p. 189).

There are broad stylistic similarities between segments of the two larger groupings from Fontanile di Legnisina and some of the material from Graviscae. Category I contains a number of broadly 'egg-shaped' forms, whereas Category II tends to the 'almond shaped', and some particular resemblances can be pushed a little harder.[5] However, most cannot: the majority of types are not shared, and there are good reasons why Ricciardi prioritises display in her

---

5 Ricciardi (1988–89) lists Graviscan comparanda for the following: Category I types 8–10, 12a–b and 14; Category II types 2–4, 10, 17a, c and d, 18, 23 and 27c.

typology. It is in the class of those presented 'in the round' that her site produces its most distinctive items, objects which seem to take their inspiration more from a ceramic stylebook than anatomy and which have adopted a striking approach to their ornamentation (see Ricciardi, 1988–89, p. 179, fig. 42 for examples of the womb as a kind of 'crested' bottle or jug supported on a stand and p. 173, fig. 38 for examples where the pedestal is more integrated into the object). If the discussion was broadened to include the somewhat smaller uterine presence in votive assemblages from Tarquinii itself (Ara Regina temple, Tarquinii: Comella, 1982) and other sanctuaries around Vulci such as at the rural site of Tessennano (Unge Sörling, 1994; Costantini, 1995), the same pattern of diversity within and between deposits would be repeated at least partially. A particular variation found in some of these locations is worth noting: that of a small lateral append-age attached near the mouth of a few of these terracotta wombs (Comella, 1982, $D_{17}IV_B$, Tav. 85e; $D_{17}VIII_B$, Tav. 86c; $D_{17}IX_B$, Tav. 86e) (Figures 6.3 and 6.4).

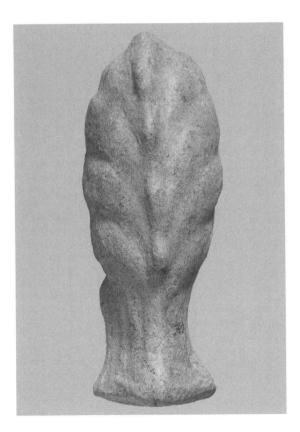

Figure 6.3 Votive womb from Tessennano (Vulci): almond shaped with vertical 'backbone', shallow furrows and small appendage on the left. High relief on flat-back: 19.6 × 7.2 cm.

Source: The Mediterranean Museum, Stockholm (10124D).

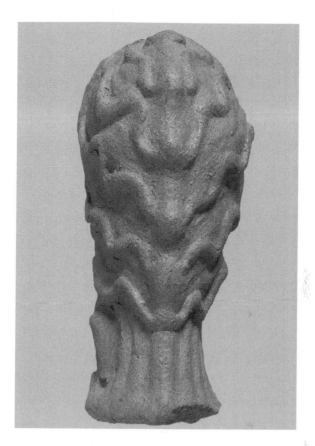

Figure 6.4 Votive womb from Tessennano (Vulci): rounded shape with vertical 'backbone' joined to transverse cording and small appendage on the left. High relief on flat back: 18.8 × 8.1 cm.

Source: The Mediterranean Museum, Stockholm (10123D).

The situation in Latium, the other main home of anatomical terracottas, is rather different. No published site has produced so many uteri, and reduction in numbers is accompanied by reduction in variety of types. Nonpublication, accidents of preservation and accessibility of sites may all have a role to play here, so it should not be concluded that such large populations of wombs never occurred in Latium. On the other hand, the Latial sample is large enough to say that the loss in diversity is not just a result of the lower numbers. The sense of variation on a single theme across this material is definitely stronger. Thus, for instance, over a hundred terracotta wombs are recorded as having been dredged out of the Tiber in Rome along with several hundred other body parts and a wider range of votive items more generally (Pensabene et al., 1980, with the

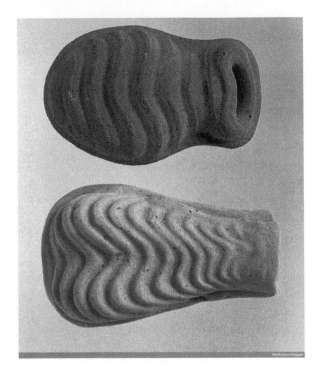

Figure 6.5 Two heavily ridged, pear-shaped votive wombs from the Wellcome Collection,
       probably originally purchased in Rome and similar to items found in the Tiber.

Source: Wellcome Library, London.

wombs at pp. 248–61 and Tav. 102–105) (Figure 6.5). Patrizio Pensabene identifies just 11 uterine types in this haul. Moreover, all of them are presented in
high relief on a base, the bodies of the womb are all characterised by transverse
ridges or lines and there is always a pronounced mouth, usually roughly circular
and heavily lipped. There is variation in the style and size of the ridging or 'ribbing', the shape of the main body, how much of a 'neck' there is and the precise
configuration of the 'mouth', as well as in the presence, or not, of an ancillary
organ. The base may also be more or less substantial, is occasionally curved on
the reverse (Pensabene et al., 1980, p. 255, n. 714) and sometimes pierced with
holes (Pensabene et al., 1980, n. 662, Tav. 102).

   A similar pattern characterises other votive deposits in Latium with any numbers of terracotta wombs. The numbers are often pretty small, particularly in
the areas of Latium Vetus nearest Rome, but the handfuls of uteri found in the
much larger anatomical assemblages at Nemi (not all published but see Blagg
and MacCormick, 1983), Ponte di Nona (Potter and Wells, 1985) and Lavinium
(Castagnoli et al., 1975; Fenelli, 1975, pp. 218–24), for example, are very much of

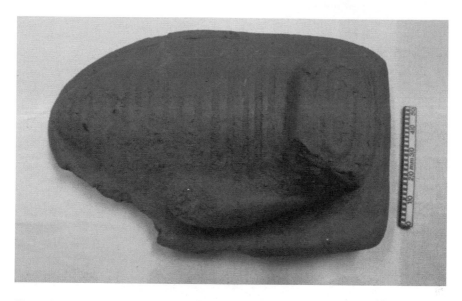

Figure 6.6 Votive womb from the Sanctuary of Diana at Nemi (Aricia): almond shaped with narrow, straight ridging, and a small appendage. High relief on a flat base.

Source: Photography by Fay Glinister (Nottingham City Museums and Galleries).

a piece in many respects. All are variations on the ridged and usually appended theme (Figure 6.6).

There are larger collections of terracotta wombs a little farther afield: from the contested territory of Fregellae, first founded as a Latin colony in 328 BC, and the more distant colonies of Luceria and Paestum to the south. Leaving these last two on one side for the moment, 56 fragmentary uteri have been found within a much larger set of anatomical *ex-votos* and other dedicatory items at Fregellae (Ferrea and Pinna, 1986).[6] Three types have been identified – all ridged with appendices (Ferrea and Pinna, 1986, pp. 137–8, Tav. LXXXI–II). It is worth mentioning that the items from Luceria (D'Ercole, 1990) and Paestum (at least those few published so far; see Ammerman, 2002, pp. 314–35) also conform to the same pattern.

The bodies of the wombs from all these sites are less rounded than most at Rome and some at Lavinium, with less drawing in at the neck, the ridges tend to be on the narrower and straighter side, like those from Nemi, and the appendages quite small and neat; but the overall sense of family resemblance shared by the votive uteri from all these locations is very strong (see Pensabene et al., 1980, n. 755, Tav. 105 for narrow straight ribbing on some items from the Tiber).

6 This means leaving on one side the modern debate about colonisation and anatomical votives, see, for example, de Cazanove (2000) and Glinister (2006) for different perspectives.

So, to sum up this brief survey: a broadly shared religious framework, a common set of votive practices, has distributed these terracotta wombs across central Italy, but the objects themselves are a bit more varied and particular. Some of this variation is specific to southern Etruria where there is the greatest typological diversity, including a few characteristically Latial 'ridged' styles (for instance, type DV14 from Graviscae is ridged and generally Latial looking: Comella, 1978, p. 179, Tav. XXXIII), whereas none of the distinctive Etruscan forms have yet been found farther south. Certain key features do, however, characterise the anatomical *ex-votos* that most readily form a coherent, unified group amongst those identified as uteri, which are also all of a roughly comparable size. They are the combination of a main body – almond-, pear-, egg-shaped or whatever – neck and, most especially, mouth: the opening is almost universally emphasised in a range of configurations. Some kind of lateral appendage is also common in Latium and found farther afield. The main body also always has a kind of structure as well as its shape. It is never left smooth and plain, but is ridged, furrowed, harnessed or crested, amongst other things. These features and their possible meanings must now be examined further.

A rough map: bodily objects

An obvious first question to ask is how far these terracotta offerings resemble real human uteri. The answer is not determinative. There are perfectly legitimate reasons why a votive womb might not look like its flesh-and-blood equivalent, even when surrounded by other votive body parts which do usually (but not always) imitate in an idealising way their living models (for examples of intentionally schematic, nonrealistic terracotta body parts, see D'Arcy Dicus, 2012, pp. 158–203) and, indeed, similitude might be accidental. However, the comparison is worth exploring briefly, especially since particular claims have been made for the realism of the *ex-voto* wombs. Jean Turfa, whose indispensable work on Italian – mainly Etruscan – votive objects and practice has already been much referred to, makes this point on several occasions. Whereas external parts conform to Hellenistic sculptural styles, she says, and other internal organs are patterned on animal viscera, simplified and schematised, the uteri display 'a better knowledge of human anatomy' (Turfa, 1994, p. 227). They do really 'resemble their human models' (Turfa, 2012, p. 169). They are 'rationalized versions of pregnant, laboring, human uteri' (made symmetrical by the artist) sometimes with additional, perhaps pathological, features (Turfa, 2004, p. 361; also Turfa, 2006a, p. 104; 2012, pp. 169–70).

Things are, however, not so clear cut. Comparing the ancient evidence to modern images of 'their human models' is productive but through the recognition of differences as well as similarities between the two arrays in terms of both representational form and content. These similarities certainly strengthen the basic identification of the items but, read in conjunction with the divergences, also underline the specificities of the ancient representational project, the way attention is being drawn to certain, more distinctive, features of these objects, these offerings to the gods. It is worth stating at this point that two silver uteri are epigraphically recorded as having been dedicated to Artemis on Delos in 145–4 BC (van Straten, 1981, no. 25e, p. 128), so the gift of these organs to the gods, as such, is also confirmed in writing. The island flourished as a 'free-port' and magnet for Italian (and Greek) merchants from 166–87 BC, and the influx certainly included families from central Italy (Rauh, 1993, pp. 47–51), so these should be taken as Italian dedications.

Today the uterus is usually displayed as a unit together with the fallopian tubes, ovaries and vagina, and there is a preference for the sectional view reveal- ing the internal structure as well as aspects of the exterior conformation. This emphasises that choices are always made in representing parts of the intrinsically messy and joined up somatic interior, in whatever context. Modern representa- tions are also mostly found in an informative, didactic context which has its own norms. Go back a century or so, however, and the line drawings of anatomical textbooks are more inclined to show an external view, a covered womb and attachments, and something more familiar begins to emerge in the centre of the picture (Figure 6.7).

Indeed, the nongravid human womb is still described as 'pear-shaped', for example in the *Oxford Concise Medical Dictionary*, and it may roughly maintain that figuration as it expands in pregnancy. The uterus has a 'base' (*fundus*), 'body', neck (*cervix*) and mouth, or to be precise two mouths at either end of the cervix, which are complex, multilayered formations. Still, though very thick and power- ful, the walls of the healthy uterus are always depicted as smooth; there are no ridges, furrows, harnesses or crests. Various protuberances can be produced by

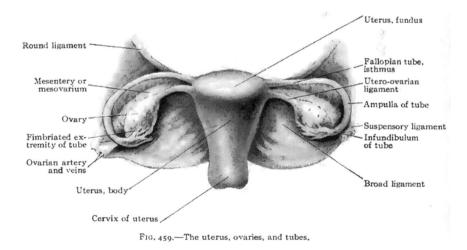

FIG. 459.—The uterus, ovaries, and tubes.

Figure 6.7 Anatomical drawing of the uterus, tubes and ovaries from an early-twentieth-century textbook.

Source: Gwilym G. Davis, 1910. *Applied Anatomy*. Philadelphia: Lippincott, p. 456, fig. 459.

certain kinds of fibroids, for example, but they entirely lack the regularity which characterises so many Etruscan uterine forms (see Turfa, 1994, p. 227 for the suggestion that the 'protuberances on various Etruscan votive wombs represent fibroids'; also Turfa, 2012, pp. 169–70).

Before considering these specific features in more detail, however, and thinking about the structuration and patterning thus highlighted in the ancient material, one other basic (and related) issue must be dealt with. This is the question of the anatomical knowledge around at the time in central Italy: the information and understandings available to, and held by, the craftsmen and suppliants at sites such as Graviscae and Lavinium. For these circumstances, this context clearly affects matters of interpretation and has an impact on the ways the votive wombs can and should be read. Representational expectations – traditions and purposes – combine with a range of representational resources – material and conceptual, technical and epistemic – to shape the selections made in manufacturing objects for offering to the gods, and in making such offerings themselves, to shape the choices made between the possibilities available.

The scholarly consensus is that human dissection (and vivisection) was a limited phenomenon in the classical world, practised only in Alexandria in the first couple of decades of the third century BC (von Staden, 1989, pp. 138–53; Nutton, 2013, pp. 130–41; Decouflé, 1964 argued for some [special] Etruscan dissection, but this claim has not been much repeated; see Haumesser, this volume). While the texts produced by key figures in these developments certainly were to circulate widely, including Herophilus's descriptions of the female generative organs, when they went west is uncertain and unlikely to be within the timeframe relevant here.[7] Learned Greek medicine – including its newer Alexandrian elements – first came to Rome in a serious and substantial manner with Asclepiades of Bithynia towards the end of the second century BC (Rawson, 1982; Flemming, 2012, pp. 66–75). His impact may not have been quite so revolutionary as is reported in the sources, but it is hard to trace any awareness of the various Hellenistic medical innovations in Rome, or elsewhere in Italy, before his arrival.

Dissection is, of course, only one possible source of anatomical knowledge, especially in a world in which blood and guts were much less concealed from view than they are now. The insides of various animals will have been most familiar through butchery and sacrifice, but injury, death and just poking around will all have contributed to a general grasp of internal human anatomy too. This last point is of particular relevance to the uterus which is, unlike other hidden organs, reachable from the outside in the normal course of events, does dramatically appear on the outside through prolapse, much less normally, and makes its main function pretty obvious.

---

7 von Staden (1989, pp. 165–9) suggests that Book 3 of Herophilus's *Anatomy* covered the reproductive organs (male and female), including his discovery of the 'ovaries', which he called 'testicles' (literally 'twins/*didymoi*') on the male model, and their related tubes.

Turfa makes a further argument which helps to explain what she sees as the particular accuracy and human specificity of the womb's votive representations in comparison to other internal organs. She suggests that the early practice of post-mortem caesarean section, as reputedly mandated by Roman regal law, would have provided extensive observational, even exploratory, opportunities: that, effectively, a somatically localised form of human dissection occurred in Italy from the earliest times (Turfa, 1994, pp. 229–32; 2012, p. 170). The evidence (one reference preserved in Justinian's *Digest* 11.8 from an Antonine jurist) for actual legislation by any king of Rome forbidding the burial of a dead pregnant woman before an attempt had been made to cut the potentially living child out of her is, it has to be said, shaky (as is, indeed, all evidence for the period). Still, together with the various reports of successful post-mortem deliveries in the Republican period (see, for example, the famous and much misinterpreted passage in Pliny, *Natural History* 7.47) and the strongly pro-natalist attitudes and actions of the Roman state more generally, this juristic citation does suggest that such endeavours were customary and that the custom was longstanding. So in the case of a pregnant woman who died almost at term, who may even have died trying to give birth, the presumption would be that efforts should be made to deliver any baby which had a chance of life before burial, rather than taking the reverse approach, which would be to prohibit interference with the corpse and prioritise funerary rites. It may even be that this custom was common to the communities of central Italy rather than just restricted to Rome where all the evidence comes from. There is no reason to think, as Turfa does (2012, p. 170), that this measure originated in Etruria, but more general cultural sharing is always a possibility. However, it is hard to imagine that there would be many such cases regardless, and emergency attempts at post-mortem delivery are not going to produce detailed knowledge and understanding of the formation and working of the human womb either. At most these practices would strengthen the sense of familiarity with this part of the body, with the uterus and its carrying capacity, but they can have added nothing qualitatively different, nothing more systematic or precise to the general picture.

In thinking about how these various glimpses and touches, ideas and comparisons might be put together, how internal bodily arrangements and processes might be envisioned, there is a further set of evidence which is also worth considering. That is early Greek medical literature, the writing of the late fifth and early fourth centuries BC, which was to become called Hippocratic, attached to the name of the most famous physician of the classical Greek world, Hippocrates of Cos (Nutton, 2013, pp. 53–71). This is a literature which deals with this problem – of imagining the depths of the human interior, mapping functions onto organs – in both a global sense and in particular relation to women's bodies, women's generative bodies (King, 1998, pp. 21–39). This is, of course, something of a stretch. It would be preferable if a wider range of texts composed in Italy before the first century BC survived and that those which did made more than passing mention of women's wombs. Plautus, for example, in the *Amphitruo* (5.1.40) and *Aulularia* (*The Pot of Gold* 4.7.10) uses the word 'uterus' only in conjunction with the pains of birth. Still there are possible points, even zones, of contact between Hippocratic medicine and Hellenistic central Italy which make this move more than just a grab for the nearest available literary descriptions of the human womb.

The first point to make is about the production and circulation of Hippocratic texts and ideas in a Greek world which included southern Italy and Sicily. Elizabeth Craik (1998, pp. 32–3) has suggested a western Greek origin for the Hippocratic treatise *Places in Man*, for example, perhaps as part of wider Italian and especially Sicilian participation in the burgeoning medical debates enacted in Hippocratic writings, the expansion and thickening of medical discourse in the Classical period more broadly. Transfer northwards of these developments is, of course, not assured but certainly possible from the fourth century onwards. The second point is that many Hippocratic authors start from common assumptions about human beings and the world, about the ways bodies work, which they elaborate and explain, rationalise and theorise to create arguments which would then be considered much less obvious and taken for granted. That 'folk tradition' is an important ingredient of Hippocratic medicine, that it builds on shared foundations, on popular beliefs, at the same time as critiquing them, was something first drawn attention to in the scholarship by G.E.R. Lloyd (1983), and it has often been explored and emphasised since. Many of these shared commitments about the world are, moreover, common to a wider Mediterranean community, like, indeed, votive practice and the basic presuppositions about gods and men that inform it. The ideas in Hippocratic texts about what a woman's womb looked like and what it did, about its structure and functioning, have therefore a reasonable chance of both having reached central Italy from the fourth century BC onwards and, perhaps more importantly, of already being there in some form. So a survey of the main points has something to offer here, albeit in a somewhat indirect sense. It also has to be said that even the Hippocratics – including Hippocratic gynaecology – fall short of a sustained description of the human uterus. The womb is discussed rather vaguely and variously and largely incidentally. It is the focus of greater therapeutic attention than analytical consideration.

Still, a reasonably consistent picture of the basic shape and structure of the human uterus emerges across the texts of the Hippocratic Corpus (Dean-Jones, 1994, pp. 65–9; King, 1998, pp. 33–5). The most programmatic statement is in *On Ancient Medicine* (22.2–4) where the bladder, head and womb in women – or wombs (*hysterai*) in the plural – are assimilated, in formation, with cupping vessels.[8] Like those instruments these organs are hollow and taper from broad to narrow, which means they attract moisture particularly powerfully and are best able to retain it. Elsewhere there are comparisons between the uterus and a wineskin (*askos*: *On Diseases of Women* 1 61 and 2 170) or a jar/vase/cup

---

8 The plural usage is discussed in antiquity (Galen, *On Anatomical Procedures* 12.2; Aristotle *Generation of Animals* 716b33) and today. Whether it is meaningful or not and in what way remains debated.

(*lekythos*: *On Diseases of Women 1* 33; *arystêr*: *On Seed* 9) as containing vessels that may or may not expand as they should and, of course, always narrow towards the opening. A slightly more complex impression of uterine shape, or perhaps structure, is suggested by the occasional reference to the womb having 'horns' (*kerata*: *Superfetation* 1) or 'cotyledons' (*kotyledones*: presumably of the womb, though this is not entirely clear, *On Diseases of Women 1* 58) and by mention of uterine 'sinuses' (*kolpoi*: *Nature of the Child* 31) usually as part of trying to explain multiple births. But it is accessible containment that is most emphasised in all this imagery and discussion within a single whole.

The vast majority of references (mostly therapeutic) are thus to a womb which consists of a hollow main body that narrows to a neck and most importantly a mouth, or mouths, as again the singular and the plural seem pretty interchangeable. The plural could be referring to the inner and outer openings of the cervix, those of the cervix and the vagina or again be just a way of generalising (King, 1998, p. 35). All these parts need to be properly aligned and shaped, and of the right qualities, in order for conception to occur, for the pregnancy to be brought successfully to term and for birth to proceed reasonably straightforwardly (Flemming, 2013). One of the key qualities in all this is flexibility. Initially of the mouth of the uterus, which must not be too soft and floppy nor too hard and tight, but resilient enough to be open in such a way as to allow seed in but not let it straight out again, and then to close around the male and female seed in the womb and stay closed for the next nine months or so. Similarly the womb itself must be able to expand as the foetus grows, or there will be regular miscarriages or stunted children. There is, however, no notion of any particular musculature of the womb either in itself or as involved in this expansion or the subsequent contraction. Indeed, there is no notion of uterine contractions at all since the Hippocratic model of birth is one in which, like a chick in an egg, the foetus runs out of food and then fights its way out to find more; the woman's role is basically passive, she suffers pain but does not labour (*Nature of the Child* 30; Hanson, 1990; Dean-Jones, 1994, pp. 221–5). These latter points stand in contrast to some of the readings of the votive wombs mentioned earlier. Turfa's (2004, p. 361) view that they mainly represent the 'pregnant, laboring' uterus is a widely held one, and it usually comes with the assumption, or assertion, that the ridges on the 'ridged' types of *ex-voto* denote the muscles necessary for this work (Ammerman, 2002, p. 325). Indeed these assumptions are so common that this type is sometimes referred to as 'muscled' (for example, Pensabene et al., 1980, pp. 248–9). Turfa (1994, p. 227) has also extended this understanding to more of the Etruscan styles, allowing any kind of transverse band to be interpreted as a muscle.

Before dealing with the details, however, it is worth stressing the central point of this summary. The main reason why the Hippocratic writers discuss the womb is for generative reasons – in particular reproductive failure, which is essentially all about the uterus, its mouth and wider somatic environment: all eminently treatable conditions (Flemming, 2013). But womb and procreation are also essential to female health more broadly. A healthy woman is a generative

woman and vice versa: nonparticipation in the reproductive processes of marriage, marital intercourse and pregnancy may well make a woman ill (the Hippocratic treatise *Diseases of Young Girls* is the most blatant in this respect),
and the cure may lie in doing these things, particularly becoming pregnant
(see Hanson, 1990). That the uterus itself is the cause of many ailments is a
related idea and, indeed, *On Places in Man* claims that wombs are the cause of
all female diseases. Indeed, it is this part's movement 'from its proper place' –
forward or backwards – that produces a range of symptoms (*On Places in
Man* 47). More dramatic movements of the uterus are envisioned in perhaps
the most famous – or notorious – of Hippocratic gynaecological maladies
or set of maladies: those engendered by the 'wandering womb' (King, 1998,
pp. 214–21; also Dean-Jones, 1994, pp. 67–77). The uterus can dry out,
particularly in the absence of regular watering in heterosexual intercourse,
and will then go elsewhere to find the moisture it requires, thus disrupting
the workings of the body, increasingly severely. The most classic symptom of
this dislocation is '*pnix*', suffocation, but there are many more depending on
where the womb transfers to, and death can result. Mobility of the uterus is
also elaborated on by Plato in the *Timaeus* (91B–D) and has a rich history in
later medical writings as well as in classical magical traditions (King, 1998,
pp. 221–41; Faraone, 2011).

Generation and female health (as essentially congruent) are what brought
women's wombs into classical medical discourse, gave them a significant if not
exactly star role, and it is likely that the same crucial concerns produced the
votive wombs in such numbers too. Now the question is whether dialogue
between the two – between texts and objects – within the wider cultural and
religious framework also sketched out can generate some more specific insights.
Is it possible to say something more concrete about why the *ex-votos* take the
form they do, which is to say that they both resemble and do not resemble the
body part they represent as envisioned then and indeed now? They were certainly recognisable, identifiable by both immortals and mortals, but did something more than that too. Mutual recognition is then the basis for the more
specific elements of the transaction with the divine which is being instantiated
and commemorated: attention is being drawn to some more particular aspects
of women's wombs.

Conclusions: bodily objects in a religious framework

On this reading it is the features of the votive wombs which exceed their basic
form, exceed what everyone knows about uterine shape and substance, which
are significant. The engagement with the divine that these objects are all about
requires recognisability and then allows for different thematic emphasis. The
items offered must resemble the part in which the gods' involvement is sought,
but can also draw attention to some particular aspect, quality or condition of
it. Most obviously the particular characteristics in question would be the ways
the essential cupping vessel or pear-shaped configuration – a larger main body

which narrows to a neck and mouth – is structured: with ridges, furrows, harness, crests or whatever. The emphasis on the opening of the womb – on the 'mouth' or 'mouths' – is also probably even greater in terracotta than text.

The argument here will be that several of these key features do make particular sense against the background just sketched out. The votive wombs can be seen as materialising some particular concerns about generation and health, about the well-functioning uterus, which have been highlighted in this discussion. It does not provide explanations for everything by any means. The striking variety in uterine representation is something which requires further discussion in itself, along with other questions relating to the appendage so often found as part of the votive package and the items inside some of them. There is no space here to cover these issues, further engagement must be deferred (although in the meantime see Fenelli, 1975, pp. 220–4; Turfa, 1994, p. 227; Schultz, 2006, pp. 110–14 on the uterine appendages). Still, several important themes emerge on the basis of the analysis so far and help move the debate forward in various ways. There is, in addition to the consistent emphasis on the mouth of the womb, considerable focus on the overall flexibility and stability of the organ, on its proper position and alignment across a wide range of forms; indeed all these points often come together.

Flexibility is perhaps most clearly expressed in the Latial ridged styles, but it is also manifest in a wider range of the furrows, cords and bands found on and in the uterine surface. The point was already made that the assumption that these ridges are muscles, the labelling of this form as 'muscled' and the idea that it is the 'labouring' or just laboured uterus which is being represented is at odds with the understandings of the womb and the process of birth found in ancient Greek medical texts. This could, of course, be an area where perspectives were not shared between the eastern and western Mediterranean, and a distinct but otherwise lost Italian tradition is here on display. On the other hand, the objects themselves, if viewed without modern presuppositions, do not obviously display actual labour, are not manifestly showing contractions or the flaccidity which follows such efforts. Rather they all embody, in all their diversity, a kind of potential plasticity: a poised tension that would allow, and crucially enable, expansion and/or contraction of the whole vessel rather than being about action within its walls. That is the kind of enlargement through pregnancy and then shrinkage back to roughly their original size after birth envisaged in the Hippocratic Corpus but which is also an obvious issue of importance and wonder more generally. The womb has to be the sort of thing that can expand and then contract repeatedly and appropriately. It has to be able to do that more effectively, more powerfully and with better timing than a wineskin or indeed anything else that might be considered on analogical terms.

Stability is represented in the regularity of the ridges, in symmetry and sturdiness more generally but perhaps most strongly in those Etruscan forms which have more distinct, widely spaced bands and cords, some of which appear to place the body of the uterus in a kind of 'harness'. These structures could be keeping the womb in its proper place, not allowing it to move forwards or backwards, let alone take off towards the head. Or they might be maintaining the proper alignment, proper positioning of the organ in its somatic setting more broadly: as well as allowing expansion and contraction, illustrating resilience and capacity in general. It is correct alignment and a properly formed opening, moreover, which is most emphasised by those votive uteruses presented in the round and on a stand. To the modern eye these are somewhat disturbing in their display: a disembodied womb on a podium, horizontal when it should be vertical, too carefully crafted and symmetrical with a gaping mouth, not to mention the decorations. These last features remain puzzling but influenced by the presentation of votive vases, the rest makes sense. The gape is, moreover, controlled, perfectly round or tensed in a four- or three-fold configuration. It invites entrance into and exit from the main body of the womb. There are no impediments, deviations, here; the path in and out is clear.

Read alongside early Greek medical discourse, therefore, the form of these terracottas can be seen to engage with a set of broad social and familial concerns, both generally and more particularly. That is in relation to both the overall identity of the objects and their specific shape and structure. The particularities of this engagement should not be pressed too hard. Divine assistance has been brought to bear on ensuring uterine flexibility and stability, proper positioning and operation, all of which are crucial to generative success and female health. A range of transactions with the gods might therefore have produced these offerings. They might form part of a standard preparation for childbearing: asking for help in ensuring a fit, generatively capable uterus or for a child (which would be the point of a healthy womb anyway) in a general sense. Or the request for assistance might have been in response to specific problems in conceiving, carrying to term or giving birth more specifically. There might have been particular worries about a mobile womb, certain symptoms which suggested movement, or it might again be about a healthy, stable, functional uterus more broadly. Pregnancy is a way of anchoring the womb, after all, just as its movement may thwart attempts at conception. Any of these would work, which may be the point. And in all cases the image of the womb dedicated to the deity conforms to the idealising style seen right across the overall population of anatomical votives.

The Greek medical writings have something concrete to offer, therefore; these are places where text and object come together in suggestive ways. They do not provide all the answers by any means, and nothing is definitive, but what is more clearly and usefully opened up is a way of thinking about the votive wombs which is more than simply realist, where the only interpretative moves are in relation to the realities of the human body – healthy and diseased – as currently envisaged. Further work is needed, but a more symbolic and integrated approach which emphasises the votive nature of these objects, their religious setting and function as much as the anatomy, and which allows for the two to coalesce in ancient rather than modern patterns, will greatly assist in the enterprise.

7 Ritual and meaning

Contextualising votive terracotta infants in Hellenistic Italy[1]

Fay Glinister

Swaddling, wrapping a baby to restrict its movement, is an ancient childcare practice still common in many countries today (Russell, 2014). The normality of the custom across the ancient world is highlighted by the fact that comment was made when babies were *not* swaddled, as at Sparta where 'they reared infants without swaddling bands, and so left their limbs and forms free to develop' (Plutarch, *Lycurgus* 16.2–3) and among the Scythians, whose bodies were characterised as flabby and squat precisely because they did not swaddle infants (Hippocrates, *Airs, Waters, Places* 20). In Hellenistic-period Italy the custom is attested by terracotta votive statuettes representing infants wrapped in bands of fabric. They form part of a category of votive offering which also includes terracotta models of human internal and external body parts, veiled and unveiled heads and statuettes of humans and animals (one of three votive categories identified by Comella, 1981).[2] They are found primarily (but not exclusively) in the regions of Etruria, Latium and Campania, and most are dated broadly from the fourth (or more often third) to second centuries BC.[3]

Etrusco–Latial–Campanian votive offerings are usually mould-made. In the case of swaddled infant votives, they may be formed from separate moulds for the front, rear and face. Details, especially relating to the swaddling bands, face and hair, may be added in freehand. The infant is always portrayed firmly wrapped, but the votives differ greatly in size and style, with many variations occurring even among examples from the same site, as is the case with those from Veii (Comunità) published by Bartoloni and Benedettini (2011). Sometimes the

1 This chapter forms part of the Wellcome Trust's 'Generation to Reproduction' project at Cambridge University. I acknowledge their support with many thanks, as well as that of Rebecca Flemming.
2 Comella identified two other votive categories: an Italic group (primarily bronze figurines of humans and animals) and a Magna Graecian/Sicilian group (primarily terracotta statuettes and busts).
3 The earliest perhaps date from the fourth century BC. There are two examples at Capua dated to the late fourth century BC (characterised by a conical hat) and third century BC examples at Lavinium and Satricum. This chapter leaves to one side swaddlings which appear as part of kourotrophic (mother/nurse/goddess and child) statues and statuettes (such as those found at Fondo Patturelli) which may or may not form part of an allied ritual tradition. They seem to me to be distinct from the swaddling votives in which the baby appears as an individual, not as part of a unit.

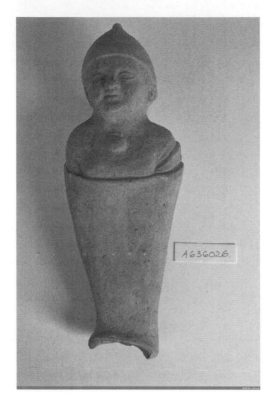

Figure 7.1 Infant with smooth swaddling clothes, Wellcome Collection/Science Museum, London, inv. A636026.

Source: Wellcome Library, London.

baby wears a cap or else its head may be shrouded by a veil. Sometimes feet poke out from the swaddling bands. In some cases the clay is modelled so as to accurately portray the swaddling material, which is often shown extending as far as the neck, although in examples from Campania the wrapping sometimes ends at the chest. In other cases the swaddling fabric is indicated by marks scored with a modelling tool. Some examples (such as Science Museum, London, inv. A636026; Figure 7.1) have simple, smooth sausage or pot-shaped bodies onto which swaddling bands were perhaps originally painted (Graham, 2013, p. 224). Like the other votives with which they are associated, the swaddled infants seem designed to be put on display in a sanctuary, either standing or laid down: in some examples the baby's feet rest on a base for support, but others have flattened or unmodelled backs, or feet incapable of bearing weight, and must have been placed in the supine position.

Inscribed Etrusco-Latial-Campanian votives of any sort are extremely rare, and of the handful of examples none are swaddlings.[4] Literary references to anatomical votives are also almost entirely absent from ancient authors, an exception being Augustine's mention of offerings of models of male and female genitalia (probably drawing on Varro and incidentally reflecting the Hippocratic belief that both males and females generated seed or semen):

> *Liberum a liberamento appellatum volunt, quod mares in coeundo per eius beneficium emissis seminibus liberentur; hoc idem in feminis agere Liberam, quam etiam Venerem putant, quod et ipsam perhibeant semina emittere; et ob haec Libero eandem virilem corporis partem in templo poni, femineam Liberae.*
>
> They think that Liber was named from 'liberation', because through his favour males during intercourse are 'liberated', by ejaculating semen. Similarly they say that Libera (whom they believe is the same as Venus) does the same thing for women, as they too emit semen; and for these reasons the same body part is dedicated in a temple – the male's to Liber, and the female's to Libera.
>
> (Augustine, *City of God* 6.9)

The dearth of other evidence makes us reliant on examining the various votive models themselves and the contexts in which they were found to try to understand the motives that lay behind their dedication. Where and to which deities were they offered, who dedicated them and why? This chapter aims to offer some speculation on avenues of research which may provide insight into this type of offering and its place in the wider practice of votive religion in Hellenistic Italy.

Space and place

We can begin with a survey of the kinds of sites where these dedications have been found. Although concentrated in Etruria, Latium and Campania, swaddled infant votives are also attested in the territories of a number of Italic peoples of the Central Appenines, for example, at Corvaro in the territory of the Aequi (Reggiani Massarini, 1988, p. 51). Several examples have been discovered in the hills around the Fucine Lake, notably at Grotta Maritza near Ortucchio, where there are at least 10 fragments belonging to swaddled infant votives dated to the third century BC (Terrosi Zanco, 1966, pp. 279–80, figs. 10–11, nn.10–12; Miari, 1997, pp. 103–11; Cairoli et al., 2001, pp. 132–4, nn. 22–6). At least one of these swaddlings comes from the same mould as an example from Luco dei Marsi approximately 15 km away, where the sanctuary of Angitia (Lucus

---

4 Two uteri to Vei (Demeter) at Fontanile di Legnisina, a knee at Veii (Campetti), another knee at Tarquinii (Ara della Regina) dedicated by a man, perhaps to Artemis, and a heart dedicated by a woman to Minerva at Lavinium. For references see Turfa (2004, p. 363, nos. 301–4).

Angitiae) may have housed a local centre of production (Cairoli et al., 2001, pp. 264–5, nn. 28–9). Another fragment of a swaddled infant was found at the Grotta di Ciccio Felice outside Avezzano (Terrosi Zanco, 1966, p. 282). Votive babies are also found in a few outlying areas, notably Luceria in Apulia (D'Ercole, 1990; Mazzei and D'Ercole, 2003, p. 275) and Pisaurum in Picenum, which is the findspot of some odd wormlike swaddlings as well as a better attested type (Di Luca, 1984, figs. 22–3). Swaddled infants also occur at several Sicilian sites (including Morgantina, Selinus and Tindari) and notably at Meligunis Lipara on Lipari (Bernabò Brea and Cavalier, 2000, pp. 122–4).[5]

In all of these areas the diversity of the locales in which swaddled infant votives have been found is striking (and is one reason why it is hard to comprehend the kinds of rituals which surrounded them). Thus, many examples come from remote rural sacred sites on hills or in caves (as in the Fucine region). They are often found near rivers or springs, as at Saturnia (Fontebuia) (Minto, 1925, pp. 604–5). Some appear in coastal sanctuaries like Graviscae and Punta della Vipera (Comella, 1978; 2001). Others come from sites which could be classed as boundary sanctuaries like that at Ripa Maiale in the Monti della Tolfa, identified by Zifferero (2002) as one of a series of cult sites forming a sort of sacred border between the cities of Caere and Tarquinii. Some are found at cult sites near cemeteries: at Fontanile di Legnisina outside Vulci (dedications to Uni and Vei are known here) (Ricciardi, 1988–89) and at the Celle sanctuary at Falerii (attributed to Juno Curitis) (Comella, 1986). Many swaddled infant votives come from contexts associated with the urban sphere, including great monumental sanctuaries such as that in the vicinity of the Ara della Regina temple on the city plateau at Tarquinii (Comella, 1982, pp. 18–22; the material seems to date to the second century BC) or the Comunità deposit at Veii (probably the city's *arx* and a good candidate for being the site of the famous temple of Juno Regina) (Bartoloni and Benedettini, 2011, pp. 403–12). Some come from smaller urban and peri-urban shrines as at Vulci (Porta Nord), the findspot of some of the finest and most charming examples (Pautasso, 1994). Finally, some have been found at major extra-urban sanctuaries such as the theatre-temple complex of Castelsecco, 2 km from Arretium (Maetzke, 1982–84).[6]

5 Of course, the distribution data are fragmentary. We cannot take account of unprovenanced votives in museums such as those in the Allard Pierson Museum, Amsterdam (inv. 8900) or the University of Pennsylvania Museum of Art and Archaeology (Turfa, 2005, n. 273). A number of unprovenanced examples are housed in London in the Wellcome Collection (e.g. inv. A636026); based on their distinctive typologies it seems likely that some came from Campania, possibly entering the collection in the 1860s from excavations at Cales; others may derive from the Oppenheimer Collection created by Louis Sambon in the early 1890s in Rome and Etruria and purchased for Sir Henry Wellcome in 1910. For more on the Wellcome Collection see chapters by Haumesser and Grove, this volume. A very similar example is held by the Antikensammlung, Giessen (inv. T III–2).

6 At its height in the second century BC, but with much earlier origins; significant numbers of swaddlings have been found here. There are also two terracotta swaddled infants in the collection of Vincenzo Funghini, who was involved in excavations of the site in the 1890s; many have been found more recently (now in the Museo Archeologico Nazionale, Arezzo). Swaddled infant votives have also been found at Piazza/Piazzetta S. Niccolò in Arezzo (Zamarchi Grassi, 1989).

Findspots with significant numbers of swaddlings include Fregellae in Latium with 16 examples (Ferrea and Pinna, 1986).[7] Around 50 are known from Minturnae on the border between Latium and Campania (Mingazzini, 1938). In Etruria, 13 come from Bomarzo (Pianmiano) (Baglione, 1976) and 28 from Graviscae (Comella, 1978; according to Comella, 1982, p. 22, they come from the same workshop as swaddlings in the Ara della Regina deposit). At least 63 have been found at Castelsecco with others known from Arretium itself (Maetzke, 1982–84, fig. 21; Scarpellini, 2001, p. 182, n. 4). Pautasso reports 47 swaddled infants from the Porta Nord sanctuary at Vulci (1994, pp. 33–44), and further examples from this sanctuary may now have been identified (Moretti Sgubini et al., 2005, p. 259). These seem to have been produced by more than one workshop. Thirty of them portray an infant with spiral swaddling bands, often with a *bulla*; another group comprises more naturalistic infants characterised by a plump, smiling, veiled face which resembles a late second century BC head from the Ara della Regina (Pautasso, 1994, p. 35). One further site must be mentioned: Paestum, where swaddled infants apparently numbering in the thousands were found at various shrines in the city. Apart from 24 swaddlings from Santa Venera barely any of these have been published (see Greco, 1985; 1988, p. 79, mentioning a figure of six thousand swaddlings and uteri; Ammerman, 2002, p. 315, n. 7 gives further references).[8]

It is often assumed that swaddled infant votives are found *in quantity* right across the Etrusco-Latial-Campanian area, but the distribution map is rather deceptive, and their dedication is actually a relatively restricted phenomenon. Of sites at which anatomical votives have been found less than half also include finds of swaddled infants (counting individual findspots within a single settlement as separate sites). Within most deposits swaddlings are considerably less common than, say, votive heads or anatomical offerings such as feet, arms or eyes. In fact, it is mostly a case of one or two swaddled infants per site. Except at Vulci (Porta Nord) where the majority of the terracotta votives seem to relate to infants (Paglieri, 1960, pp. 81–2) they never comprise a significant percentage of a votive deposit even where the site includes (what we presume are) fertility-related offerings such as uteri with which we might expect to see swaddlings associated. Thus there are no swaddlings from Veii (Porta Caere) even though terracotta reproductive organs make up the majority of anatomical votives here, and although Pyrgi was a cult centre for a fertility goddess (known from inscriptions: Uni/Eileithyia/Leucothea), few swaddlings (or indeed uteri or genitalia) are found here compared to more general anatomical types and

---

7 I aim for accuracy, but many figures must remain approximate. Different publications sometimes give different statistics by counting, for instance, fragments as representing whole examples or by interpreting (or discounting) damaged infant heads as swaddled types. Archival research also sometimes uncovers additional votives.

8 A Roman colony from 273 BC, Paestum seems to represent a case apart in terms of location and sheer number of votives, which were found in both suburban and extra-urban sanctuaries: Giardino Romano, Tempio Italico and Santa Venera (immediately outside the city walls).

statuettes. Comella (1981, p. 763) reports just three swaddling votives, six uteri plus nine fragments, and three examples of male genitalia plus four fragments.

In most cases swaddlings are attested in very small numbers, even in large deposits. So for example at the Ara della Regina, a very substantial deposit with many fertility-related anatomicals (including 233 uteri and 89 phalli), there are only 25 swaddlings as opposed to around 300 heads and 200 feet (Comella, 1982, pp. 221–3). Even at Graviscae, in a cult setting (room M of building γ) with an inscribed dedication to Uni and where scholars see a rare example of 'specialisation' of votive material, there were 22 swaddlings compared to 145 uteri, and there were also offerings of statuettes, feet and hands, so specialisation only went so far (Fiorini, 2005, pp. 68–70, who notes that the area seems to have been abandoned by the start of the second century BC).[9]

In summary, although in a few cases like Graviscae swaddled infants appear in deposits with an elevated number of fertility-related votives – which *may* suggest an emphasis on maternity and fertility at these sites – it seems that they were not associated with fertility and reproduction per se, as they more typically form part of general votive complexes alongside anatomical offerings such as legs or hands and other *ex-votos* such as statuettes, pottery, coins and so forth. In most cases, therefore, votive assemblages do not offer much in the way of illumination when we come to consider the contexts in which swaddled infant terracottas were dedicated.

Chronological issues

A further issue to contend with is the chronology of terracotta votives (problematised in this volume by de Cazanove who views the dating in general as overly early; see de Cazanove, 2015a). Despite the best efforts of scholars engaged in cataloguing them their dating remains in most instances highly tenuous. Most terracotta swaddlings can only be given a generic 'third to second century BC' date based on the analysis of mould series or of stylistic features such as hairstyles.[10] Exceptional sites such as Graviscae or Pyrgi apart, few can be securely

9 If the rite I posit in this chapter was so important to the community, should we not find more? Not necessarily. In ancient Italy votive religion was a choice, not an obligation, and the form of offering could be flexible. Some worshippers may have marked the ritual simply by sacrificing or else by making an offering of a swaddling in a material other than terracotta (such as wood, wax or even straw). It is even possible that votive babies were created out of foodstuffs similar to the bread and cakes in the form of swaddled infants given as gifts to brides and new mothers in parts of early modern Germany. Finally, it is also possible to envisage the dedication of actual fabric bands.

10 For example, infants with a curl on the forehead such as those at Rome (Pensabene et al., 1980, p. 215, Tables 90–94) and Pyrgi (Bartoloni, 1970, p. 560, fig. 411.1) are seen as influenced by the Eros of Lysippus and dated to the first half of the third century BC (Pensabene et al., 1980, p. 222).

dated on the basis of excavation data. Moreover, even in these cases it is really the final deposition of material from the site which is datable, not the moment in time when the votive was dedicated. Votives may have been displayed in a sanctuary for extended periods before being cleared away into pits, as seems to have been the case at Vulci (Porta Nord), which coin finds suggest was only closed in the Domitianic period (Pautasso, 1994, p. 91 and p. 108, n. 407).

The inability to closely date most swaddling votives and the need for ongoing work to clarify manufacturing and distribution networks makes it impossible to pinpoint a specific place of origin for the genre as a whole. However, the distribution data (numbers of votives and findspots) highlight the strong presence of swaddlings in Etruria, and by contrast their somewhat more limited occurrence in Rome and its hinterland, despite the existence there of large and otherwise representative votive deposits. So, for example, no swaddled infant votive types are to be found in the substantial and well-published Latin deposit of Ponte di Nona (Potter and Wells, 1985). Of course, the statistics rely on material which is sometimes a chance find or which comes from very old or poorly published excavations, but even allowing for this and other issues of preservation and recovery, it is particularly noteworthy that the swaddled infants from the city of Rome itself do not stand out in terms either of quantity or of especially early date. The so-called 'Minerva Medica' deposit on the Esquiline includes only one swaddled infant (Gatti Lo Guzzo, 1978, p. 145, type Z1 dated to the second century BC). About 25 have been found in the Tiber, and these are often presumed to have come from the Tiber Island sanctuary to Asclepius, but none at all are attested in the Pons Fabricius votive group found nearest the island (Pensabene et al., 1980, pp. 215–23). These are not high figures for a city of such magnitude. It therefore seems that Rome was but one participant in a wider cultural trend.[11] Its origins remain to be identified but it is perhaps noteworthy that, leaving aside Paestum, the largest concentrations of swaddlings are found in Etruscan centres, in numbers which elevate going northwards.

Motive and meaning

We come now to consider the motives and aspirations of the worshippers who dedicated swaddled infant votives. Who dedicated them and why? Can the offerings be seen as representing successful outcomes (live births, healthy children) for dedicants, or can other explanations for their deposition be posited? And are these explanations valid for specific communities or more widely within Central Italy? For Turfa and Becker (2013, p. 866), 'the scores of votive models

---

11 It is still a widely held view that terracotta votive types can be used to mark the spread of Romanisation (de Cazanove, this volume), but I maintain that the role of colonisation in their spread has been overplayed. In a forthcoming article I will examine the evidence of earlier votive forms and argue for the importance of the 'long view' in understanding processes of cultural and religious change in Archaic and Republican Italy.

of swaddled infants testify to the happy outcome of many births'. But not all scholars connect swaddled infant votives with children and childbirth. Smithers (1993, p. 29) suggests that they are associated with the 'perpetuation of the family' (hence their association with healing- and fertility-related votives) and that they represent 'a request for the safe passage of a child to the afterlife'. He points to a votive in the Getty Museum holding what he interprets as a pomegranate, symbolic of death, rebirth and immortality (Smithers, 1993, fig. 22). In a similar vein, Fridh-Haneson (1987) argues that swaddling votives symbolise the reborn adult initiates of an Orphic mystery cult involving rebirth to eternal life by means of divine adoption. Her primary evidence is the presence in south Italian graves, alongside Orphic texts, of statuettes of women holding infants (*kourotrophoi*). She is also influenced by swaddled votives from Lavinium whose facial features resemble youths or adults (Fridh-Haneson, 1987, p. 74, fig. 9). Examples of these are published by Fenelli in the exhibition catalogue *Enea nel Lazio* (Anon., 1981, D 125–7, pp. 208–9); she refers to numerous similar votives from the sanctuary and tentatively suggests a chthonic connection (*contra* Torelli, 1984, p. 9, n. 17). Other examples of mature-looking swaddlings can be cited, including some from Teanum Sidicinum (Loreto) (Johannowsky, 1963, fig. 12e) and in particular an oddly flattened votive from Falerii (Vignale, third to second century BC, Villa Giulia inv. 7359). The great majority of swaddlings, however, have chubby infantile faces and it seems unlikely that there is a specific cultic aspect to ones which are adult in appearance. Instead, they are likely to be the result of simple artisanal practicalities such as the availability of moulds (see Guarnaccia, 2001, p. 97 for the suggestion that the circulation of mould series for swaddlings can sometimes be linked to the circulation of matrices for male and female votive heads). There are several examples of mould series crossing typological boundaries: a female statuette from Veii (Campetti), for example, was reworked into a swaddling by wrapping a sheet of clay round the figurine and incising lines in it to represent cloth bands (Vagnetti, 1971, Table XLVII, M II).

The theories of Fridh-Haneson and Smithers have not been widely taken up. So if we set aside the idea that swaddled infant votives were used in some sort of cult involving rebirth, what might they represent instead? The fact that they are frequently found together with anatomical votives has encouraged many scholars to see them as connected with the healing of a sick child. This would not be surprising in a world in which young children were particularly vulnerable and high infant mortality was a fact of life. There is no obvious evidence of medical problems on extant votive babies, but that is explicable if they were offered after a cure and symbolised the healed child. Swaddlings have also been seen as representing a general request for the ongoing maintenance of good health: thus, considering examples from Veii (Comunità) with older infant faces, Bartoloni and Benedettini (2011, p. 403) suggest not a request for the immediate protection of the baby but rather a generic propitiation for the person's future. Given that reproduction was a prevalent concern for the peoples of ancient Italy, the votives have also been connected to a request for divine aid with conception or thanks for a pregnancy, with the swaddling symbolising the anticipated child.

Yet in the strictly reproductive context votives such as uteri seem more pertinent dedications (Graham, 2013, pp. 219–23; Flemming, this volume), and it is easier to imagine swaddlings representing a living child, like the wax votive *Fatschenkinder* of early modern southern Germany given in thanks for a successful birth.

At the most generic level, swaddling *ex-votos* are to be located within the sphere of fertility, broadly defined: they obviously represent familial concerns for young infants and were offered as part of a strategy to secure divine protection. As de Cazanove (2008) has shown very clearly, terracotta offerings of infants are best seen as payments of a chain of vows that accompanied the child through the early stages of its life. In the absence of literary or epigraphic evidence, it is difficult to identify any specific life events or rites of infancy which prompted their donation, but what follows will attempt to locate one possible explanation and consider why the dedication of these offerings might represent an important moment both in the life of the child and of the community it inhabited.

Forming citizens

In the modern West the renewed popularity of swaddling is associated with the belief that swaddled infants sleep better and cry less – and numerous studies have indeed documented more tranquil behaviour and longer sleep periods for swaddled children (Franco et al., 2005; van Sleuwen et al., 2007). However, the primary ancient source for the practice, the *Gynaecology* of the second century AD medical writer Soranus, recommends swaddling for quite another reason: to mould the child into the correct shape. 'Swaddling clothes', he says, 'serve to provide firmness and an undistorted figure; we deem it appropriate to loosen them when the body has already become fairly firm and there is no further fear that any of its parts may become deformed' (*Gynaecology* 2.42). Similar theories appear in Galen (also second century AD) who warns of potential malformations of malleable newborn bodies caused by incorrect forms of swaddling (*On the Causes of Disease* 7.28–9 Kühn).

In order to achieve a proper shape Soranus (*Gynaecology* 2.14) prescribes that strips of woollen cloth be wound over the baby's hands and fingers, then over the arms. Each leg is to be wrapped separately down to the tips of the toes. Finally, with arms at the sides and feet together, the baby is to be wrapped with a wide cloth from chest to feet and the head bandaged round.[12] No swaddled votive types can be shown to comply fully with Soranus's elaborate system of

---

12 Ironically, modern clinical studies have identified swaddling in the manner Soranus recommends, with legs in extension and adduction, as a risk factor for the development of hip displasia and early-onset arthritis (Storer and Skaggs, 2006). Given that a child's natural bodily functions would have required the swaddling bands to be changed regularly, the complex and time-consuming method described by Soranus is likely to have been restricted to households wealthy enough to have a dedicated childcarer, whether a slave or a paid nurse. Soranus does, however, also suggest slightly less complex forms of swaddling.

individually wrapped limbs, but many exhibit a careful, realistic form of wrapping evidently drawn from life, with the swaddling fabric stopping below the neck to reveal the edge of an undergarment, and their heads are mostly covered. Infants from southern Italy often wear a cap but otherwise they are commonly veiled by the end of their swaddling blanket – not to be seen as an indicator of the Roman origin of the dedicants but merely as normal swaddling practice (see Glinister, 2009 on veiling and ethnicity in the ritual context).

The children that votives represent must be in the earliest phase of infancy, up until the putting aside of swaddling clothes. But the fleshy, alert, beaming faces of the more realistic votives do not resemble newborn babies; they look much more like infants around the two- or three-month-old mark who have put on weight and begun to smile responsively (cf. Graham, 2014, pp. 29–30; the presence or absence of hair is not a relevant factor in attempting to assess a baby's age). Given that our literary sources belong to quite different time periods and cultures, it is no surprise to find disagreement on how long swaddling was to be continued. Plato (*Laws* 7.789e) in the fourth century BC recommended swaddling until the age of two, although iconographical evidence from Greece does not appear to support such a prolonged period of swaddling, and it is hard to believe on purely practical grounds. More plausibly, a passage of Nicander (second century BC) implies that swaddling would have been long discontinued by the time an infant was teething (typically six months onwards) and could toddle:

> Let no-one unknowingly fill his belly with henbane, as men often do by mistake, or as children – who having put away their swaddling bands and hair-bindings, and finished their dangerous crawling, and now walk upright without their worried nurse beside them – through ignorance bite the stems that bear the noxious flowers, since their teeth have just erupted from their jaw, and their swollen gums itch.
>
> (Nicander, *On Antidotes* 415–24)[13]

Soranus reports that swaddling clothes were sometimes removed after 40 days, sometimes much later, but that 60 days was typically the end point. He himself recommends a flexible approach based on the physical development of the individual child. Some children firm up quickly, he says, 'because of a superior bodily structure; in others, it happens more slowly, because of a weaker physique' (*Gynaecology* 2.42). Soranus indicates that the discontinuation of swaddling was a process undertaken carefully over a period of days. One practical reason for this may be that—as many parents know—some infants grow 'addicted' to swaddling, showing distress when carers attempt to end the practice, and must be weaned gradually from it.

There is no literary evidence for any sacred ritual at which swaddling bands were put aside, but the end of the swaddling phase seems a significant point in a

---

13 I owe this reference to Laurence Totelin.

child's development. At this time the parent (a different dedicant is possible but hard to imagine) might plausibly make a dedication representing the successful completion of a life stage (Crawford-Brown, 2010, p. 5; Graham, 2014, p. 40 suggests that votive statuettes of children were offered after weaning, another crucial life stage, to confirm the child's place in the community and to ensure protection for the future). Not only does it come at the end of the most dangerous period of young life, but Soranus's evidence, if admissible for the Hellenistic period, suggests that medical theorists saw the removal of the swaddling bands as the moment when the infant's human form was perfected. This idea of 'perfection' or 'completion' can be tied in to evidence from a Roman context for childhood rituals which, I will suggest, are associated with the formation of the citizen.

These rituals involve the *bulla*, a bubble-shaped apotropaic amulet which is found around the neck of many (but by no means all) swaddled infant votives. It is attested on votives from, for example, Vulci, Veii, Graviscae, Tarquinii (Ara della Regina) and Cortona (Peciano, Mulino Piegai) in Etruria and in the south at Capua and Luceria. While the *bulla* is found quite widely in Central Italy the only literary evidence for its use comes from Rome. The sources generally attribute an Etruscan origin to it. Festus (428.36L) says it was worn by Etruscan kings, and Tarquinius Priscus was supposedly the first to give his (teenage) son the *bulla* (Plutarch, *Roman Questions* 101); however, it is also sometimes dated to the time of Romulus (Plutarch, *Romulus* 20.3; Macrobius, *Saturnalia* 1.6.16). Actual examples are found in funerary contexts as far back as the eighth century BC, not only in Etruria (for example, at Tarquinii and Veii-Quattro Fontanili), but also in contemporary Latium (at Osteria dell'Osa) and Campania (for example, Cumae and Pithecusae).

Although the archaeological attestations of the *bulla* demonstrate that it was a cultural element shared by various peoples of central Italy, the evidence for its gender specificity is rather more complicated. Some have been found in graves attributed to women (Biancifiori, 2012), and at Lavinium (Eastern Sanctuary) the *bulla* appears on a fourth to third century BC votive statue which has been identified by some as a girl (D 239; Migliorati in Anon., 1981, p. 254; Weis, 2014, p. 301, n. 42; see also Torelli, 1984, fig. 11, who regards the statue as a male). On comparable statues from Veii (Portonaccio) *bullae* appear only, as far as I am aware, on indisputably male examples (Baglione, 2001).

The sole reference in literature to a female with a *bulla* occurs in a play by Plautus (*Rudens* 1171). In this, Palaestra's possession of a *bulla* and other jewellery given to her by her father proves her free birth and secures her escape from slavery. Because the play, however, has a Greek context (it is based on Diphilus' *Epitrope*) it has been suggested that the term *bulla* may simply be a translation of the Greek original's *perideraion*, 'necklace' (for the debate see Gabelmann, 1985; Goette, 1986; Palmer, 1996; 1998[1989]). Aristotle (*Poetics* 1454b) describes such scenes of discovery by means of *perideraia* as among the least artistically pleasing dramatic devices. In a comparable recognition scene in *Epidicus* (639–40) Plautus uses the word *lunula* for a golden token which establishes a lost girl's origins. In the only other literary reference to *lunulae* they are defined by Isidore as 'female ornaments in the shape of the moon (*luna*), small hanging gold bubbles' (*Etymologies* 19.31.17). Despite the strong likelihood that Isidore's explanation ultimately derives from a late Republican antiquarian gloss of *Epidicus* itself, modern scholars widely consider the *lunula* to be the female equivalent of the *bulla* (Dolansky, 2008).

On balance, the association of the *bulla* with males (and with masculine values), at least at Rome, is far stronger than it is with girls, whereas Idisore's definition of the *lunula* may be compared to necklaces on votive swaddlings from Saturnia (Fontebuia: Minto, 1925, coll. 603–5, fig. 6) and Tarquinii (Ara della Regina: Comella, 1982, Table 4a). There is also an example in the Wellcome collection (A636023; see also Figure 7.1). These necklaces have multiple ornaments comprising a central *bulla* flanked by crescent- or heart-shaped amulets. Different again are examples from Paestum (Giardino Romano) which, although they are regularly assumed to represent 'Roman' religious forms, are stylistically unusual, with multiple amulets hanging from a diagonal strap across the body (Torelli, 1999, pl. 16–17). Torelli (1999, pp. 74–6) identifies this as a *lorum* and argues that it demonstrates the low status of the colonists here.[14] Certainly, Juvenal (*Satire* 5.164–5) explicitly contrasts the 'Etruscan gold' (*bulla*) with the *lorum*, the knotted leather strap worn by the poor (he means poor *citizens*), but Pliny (*Natural History* 33.4.10) simply describes the *lorum* as being worn in earlier days by those below equestrian status. Paestan swaddlings also wear a distinctive conical cap, which Torelli identifies as the *pileus* of freed slaves. But the cap does not look much like, for example, the *pileus* on the coin issued by Brutus after Julius Caesar's assassination (*RRC* 508/3). It *does* look like the cap on swaddled infants at Capua (Bonghi Jovino, 1971, Table XXXVII, nn. 51–2) as well as Greek images which Ammerman (2007, pp. 146–8) points out usually depict children of citizen status, sometimes even heroes. Note also the parallel between the Paestan examples and the cap worn by the swaddled twins Aeolus and Boeotus shown in Figure 7.2, an Apulian volute krater of c. 330–20 BC attributed to the Underworld Painter (Michael C. Carlos Museum, Emory, inv. 1994.001). Most likely the cap is simply standard southern Italian infant dress, not a marker of low status.

Some infants lack any ornamentation (for example, swaddlings from Lavinium, Satricum, Graviscae, Tarquinii, Castelsecco and Pisaurum), whereas at some sites both ornamented and nonornamented types can be found (as at Vulci, Veii, Luceria and Rome, in both Tiber and Minerva Medica votive groups). One possibility is that terracottas without ornamentation were once 'dressed' with an actual *bulla* or other necklace (just as some infant votives with smooth jar-shaped bodies might once have been swaddled with cloth strips) or that ornamentation painted onto the terracotta has eroded over the centuries (Graham, 2014, p. 32).

---

14 Asconius (*ad* Cicero, *Against Verres* 2.1.152) says that those of freed status were granted a leather *bulla* (*simul cum praetexta etiam bulla suspendi in collo infantibus ingenuis solet aurea, libertinis scortea, quasi bullientis aquae, sinus communiens pectusque puerile*), but the date of this is not certain.

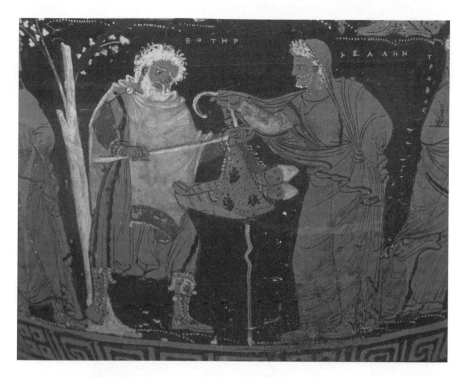

Figure 7.2 Apulian volute krater of *c.*330–320 BC, attributed to the Underworld Painter. Michael C. Carlos Museum, Emory, inv. 1994.1.

Source: © Michael C. Carlos Museum, Emory University. Photo by Bruce M. White, 2005.

It could also be argued that infants without a *bulla* are female. As skin tones were conventionally rendered in red for males and white for females, a study of paint or slip traces on the faces of surviving votives might assist in identifying an infant's gender. Slight traces of colour are visible on a number of examples (for instance, D'Ercole, 1990, p. 125) but analysis of a large sample, comparing skin tone with the presence or absence of the *bulla*, could decide the matter.

Gender distinctions may also have been highlighted by use of particular styles of swaddling. Beaumont (2012, p. 52) claims that 'in visual terms swaddling renders the infant genderless to the onlooker', yet in the drive for the perfection of the human form medical theory and practice as embodied by Soranus encourages visibly gendered forms of swaddling. In his instructions for moulding the child to perfect its body Soranus advises that male and female children should be wrapped differently. He says, 'in females bind the parts at the breasts more tightly, yet keep the region of the loins loose, for in women this form is more becoming' (*Gynaecology* 2.15). Compare his near contemporary Galen, who complains how wet nurses damage the bodies of baby girls by binding them in a way that makes the hips and thighs larger than the chests (*On the Causes of Disease* 7.28–9 Kühn). Although we cannot directly marry Soranus's instructions with our much earlier swaddled infants, we should certainly bear in mind the possibility that gender-specific wrapping styles were used for infants (and their votive counterparts) during the Hellenistic period. Again, this requires a wider analysis of the votive material.

As we have seen, the archaeological evidence for the *bulla* is not entirely clear cut, and it is likely that its use and meaning fluctuated over time (for one interpretation of changes of meaning see Haack, 2007a). During the period in which swaddling votives were being dedicated, however, the literary sources suggest that the *bulla* was restricted to *ingenui*, freeborn boys (see, for example, Plutarch, *Roman Questions* 101; Goette, 1986; Palmer, 1998[1989]). Indeed, until the end of the third century BC it seems to have been further restricted to the elite (as noted earlier, Pliny ascribes it to those of equestrian rank).[15] That the *bulla* remained a marker of high status is also implied in Statius' comments on the social background of his father (*Silvae* 5.3.116–20). There is a strong possibility, therefore, that the *bulla* on a swaddled infant *ex-voto* was emblematic of both the gender and the social status of the child it represented (see also Comella, 1982, p. 226). More specifically, it can be argued that the *bulla* marked that child's citizen status.

The *bulla* was given to a Roman child at a naming ceremony performed on the *dies lustricus* (Plutarch, *Roman Questions* 102). This rite, concluding the first week of life, is often described as the child's 'social birth'. Children given a name and placed under divine protection (symbolised by the *bulla*) enjoyed a publicly recognised social existence. It was an important moment not only for the family but more widely for the state, whose social and political continuity was entirely dependent on new members joining the citizen body. In fact, its importance to the public sphere can be demonstrated by the custom described by L. Calpurnius Piso Frugi, writing in the later second century BC. To record each birth a coin was deposited in the treasury of Eileithyia (whom Dionysius identifies with Juno Lucina). This was paralleled by the deposition of another coin in the treasury of Juventas to record a child's coming of age. Piso attributes the origin of the custom to Servius Tullius, as institutor of the census at Rome, explaining that thereby Servius 'would know each year how many people there were in total, and which were of military age' (F16 Cornell = Dionysius of

---

15 When in 210 BC money to outfit the Roman fleet was desperately required, the senators are said to have sacrificed their wealth but retained the *bullae* of their sons (Livy 26.36.5). A speech of Scipio Aemilianus (129 BC) bemoans an elite boy dancing like a little slave while wearing his *bulla* (*Oration* 30.10 = Macrobius, *Saturnalia* 3.14.7). In the 70s BC Sertorius gave golden *bullae* to the sons of the Iberian elite (Plutarch, *Sertorius* 14.1–3). The *bulla*'s special association with elite boys, however, did not preclude its use in other contexts, perhaps with different meanings (it could be worn by animals, for example).

Halicarnassus 4.15.5). Piso had held the censorship himself, and his explanation sounds like a pragmatic rationalisation of the custom, but it shows that both the start and conclusion of childhood were marked by parallel rituals conducted by the family but very much in a public context.

An etymology which can be traced back as far as Varro derives the word *bulla* from Greek *boulê*:

> The golden *bulla* was the distinguishing mark of boys wearing the *toga prae-texta*; it used to hang on their breast, to indicate that their youth needed to be governed by the counsel of another (indeed, *bulla* is derived from Greek *boulê*, or 'council' in Latin); or else it was because the *bulla* touches the part of the body, i.e. the breast, in which by nature counsel dwells.
>
> (Paulus-Festus 428.38L)[16]

The etymology itself is a somewhat facile construction (it is dismissed by Plutarch, *Roman Questions* 101, who instead offers interpretations of the *bulla* linked to the idea that it protected the child). Nevertheless, it shows that ancient authors saw the *bulla* as belonging to members of the community who were somehow unformed or incomplete, who still required the counsel of others. The idea is backed up by the fact that the *bulla* was worn until the teenager exchanged his *toga praetexta* for a man's *toga virilis*, at which point the *bulla* was placed in the household shrine as a dedication to the Lares.[17] Only when the boy gave up his *bulla* did he truly become a man and a citizen. Then, dressed in the white toga of the freeborn adult citizen, the boy went to the Capitol to sacrifice and (modern scholars suggest) was enrolled on the list of citizens. Accompanied by family members and friends as witnesses to the rites, the boy/man moved symbolically and actually from the domestic to the public sphere. In the Roman context, therefore, the *bulla* protected and marked out those in a liminal pre-citizen state, simultaneously symbolising their potentiality as future citizens. The evidence does not allow us to apply this theory without question to a non-Roman context, but the existence of rituals allied to the development of children into citizens is also perfectly plausible in, for example, an Etruscan setting. Recent research has emphasised that Etruscan society during the Hellenistic period was more egalitar-ian than previously thought (Kron, 2013, p. 63), and hence is likely to have placed more importance on citizens as crucial constituent parts of the city-state.

---

16 *Bulla aurea insigne erat puerorum praetextatorum. Quae dependebat eis a pectore ut significaretur eam aetatem alterius regendam consilio (dicta est autem bulla a Graeco sermone* boulê, *quod consilium dicitur Latine), vel quia eam partem corporis bulla contingat, id est pectus in quo naturale manet consilium.*

17 See, for example, Persius (5.30–1). A comment by Propertius (4.1.131–2), 'When the *bulla* was removed from your innocent neck and you put on the toga of manhood in front of your mother's gods' (*mox ubi bulla rudi dimissa est aurea collo, matris et ante deos libera sumpta toga*), may suggest a special connection with the *Lares* of the child's mother, which deserves further exploration. On the toga see Davies (2005); Dolansky (2008).

One final aspect must be considered when assessing the possible connection of swaddled infant *ex-votos* with citizenship: the deities to whom they were offered. In most cases the deities remain unknown or their identity speculative, often based purely on the typologies of votives found at a site. But where there is epigraphic evidence, amongst other candidates some names crop up repeatedly. There are dedications to Juno/Uni from Vulci (Fontanile di Legnisina), Caere (Manganello) and Falerii (Celle). Mater Matuta/Leucothea is attested at Cales. At Teanum the Sidicine sanctuary of Loreto may have been dedicated to Pupluna (for the swaddling from this site: Museo Archeologico, Teanum Sidicinum, inv. 292346; Sirano, 2007, p. 23). Although deities such as these are often described simply as 'fertility' goddesses, it is striking that their range of responsibilities is much broader than that. Often they appear to be poliadic deities, ensuring the development and security of the whole community, whose building blocks were precisely the fertility of individuals and families. On the other hand, it is worth remembering that a number of the contemporary bronze statues of toddlers found in Etruscan sanctuaries are inscribed to *male* gods, including Silvanus and Tec Sans, that is Sancus (the latter on the famous Putto Graziani in the Vatican, inv. 12107). When looking at swaddled infant votives, therefore, common gender assumptions regarding dedicators (as female) and dedicatees (as goddesses) may require revision.

Conclusion

The making of an offering to mark a 'deal' struck between worshipper and deity is an enduring ritual practice which played a major role in ancient religious practices. The votives of infants examined here demonstrate that the well-being and progress of children was a cause for both family and community concern. They can be seen to celebrate the safe conclusion of the dangerous 'pupal' phase during which the child's body had been moulded by its swaddling bands into the 'perfected' body – not just of the human being, but of the proto-citizen, symbolised and protected by the *bulla*. The swaddled infant *ex-voto* thus represents one of a series of life stages through which the child passed on the journey to full citizenhood.

8   The foot as *gnōrisma*

Sara Chiarini

In order, then, that it should not go rolling upon the earth, which has all manner of heights and hollows, and be at a loss how to climb over the one and climb out of the other, they bestowed upon it the body as a vehicle and means of transport. And for this reason the body acquired length, and, by God's contriving, shot forth four limbs, extensible and flexible, to serve as instruments of transport, so that grasping with these and supported thereon it was enabled to travel through all places, bearing aloft the chamber of our most divine and holy part.

(Plato, *Timaeus* 44e–45a)

Introduction

Everybody has been asked at least once in life to describe the physical appearance of an acquaintance to someone who does not know that person. I dare to suppose that among the readers of this chapter the majority might reasonably have appealed to details such as stature, frame, skin colour, eyes and hair and perhaps the way that person dresses. It is difficult to imagine recalling the shape of the feet or the look of a person's shoes as key identifying marks. Yet ancient people often did precisely that: feet were among the most important signs of recognition and symbolic representation associated with an individual.

The evidence for plastic reproductions of feet (both bare and with footwear) and sketches of footprints, either traced or engraved, is attested across the ancient Mediterranean. This material served a wide range of functions. Large quantities of votive feet are found in the sanctuaries of health-related divinities as votive dedications following the healing of a mobility condition or other type of illness. Exemplary collections include the hundreds of clay feet unearthed in the sanctuary of Asclepius at Corinth, which was apparently a centre specialising in the pathologies of limbs as well as genitalia between the fifth and the fourth centuries BC (Roebuck, 1951, especially pp. 127–8 for the list of votive feet) and that of Ponte di Nona, not far from Rome, whose tutelary deity remains unknown (Potter and Wells, 1985).[1] The high concentration of terracotta limbs

---

1 Potter and Wells (1985, p. 30) note that paired feet at the site outnumber single ones by a ratio of roughly 3:1. One wonders whether this prevalence may depend upon the synechdochic dedication of feet for more general ambulation diseases rather than specifically podiatric pathologies.

at these sites has been associated with the typical profile of the suppliants who are imagined to have been predominantly farmers or, more generally, people coming from the countryside and leading a rural lifestyle in which healthy feet and limbs were essential for undertaking agricultural and pastoral activities (Oberhelman, 2014). Although this explanation may be appropriate for the majority of these cases, other reasons for the dedication of sacred images (*agalmata*) of feet, such as travel or war, should be taken into account as well. For instance, in the case of sanctuaries not linked directly to medicine and other healing practices feet may have been dedicated to thank the gods for a safe return from a long business trip or a battle (Roebuck, 1951, p. 128).

This last observation directs discussion towards the theoretical framework of this chapter, which concerns the link between the symbolism of feet and notions of space and identity by means of the notion of presence. To signal and immortalise one's presence in a sacred place, especially if getting there had required a long pilgrimage, Greeks and Romans often left sculpted feet and more frequently footprints as a token or marker of their presence (in other words as a form of *gnōrisma*). This practice was also a common method used to commemorate other places that had a special significance for one's life, such as the *gymnasium* where a youth was educated for several years. Even a sign of the presence of a divinity, placed in a dedicated temple or in the form of a personal amulet, could consist of footprints or feet. For instance, Sarapis's feet are easy to recognise due to the small bust of the god usually carved right on the top of the ankle (Guarducci, 1995, pp. 73–4), whilst another example of divine feet can be found in Artemis's footprint (*íchnos*) discovered in the Turkish village of Çomaklı and identified with the ancient city of Pogla in Pisidia (Petridou, 2009). In such cases the feet are the body part chosen to represent identity and to guarantee the presence and the protection of the deity. This chapter will develop this argument, drawing on both literary and archaeological sources that emphasise the close relationship between physical presence in a given place and personal identity as embodied by the symbolism of the foot.

Ancient literary evidence

Our starting point is a set of literary passages that evoke the role of feet as identifying marks in scenes of *anagnórisis*. The *Odyssey* provides the first and most revealing instances of recognition by means of the appearance of feet at the end of the *Telemachy*.[2] Telemachus and Peisistratus, the son of Nestor, finally reach the palace of Menelaus and Helen, where they hope to obtain some information

---

2 Although not explicitly referring to the matter of individuation, the *Iliad* also contains some interesting expressions in which *pódes* ('feet') polarise the two main mobility abilities of a warrior: to keep a firm position on the battlefield and to move quickly. Stable contact with earth and the possibility of movement on its surface are both rooted in feet. In a metonymic form, feet 'take' or 'keep' the person to/in a given place, and they look almost personified and detached from the rest of the body (for instance, Homer, *Iliad* 13.515, 15.405 and 17.700).

about the fate of Odysseus. As the two boys approach the *megaron* to meet the Spartan couple, they have not yet introduced themselves. After having taken her place on the throne, Helen takes the floor first and says to her husband:

> Do we know, Menelaus, fostered of Zeus, who these men declare themselves to be who have come to our house? Shall I disguise my thought, or speak the truth? Nay, my heart bids me speak. For never yet, I declare, saw I one so like another, whether man or woman – amazement holds me, as I look – as this man is like the son of great-hearted Odysseus, even Telemachus, whom that warrior left a new-born child in his house, when for the sake of shameless me ye Achaeans came up under the walls of Troy, pondering in your hearts fierce war.

> (Homer, *Odyssey* 4.138–46)

Helen does not need to hear the speech of Telemachus to recognise him: his appearance enables her to identify him as Odysseus's son.[3] However, she does not mention any physical detail which has led her to this assumption, nor does she give any other clue about how she successfully recognised him.[4] This task is accomplished by Menelaus, who speaks immediately after his wife and who lists five body parts which have led him to agree with Helen about the identity of the young guest in front of them. The first place in Menelaus's classification is occupied by feet, which look exactly like those of Odysseus (κείνου τοιοίδε πόδες) and which occur before other potentially more 'evident' – from a modern perspective at least – signs of characterisation such as hands, eyes or hair:

> Then fair-haired Menelaus answered her: 'Even so do I myself now note it, wife, as thou markest the likeness. Such were his feet, such his hands, and the glances of his eyes, and his head and hair above. And verily but now, as I made mention of Odysseus and was telling of all the woe and toil he

---

3 The close resemblance between Telemachus and his father Odysseus is a recurring theme in the *Telemachy*: it appears for the first time at *Odyssey* 1.206–9, where Athena in the guise of the Taphian Mentes asks Telemachus to confirm whether he is the famous son of the famous Odysseus (εἰ δὴ ἐξ αὐτοῖο τόσος πάϊς εἰς Ὀδυσῆος), since he strikingly resembles him in the head and the beautiful eyes (αἰνῶς μὲν κεφαλήν τε καὶ ὄμματα καλὰ ἔοικας ‖ κείνῳ) – note that only head and eyes recur here as special bearers of the likeness. A further occurrence of the motif is *Odyssey* 3.122–5, this time with Nestor in the part of the interlocutor of Telemachus. An interesting detail of this second passage should be taken into account: the only distinguishing feature of Telemachus explicitly mentioned by Nestor – which also lets him recognise the boy – is his rhetorical proficiency. Although this is an intellectual and not an aesthetic feature, we find the formulaic expression σέβας μ'ἔχει εἰσορόωντα ('amazement holds me, as I look'), which is also present at *Odyssey* 4.142. This formula suggests the traditional nature of scenes of *anagnōrisis* in the epic diction and its connotation as a basically visual experience.

4 Commenting on these verses, Athenaeus (190e) ascribes a peculiar talent for recognising parental similarities to women, being always concerned with monitoring each other's 'virtue': πάνυ γὰρ αἱ γυναῖκες διὰ τὸ παρατηρεῖσθαι τὴν ἀλλήλων σωφροσύνην δειναὶ τὰς ὁμοιότητας τῶν παίδων πρὸς τοὺς γονέας ἐλέγξαι ('Indeed women are exceptional in spotting the analogies between children and their parents thanks to their guard over each other's virtue').

endured for my sake, this youth let fall a bitter tear from beneath his brows, holding up his purple cloak before his eyes'.

(Homer, *Odyssey* 4.147–54)

Another passage from the *Odyssey* is probably better known since it belongs to the famous scene of the dialogue between Odysseus disguised as beggar and Eurycleia his former wet nurse. Penelope has asked Eurycleia to wash the anonymous guest's feet, and the servant approaches the beggar with these words:

Therefore will I wash thy feet, both for Penelope's own sake and for thine, for the heart within me is stirred with sorrow. But come now, hearken to the word that I shall speak. Many sore-tried strangers have come hither, but I declare that never yet have I seen any man so like another as thou in form, and in voice, and in feet art like Odysseus.

(Homer, *Odyssey* 19.376–81)

In contrast with the first passage from the *Telemachy*, the *anagnōrisis* has not yet taken place: Eurycleia does not say that the person in front of her is, or might be, Odysseus, but simply states the resemblance between the beggar and Odysseus, especially with regard to his build, his voice and, importantly, his feet.[5] The identification cannot yet happen for it must be provoked by the scar on Odysseus's leg, according to the mythical tradition. In any case, feet are combined once again with two other external physical markers, which appear much more effective to our modern sensibilities. It should be kept in mind, however, that feet hold an outstanding role in the whole episode because of the foot-washing scene, and that the noun for 'foot' (πούς) occurs three times within 12 lines. Odysseus guesses that there is the risk of being recognised and tries to avoid it by pretending to have already been mistaken with Odysseus by many other people, but as soon as Eurycleia gets closer to Odysseus's feet in order to wash them there is no way out for him. She notes the unmistakable scar which the young Odysseus caused himself during a hunt on Mount Parnassos. However, it is significant that in the two Homeric scenes of *anagnōrisis* the only physical trait which occurs in both instances are feet: this cannot be by chance, and it must be grounded in deeper anthropological issues than the mere fact that in antiquity feet might have been more exposed than today as a result of more open models of footwear (Lacroix and Duchesne, 1862; Peacock, 2005; Blundell, 2006). That this is a trivial and weak argument will be demonstrated later with the support of further evidence, which together reveals the deep symbolic value of feet within ancient culture.

---

5 Ferrari (2001, p. 681 n. 49) notes the formulaic combination of body (δέμας) and voice (φωνή or αὐδή) (compare Homer, *Iliad* 13.45, 17.555 and 22.227; *Odyssey* 2.268 and 2.401). This emphasises the choice of feet as a third element of the series. Thus the mention of feet in our main passage might disclose the forthcoming scene of foot washing and the consequent *anagnōrisis*.

Not only did the direct examination of feet facilitate the process of recognising a person, the tracks left by feet also fulfilled the same function, albeit in a more indirect manner and even in the absence of the identified person. The identification of footprints left in soil is another traditional theme that appears across a number of different literary genres. It is found, for example, in Book 13 of the *Iliad* when Poseidon disguised as Calchas visits the Aiantes and urges them to arrest Hector's fury. The god touches the two heroes with a sceptre and then disappears. The Locrian Ajax realises immediately that it could not be the soothsayer and says to his companion:

> Aias, seeing it is one of the gods who hold Olympus that in the likeness of the seer biddeth the two of us fight beside the ships – not Calchas is he, the prophet, and reader of omens, for easily did I know the tokens behind him of feet and of legs as he went from us; and plain to be known are the gods – lo, mine own heart also within my breast is the more eager to war and do battle, and my feet beneath and my hands above are full fain.
>
> (Homer, *Iliad* 13.68–75)

Note that, according to the last line, the courage instilled by Poseidon in the two warriors becomes visible through feet and hands. Ajax, son of Oileus, is not able to indicate exactly which of the Olympians he has just met, but the form and the breadth of the footprints make him sure that the visitor could not have been Calchas but rather a divinity (on the human capability to recognise the presence of a divinity, see the commentary on this passage by Eustathius *ad Iliadem* 13.71 [3.441.7–13]).

That footprints are the most reliable signs left by a god, which enable men to identify him, is stated also in the dialogue between Kalarisis and Knemon in Heliodorus's *Aethiopica*. Knemon asks how someone can be sure to have met a divinity in the real world and not during a dream. Kalarisis begins his answer by quoting the passage from the *Iliad* discussed earlier, before commenting on its meaning. Kalarisis's opinion is that disguised gods cannot escape the careful gaze of wise men:

> The gods and other heavenly powers, Knemon, coming and going from us, change themselves seldom into the likeness of other creatures, but commonly into men, that we, supposing by the likeness of their figure that what we saw was a dream, may be so beguiled. But although the rude and profane people know them not, yet can they not escape the wise man. He will know them either by their eyes, in that they look steadfastly and never shut their eyelids; or better still by their gait, in that they move not their feet nor set one foot before another, but are carried by some force and unchecked power through the air, rather sliding through than striding over the winds.
>
> (Heliodorus, *Aethiopica* 3.13)

Accordingly, two main features disclose the divine nature of an individual: the stillness of their eyes and, still clearer, their gait. The supernatural and aerial force carrying the gods provides their step with an unmistakable character and consequently extends also to their footprints. Indeed, the text continues:

> Wherefore the Egyptians make the images of their gods with their feet joined together and not separated asunder. Which thing the skilful Homer, like an Egyptian and one well instructed in the holy doctrine, secretly and closely signified in his verses, leaving them to be understood by such as had the power. Of Pallas he speaketh thus: 'Also her terrible eyes did glister as she looked.' And of Poseidon thus: 'His footprints as he went easily I knew' – meaning that he went, as it were, with a swimming gait; for the word 'easily' goes with 'went,' not, as some folk wrongly have imagined, with 'I knew'.
>
> (Heliodorus, *Aethiopica* 3.13)

Other instances of this motif can be found in the *Histories* of Herodotus. The historian describes the landscape of Scythia and asserts that 'they show a footprint of Heracles by the Tyras river stamped on rock, like the mark of a man's foot, but forty inches in length' (Herodotus, *Histories* 4.82). This footprint attested the passage of the hero in that region. In another passage Herodotus (*Histories* 2.91.3) reports that the sandal left by Perseus when he appeared to the Egyptians of Chemmis at the sanctuary dedicated to him was two cubits in length. The prosperity bestowed by Perseus on this occasion is related to the belief that divine feet made the ground they touched fertile. A similar instance can be identified in the two divine footprints – the bigger one belonging to Dionysus and the smaller to Heracles – preserved on an isle beyond Heracles's pillars which attest their passage there (Lucian, *A True Story* 1.7). Moreover, in the life of Commodus from the *Historia Augusta* (*Commodus* 16.2), the outgoing footprints of the gods in the forum are interpreted as an ill-omened sign.

Epic is not the only literary source for the highly physiognomic function of feet in the Greek world: tragedy provides some interesting evidence as well. In particular, Aeschylus presents a scene of *gnōrismós* at the beginning of *Libation Bearers*, when Electra identifies her brother Orestes at their father's grave:

> But I invoke the gods, who know by what storms we are tossed like seafarers. Yet if I am fated to reach safety, a great stock may come from a little seed. And look! Another proof! Footprints matching each other – and like my own! Yes, here are the outlines of two sets of feet, his own and some companion's. The heels and the imprints of the tendons agree in proportion with my own tracks. I am in torment, my brain is in a whirl!
>
> (Aeschylus, *Libation Bearers* 201–11)

Unlike the Homeric instances discussed earlier, this passage has been the subject of many commentaries concerning the plausibility of the means of recognition that it describes. This debate originated in the rationalistic and polemical treatment of the corresponding scene by Euripides in his tragedy *Electra*. The three signs (τεκμήρια) through which Electra recognises her brother, detached from her as a newborn – the lock of hair, the footprint and the fringe of clothing – do not follow a logic of realism; rather as Paduano (1970) has explained, they follow the principle of the ancestral blood bond within the same *génos*. In the case of the 'second sign' (δεύτερον τεκμήριον), it is obvious that Aeschylus could not have truly believed that Orestes's footprints corresponded with those of his sister. These verses are not concerned with the question of realism or likelihood: the fantastic dimension of myth and fiction dominates over any rationalistic argument. In any case, the focus of this chapter prevents any detailed engagement in such debate and aims instead at some remarks concerning the role of feet in identification. First, the same tradition observed in Homer must lie behind this source, and, second, the fact that it might sound almost paradoxical that the footprints are a more reliable sign of recognition than physical presence itself. When Electra stands in front of her brother claiming his identity, she becomes more sceptical and finds it more difficult to recognise Orestes from his immediate presence than from his mediated signs.[6]

The Euripidean elaboration of Orestes's *anagnṓrisis* on the part of Electra reveals the radical change of mentality between the two authors. Euripides clearly harks back to the Aeschylean version, but his aim is not to contend personally with his predecessor. Rather, he wants to stress the decline of archaic values on the one hand and, on the other, the rise of a sophistic culture to which he is not merely subjugated, as is shown by the ironic features of the hyperintellectualistic and intricate answer of Electra to the old man inviting her to compare her feet with the footprints left at her father's grave:

Old man: Then stand in the footprint and see if the tread of the boot will measure with your own foot, child.

Electra: How could there be an imprint of feet on a stony plot of ground? And if there is, the foot of brother and sister would not be the same in size, for the male conquers.

(Euripides, *Electra* 532–7)

This scene takes place in a completely different location from the Aeschylean one: Electra has been married to a man of low rank and lives away from the palace. The old man invites her to visit her father's grave to check if the footprints impressed there do really belong to her brother Orestes as he has already conjectured. The reference to *Libation Bearers* is evident: Electra should prove if her feet are of the same size (σύμμετροι) as the footprints on the ground. Apart from the impossibility that Electra will be able to reach the place where her

6 The metaphor of feet pressed on the ground as a clue to the presence of Orestes returns in Aeschylus, *Libation Bearers* (691–9) within the dialogue between Clytemnestra and Orestes disguised as a foreigner. As the stranger tells the queen that Orestes has died, she swears at the hostile fate ceaselessly plaguing the *genos*, even if its members are kept away from the crimes of the family. Clytemnestra declares 'And now Orestes: he was indeed prudent in keeping his foot out of the mire of destruction' (Aeschylus, *Libation Bearers* 696–7).

father lies, her answer is a crude rationalistic critique on the absurdity of being able to identify the footprints of her brother simply by superimposing her own feet. Female feet can never coincide with male ones even if the two persons are relatives. As Paduano (1970) correctly explained, the critique is not directed personally at Aeschylus as if he really meant that Electra had recognised the presence of Orestes because her feet were a perfect match with the footprints. Instead, the whole Aeschylean passage needs to be read in a less literal and more mystical way: as already noted, the *anagnōrisis* of the *Libation Bearers* is embedded within the archaic philosophy of *génos* which defines the entire production of Aeschylus, while Euripides experienced the decline of such a system of values and the emergence of the sophistic method in cultural debate. Apart from the critical attitude of Euripides towards such an irrational and almost religious idea of familiar links, the value of this passage for the present inquiry lies rather in its indirect evidence of the ancient and deep-rooted custom of considering feet an important marker of identity.

In addition to the instances presented earlier, many other sources deal with the peculiarity of the feet of a god or hero as a distinctive trait. The monosandalism of Dionysus, Hermes, Jason, Persephone and Perseus; the lameness of Hephaestus, Oedipus and Lycurgus; and the heel as the weak point of Achilles are all well-known mythical-folkloric motifs. They have all been the subject of many anthropological and cross-cultural investigations which cannot be reviewed here (for example, Brelich, 1955–57; Yche-Fontanel, 2001; Ginzburg, 2008, pp. 206–75; more specific studies include Fauth, 1985–86; Byl, 1993; Petrone, 2004). For the present inquiry it is enough to keep in mind the existence of these further sources in order to embed the specific topic of the role of feet in the statement of individual presence within a broader cultural panorama. Only one final observation concerning the subject of the naked foot needs to be highlighted, for it concerns the relevance of the direct contact between foot and ground in ancient civilisations. Several French scholars have already explained this as physical and symbolic link between men and earth: discussing the monosandalism of Jason, Moreau (1994, p. 133) states that 'to put a foot on the ground is to get into contact with the earth and the lower world' (see also Martin, 2004, pp. 253–5). Earlier, Motte (1963, p. 472) gave a similar interpretation of the nudity of the feet of Socrates and Phaedrus during their walk along the bank of Ilissos: 'to put a foot on the ground can arouse a special virtue through the contact with the earth'. According to this view, contact with earth documents the presence of a person in a given space. In turn, the sign of the physical presence brings individuation. This logical chain has its material location in feet and constitutes the unifying pattern of all the evidence discussed in this chapter.

Before leaving the literary material it is important to note that the marked individuality of feet in all the sources examined here is interwoven deeply with the function of feet (and footprints) as the primary sign of the physical *presence* of a person in a given place. Two additional passages serve to stress this link further, in both of which the appearance of a character is invoked by calling his or her feet or shoes as if his or her presence could only be guaranteed by the footprints left at the point of contact with the earth: Athena in Homer, *Iliad* 23.770 and Darius in Aeschylus, *Persians* 659–62. Moreover, the occurrence of feet as a synecdoche standing for the wholeness of the person is exemplified by some common Greek sayings, including ἐκτὸς ἔχειν πόδα 'to keep the foot out' (in the sense of not being involved in something) or πόδα ἔχειν ἔν τινι 'to have the foot in something' (in the opposite sense of being actively involved) (for an overview of the metaphorical repertoire on feet, see Kötting, 1972, pp. 734–6). Having reviewed the literary evidence, we must now redirect our attention to other types of artistic materials which exploit the link between feet and presence with the aim of gathering together these different expressive forms within a common and coherent anthropological interpretation of feet as an identifying marker.

The iconography of feet in the Greco-Roman world

There is a common link between the literary sources examined earlier and the many images of feet, footprints and shoes produced in antiquity which has never been explicitly stated until now. The representation of feet and footprints consists of an astonishing number of instances from all periods beginning in Pharaonic Egypt and lasting until Late Antiquity. Throughout, these sculptures, reliefs and impressions served two main functions. First, as divine feet or footprints, they symbolised the permanent presence of a god or hero within a sacred space. Second, as human representations, they offered a durable memory of the temporary passage of a person in a given place. Both categories find their counterparts in the literary evidence presented earlier, and, in order to highlight this analogy, the following discussion focuses exclusively upon the symbolism connected with identification and presence, leaving aside more commonly discussed matters of healing in order to shed new light on alternative readings of the iconography of feet. Consequently, the many representations of feet or footprints which appear to have acted as an *ex-voto* connected *directly* with the healing of a foot illness or injury are not included (for this see Guarducci, 1942–43, pp. 335–7; Castiglione, 1970).

Reproductions of soles, either in pairs or the right foot in isolation, were left at sanctuaries by many worshippers and pilgrims who wished to immortalise their visit to that sacred place. They were carved on stone, on the floors or thresholds of temples or on votive stelai and were often accompanied by inscriptions recording the name of the worshipper. In the first systematic study of this material, Margherita Guarducci (1942–43, p. 308) speculated on the two main meanings expressed by such images: on the one hand they were to maintain a memory of the long trip undertaken – mainly on foot – in order to reach the place of worship, and, on the other, they perpetuated the presence of the pilgrim at the sanctuary even after his or her departure. The first of these stresses the symbolism of mobility conveyed by feet; the second deals with the issue of physical presence and individuality, which corresponds exactly with the function

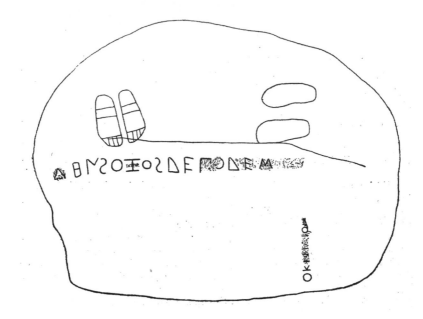

Figure 8.1 Inscribed stone by the *temenos* of Athena Sammonia, northern Crete, sixth century BC.

Source: After Guarducci (1942–43, p. 311), fig. 3.

ascribed to feet in the literary evidence examined earlier.[7] Later visitors to the sanctuary could see those footprints with their accompanying inscriptions and thus attribute to them a very specific identity.

Among the earliest examples of such 'steps' (βήματα) recalled by Guarducci – after the ancient Egyptian ones – are the soles carved on stones near the sanctuary of Athena Sammonia in northern Crete, which date from the sixth to fifth century BC. Next to these sketches were inscriptions, limited largely to the proper name of the person to whom the footprints belonged. One slightly more elaborate example reads: 'these feet are of Denios' (Δηνίō <τ>οίδε πόδες) (Figure 8.1).

Later periods, especially the Hellenistic and Roman, provide increasing numbers of such votive images in sacred contexts. For some of these later instances László Castiglione (1970, p. 128) refuted the symbolic association between foot and movement, stressing instead the link between foot and fixity of presence in a place. He suggested attributing the footprints not to pilgrims, but to priests or, more generally, to the personnel of cult. A special category of this

7 See also van Driel-Murray (1999) for a discussion of Roman shoes and distinctive hobnail patterns as a 'material projection of the self' capable of acting as a signature of the presence of an individual in a particular place.

vast collection concerns the so-called *itus et reditus*, showing two pairs of feet or shoes of the same pilgrim oriented in opposite directions. They may signify the already accomplished outward journey and the upcoming return, for the safety and success of which the worshipper also asks (Guarducci, 1942–43, pp. 318–21). Castiglione (1968, pp. 127–37) has, however, questioned this explanation and proposed to interpret the inverted footprints as a superstitious symbol of mutually annulling forces meant to protect the pilgrim from bad influences.

Sacred spaces are not the unique settings for images of feet as signs of presence and other public and educational places preserve similar finds (for Roman baths and private houses see Dunbabin, 1990, pp. 96–102; see also van Driel-Murray, 1999). Just as pupils today are used to leaving a memory of their attendance at a given school with doodles, signatures or dates on the school desks, ancient children had a similar habit. In particular, some *ephebes* drew the outline of their feet on the walls of *gymnasia*. With the same intention as the pilgrims who visited sanctuaries, these children sought to leave a long-lasting epigraphic memory of the years spent in that institution and chose their feet as an appropriate marker of both their presence and their individuality (Guarducci, 1942–43, pp. 321–2; 1995, pp. 366–71). The *gymnasium* of Cyzicus preserves one of the most interesting examples of this practice. On a marble slab covered with many inscriptions of *ephebes*, three names are inscribed in the genitive within the outline of a foot: reading from left to right Ἀκροδάμαντος, Ἀρίστωνος and Ἀπελλάδος (Figure 8.2).

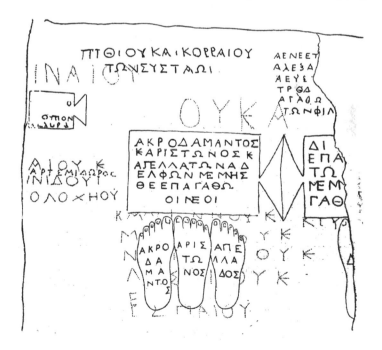

Figure 8.2 Marble slab from the *gymnasium* of Cyzicus, second century AD.
Source: After Guarducci (1942–43, p. 322), fig. 10.

The same three names appear in the central inscription of the slab above the drawings of the feet and within a *tabula ansata*. The three boys make the message implied in the footprints explicit, that is to be remembered by future generations of pupils of the *gymnasium*. The main inscription in fact reads, 'Keep a good memory, you children, of the brothers Akrodamas, Ariston and Apellas'. In comparison with the inscribed footprints left in sanctuaries, the religious aspect is missing from this example, but all other symbolic elements are present. As Margherita Guarducci (1995, p. 370) observed, the *ephebes* aim to immortalise their own physical attendance at the *gymnasium* and to be identified by future pupils.

Of course the choice to make oneself recognisable through the image of one's own feet or footprints follows not so much a logic of realism or reliability, but of the deep-rooted symbolism of presence, which has been already highlighted in the analysis of the literary passages earlier. Drawings and engravings of feet have such rough and depersonalised contours that nobody would dare to state that ancient people truly believed in the possibility of identifying a person from those sketches. However, because human contact with the earth materialises in the surface of soles, feet were evidently considered to be the most suitable body part for symbolising the presence of a whole individual, especially when the issue of recognition was not conceived absolutely, but in close relationship with the concept of physical presence in a given place. Images of feet made it possible not just to recognise somebody but to *recognise that that somebody was there*.

Human beings were, however, not the only ones to leave their traces on the ground: gods and other fantastic creatures did so too (for an overview see Bord, 2004; on feet as hints of theophanies see Weniger, 1923–24; Kötting, 1983). Epigraphy provides material comparable with the literary sources cited earlier for depictions and impressions of divine feet. These consist of both plain images of footprints and full sculptures of bare feet or shoes often of greater dimensions than human feet. Later examples are integrated with divine busts which rise above the ankle. These were also typically displayed in sanctuaries, and Isis, Serapis and Zeus Hypsistos are the three divinities for whom the largest number of instances of such representations are known (Guarducci, 1942–43, pp. 322–30; Castiglione, 1967; Canto, 1984; Rodriguez Oliva, 1987; Dunbabin, 1990, pp. 85–8; Guarducci, 1995, pp. 73–4; Takács, 2005).

If human visitors to holy places left their footprints in order to confer an eternal duration to their temporary passage, the divine inhabitants of those buildings made their constant presence visibly recognisable through the images of their feet. Moreover, such footprints could record with a permanent memorial the spot of a godly epiphany, the origins of which Castiglione (1967, p. 252) attributed to Egyptian worship, which spread subsequently across the Greco-Roman world. By entering the *temenos*, the worshipper might have encountered the divine footprints and placed their own soles over them in order to establish a direct contact with the divinity and, through that, to ensure a positive outcome for their petition (Guarducci, 1942–43, p. 323). Because many of these finds are in fact votive offerings made by humans, they are often also equipped with dedicatory inscriptions. One example, particularly interesting because of its relatively early date and uncommon provenance (most divine feet have been found in Egypt), is the well-preserved slab with the low relief of the footprints of Isis, which was found at Thessaloniki (Archaeological Museum of Thessaloniki, inv. 841) and which dates to the first century BC (Figure 8.3). The inscription running above the image of the feet dedicates the piece to the divine couple of Isis and Serapis, the Egyptian gods who were assimilated into Greco-Roman religion from the Hellenistic period onwards.

This summary of the iconographic material has led us to make the same observations as during the analysis of the poetic passages referring to feet as a means of identification and proof of the physical presence of a person in a given place (Castiglione, 1968, p. 130). Bringing together these two collections of evidence is therefore fully justified by the common anthropological issue which has been proven to lie beneath both cultural phenomena. Indeed, this is something that can be detected in almost all documented ancient civilisations from northern Europe to the Far East, and the next section aims to embed

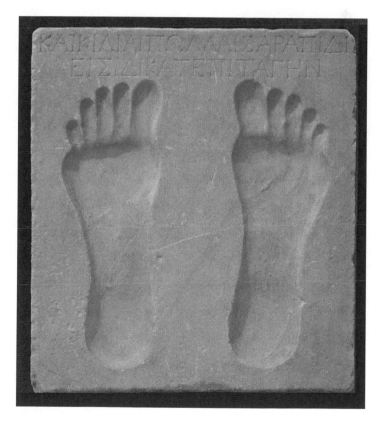

Figure 8.3 Votive plate with footprints of Isis, first century BC. Archaeological Museum of Thessaloniki, inv. 841.

Source: Gerald L. Stevens.

the motif of feet as a symbol of presence and individuality within a broader cross–cultural perspective.

A cross–cultural phenomenon

A complete report of the representations of feet in all ancient cultures is a task for which a whole book would not suffice. Therefore the aim of this section is not completeness; rather it seeks to expand the material context beyond traditional Greco-Roman boundaries in order to reflect critically on the peculiar phenomena examined in this chapter. Among the thousands of pieces which related to the many ancient civilisations of Europe and Asia, some specific examples that attest the same symbolism of *gnōrismós* and presence are highlighted here, organised according to the same partition between images of human and divine feet.

The inspection of soles or footprints as a means of affirming the identity of a foundling is a practice documented in the Near East from the Sumerian period until the Islamic age. Sumerian scribal *vade-mecums* (reference guides) for adoption deeds, known as *Ana Ittišu*, contain formulas related to the measurement of a foundling's feet on the part of the foster parents as a guarantee of the validity of the adoption. Moreover, the clay bars containing the adoption document had to be sealed with the child's footprint (although these were often reduced to mere nail imprints: Liverani, 1977, pp. 107–10). Such documents were also produced during the Akkadian kingdom (finds come mainly from Emar and a further clay imprint was found in Nippur: Malul, 2001). The custom appears to have been inherited by the Arabs who applied a technique called *qiyāfa* ('ability to detect footprints') in order to recognise the father of an infant in cases of polyandry. According to this practice, a *qā'if* (a sort of soothsayer) was appointed to identify the father by comparing the footprints of the newborn with those of the possible fathers.[8] As Liverani (1977, p. 109) correctly points out, the question of realism and concrete evidentiary value has nothing to do with this evidence, much like with all the material discussed in this chapter. These habits were pursued not as useful practical means to succeed in a *gnōrismós* but as heritage of the deep symbolic value of feet as sign of presence.

The metaphor of feet signifying the presence of a person is also attested in the Old Testament. Isaiah (Isaiah 52.7) acclaims the footmarks of the messenger of peace: 'How beautiful upon the mountains are the feet of the messenger and the preacher of peace! Announcing good and preaching peace, they are saying to Zion, "Your God will reign!"' This metaphor is also applied to God in order to express His appearance among His people: 'The glory of Lebanon will arrive before you, the fir tree and the box tree and the pine tree together, to adorn the place of my sanctification. And I will glorify the place of my feet' (Isaiah 60.13)

---

8 *Qā'if* were experts responsible for recognising parental relations from general physical traits, but feet seem to have been the most important bodily details considered. Liverani (1977) establishes the connection between pre-classical Mesopotamian sources and the Arabic ones.

and 'Son of man, the place of my throne, and the place of the steps of my feet, is where I live: in the midst of the sons of Israel forever' (Ezekiel 43.7) (for the 'footstool of God' see 1 Chronicles 28.2; Psalms 99.5; Lamentations 2.1).

These biblical passages move our attention from human to divine feet. Archaeological evidence for divine and superhuman representations of feet is not limited to the pagan figures of Greco-Roman religion, but is also attested in other ancient religious contexts. One of the earliest images of divine footprints is preserved at the north Syrian site of 'Ain Dara (Figure 8.4). The site houses a temple excavated 1980–85 and considered the closest architectural parallel to the coeval Solomon's temple of Jerusalem as it is described in the Bible (1 Kings, 7; Monson, 2000). The Canaanite sanctuary of 'Ain Dara appears to have been devoted to the goddess Ištar and was in use for approximately 550 years from 1300 to 740 BC. On some slabs of the distyle *in antis* portico are preserved four gigantic footprints (each about three feet long) oriented towards the inside of the temple: a parallel pair on the first slab of the entrance, a single left footprint on the second slab of the entrance and a single right footprint on the slab at the opposite side of the antechamber on the threshold between antechamber and main hall. These footprints have been attributed to the resident divinity, as if she had first stopped at the entrance of her temple and had then taken a stride of about 30 feet. Monson (2000, p. 26) has calculated that such a step would belong to a being around 65 feet tall. Although this evidence is unique in the archaeology of the ancient Near East, the symbolic relationship between feet, identity

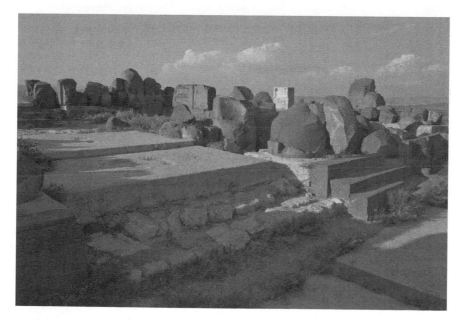

Figure 8.4 Tell 'Ain Dara, Syria: footsteps at the temple entrance.

Source: Wikimedia Commons, Author: Bertramz.

and presence seems not to have been rare in this cultural sphere, as the textual documents presented earlier demonstrate, especially the formulas of adoption.

Moving further east, Buddhist and Hindu cultures offer additional tantalising comparative material thanks to the thousands of imprints of the feet of Gautama Buddha (the so-called *Buddhapadas*) and of Vishnu (for links with the footprints of Isis and Serapis see Thomas, 2008). They abound across Asia and date from a long period between antiquity and the modern age. The earliest examples of *Buddhapadas* belong to the second century BC (Quagliotti, 1998) and often bear distinguishing marks such as a *Dharmachakra* at the centre of the sole or the 32, 108 or 132 auspicious signs of the Buddha engraved or painted on the sole. Anna Maria Quagliotti (1998, pp. 34–5 and pp. 119–20) related *Buddhapadas* to *stupas*, the commemorative monuments housing sacred bodily relics of the Buddha or other holy persons.

All of these divine footprints are the material transposition of the use of feet as synecdoche for the whole person. They also can signify either the former appearance or the continuous presence of the deity. As an object of worship, the footprint indicates the place where the deity once manifested himself or herself. As reminder of the permanent presence of the god or goddess, the footprints invite the worshipper to put their own feet over them in order to come into direct contact with the deity and consequently to achieve protection and positive influence. Together with these artificial representations of feet, natural petrosomatoglyphs of feet – peculiar cuts or holes on rocks that were considered to be footprints left by gods or heroes – were also worshipped. One of the most famous cases is that of Adam's Peak in Sri Lanka. On the mountain called Sri Pada a wide cut on the rock was identified as the left footprint of a divine figure. Its uniqueness lies in the fact that its worship is shared by four major religions. The mark was ascribed first by the Tamil Hindus to Shiva as he danced the world into creation (and the corresponding right footprint was located at Phra Sat in Thailand), Buddhists contend that during one of his visits to Sri Lanka the Buddha left his print on a sapphire now covered by the print of Shiva, Portuguese Christians claimed that the footprint was left by St. Thomas as he brought Christianity to Sri Lanka and finally Muslims contend that the footprint was left by Adam as he stood on the mountain top for one thousand years of penance after he was exiled from the Garden of Eden (Kinnard, 2000). Another well-known case of reuse is that of the *quo vadis* footprints of Jesus in Rome. The Roman marble relief originally offered by a pagan worshipper to the god Rediculus was later connected to the episode of the vision of Jesus that Saint Peter had on his escape from Rome. Apocryphal sources locate this event exactly at the intersection between the *via Appia* and the *via Ardeatina* where the marble footprints lay. When early Christians became aware of these existing imprints, they immediately connected them with that legend, and the image was made the proof of two successive *gnōrismói*.

The practices of identifying natural marks as footprints of figures from religion and folklore on the one hand and of carving artificial human footprints on the other continue into the Middle Ages and beyond, with a peculiar concentration in the British Isles and in Scandinavia. As has been observed with regard to the Greco-Roman representations of feet, the images presented in these regions are more or less detailed and range from simple contours of the sole to more precise outlines including toes and single phalanges. But all such representations are rather standardised, even though their aim is paradoxically that of guaranteeing the individuality of the worshipper or the worshipped. As already remarked, the evocative force of footprints and of representations of feet more generally lies in their deep symbolism of presence rather than in perceptual realism. This lack of interest for a logically plausible form of *gnōrismós* constitutes precisely the consistent feature which connects both the literary and the archaeological sources examined in this chapter.

Conclusion

In ancient contexts many symbolic values were ascribed to feet, including those associated with fertility, contact with the underworld, contrast between filthiness and purity, submission and so forth. Most of these topics have been investigated extensively by modern scholars, beginning with the study of Cornelius Verhoeven (1956) on the symbolism of feet in antiquity (an earlier and wider contribution was made by Nacht, 1923). In the context of his collection of mythological, literary and material sources relating to the various meanings of feet, he notes the topic of presence, but only briefly as an introduction to the themes of subjugation and violence (Verhoeven, 1956, pp. 128–32 where he insists on the aspect of verticality, which is useful to him in order to introduce the concept of submission). In those few pages he hints at the importance attributed by ancient people to the link between feet and the earth and the connected individual signs of physical presence. Unfortunately Verhoeven did not develop this observation further in terms of assessing the symbolism of presence and individualisation but, as this chapter has demonstrated, the relationship between footprints as a sign of presence in a given place and the contextual seizure of that place deserves critical attention. Indeed, moving from this theoretical premise, this chapter has suggested that it is necessary to read the literary evidence for the role of feet in the context of a *gnōrismós* on the one hand and a certain class of material footprints and feet representations on the other as parallel phenomena. They both share the same underlying symbolic conception that has been emphasised throughout: feet were understood as an identifying trait which could state the presence of a determined person in a given place. This approach recovers Verhoeven's elaboration of the topic of verticality as anthropological link between feet and presence, but it expands its value from the symbolism of possession and submission to that of individual recognition. The first trajectory of this verticality – the one developed by Verhoeven – proceeds downwards from the feet to what lies underneath them and expresses in this way the domination over somebody or something. The opposite direction moves from the ground upwards and establishes a profound link between the surface occupied by the soles and the person. This chapter has argued that the anthropological explanation of the frequent occurrence of feet as symbolic sign of individual recognition in ancient sources derives from this ideal connection. In turn, this cultural phenomenon might be linked with a cognitive issue that has been highlighted by Carlo Ginzburg (2000, pp. 166–9), when he states that the human classification system is based upon the hunter tracking the animal. As each species has a distinctive foot, we know the animal being tracked based upon its footprints. This ancient way of identification may have survived subconsciously in myths and more widely in the traditional heritage of symbols.

These observations can prove fruitful in the context of anatomical votives. Although *ex-votos* linked to requests for healing have not been the focus of this chapter, many of the examples of feet and footprints cited here were originally produced, dedicated and encountered in religious, often votive, contexts. Moreover, it has been argued that feet allowed an individual not only to assert their presence but also to communicate directly with a deity or other divine entity. Placed against this backdrop, more 'traditional' votive models of feet and lower limbs should be reexamined critically and closely as objects potentially invested with multiple meanings and as a material testimony of the relationship established between mortal and divine on the occasion of a vow or other religious performance. Given the power and diffusion of the ideas associated with presence and individual identity, it is necessary to revisit commonly held assumptions about the models of feet found at sites such as Corinth and Ponte di Nona and their allegedly univocal connection with ailments of the feet in order to shed new light on how these rather standardised objects might have been invested with the personal identity of the petitioner, and perhaps even to consider whether some may have been designed to represent direct encounters with the divine in those places.

9 The open man

Anatomical votive busts between the history of medicine and archaeology

Laurent Haumesser[1]

Hanging on the dining room wall in the Paris apartment of writer, critic and publisher Jean Paulhan was one of the most striking works by the artist Jean Fautrier, painted in the late 1920s (Figure 9.1). It shows the open belly and intestines of a naked man with closed eyes, but whether the figure is standing, lying, viewed frontally, from above or from the side we cannot tell; the painting has two differently positioned signatures suggesting that it can be viewed either horizontally or vertically (Paulhan, 1949; Paris exhibition, 1989, p. 92, no. 65; Stalter, 1989, pp. 21–2). This work seems to follow in the tradition of paintings of flayed figures and anatomy lessons but eludes immediate classification because of its symbolic dimension and enigmatic nature.[2] This ambiguity is echoed in the painting's title. Sometimes called *The Autopsy* – a title suggesting a clinical interpretation of the subject – it is generally known by the more neutral title of *The Open Man*.

This name would also be well suited to a work acquired in 2011 by the Musée du Louvre (Figure 9.2). Setting aside differences of period and culture, this acquisition presents formal analogies with Fautrier's painting and has prompted similar questions (Gaultier et al., 2013, pp. 204–5; Haumesser, 2013). This *ex-voto*, representative of votive offerings produced in Hellenistic central Italy whose purpose was essentially symbolic and religious, has nonetheless been regarded as evidence of Etruscan knowledge of anatomy and even as a model of an autopsy and a medical teaching aid. The latter interpretation is that of French doctor Pierre Decouflé, the first owner of the object, who developed a particular interest in representations of organs amongst the terracotta votive offerings of central Italy (Decouflé, 1960; 1961; 1964). His was not an isolated case: Decouflé was one of a long series of doctors who from the late nineteenth century devoted specific studies to ancient anatomical representations before archaeologists turned their attention to this field.

---

1 Text translated from the French by Sally Laruelle. © Musée du Louvre / Laurent Haumesser.
2 During the same period Fautrier painted open animal carcasses, the animal companion pieces of anatomy lessons in the pictorial tradition (Paris exhibition, 1989, p. 56, nos. 10 and 11).

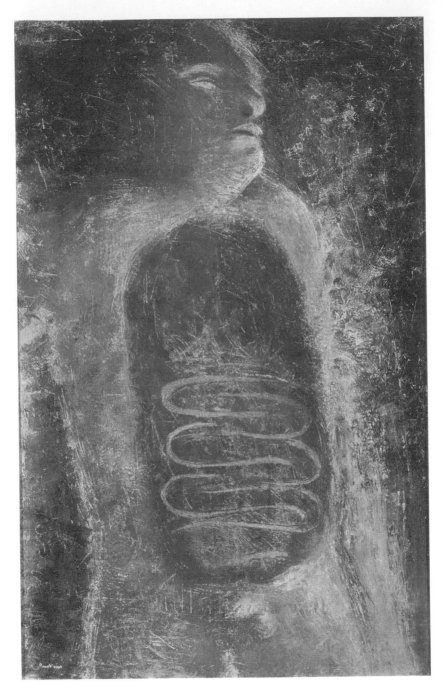

Figure 9.1 L'homme ouvert (The Open Man) by Jean Fautrier, Dijon, Musée des Beaux-arts, inv. DG 892.

Source: Musée des Beaux-Arts de Dijon. Photo François Jay © Paris, ADAGP, 2014.

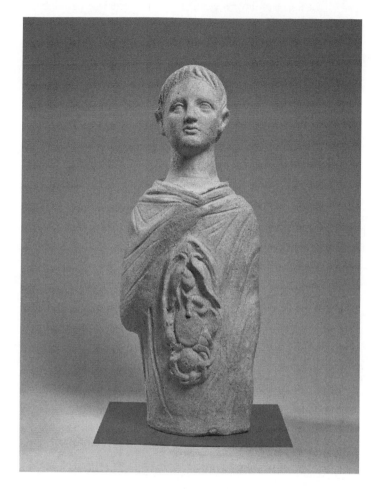

Figure 9.2 Decouflé bust, h. 68 cm. Department of Greek, Etruscan and Roman Antiquities, Musée du Louvre, Paris, inv. MNE 1341.

Source: Musée du Louvre, Dist. RMN-Grand Palais / Thierry Ollivier.

Rather than isolated limbs or organs (which are simpler and rarely display pathological features) the few similar specimens of busts that open the internal organs to display like the plates in modern anatomy books were a favourite subject of study among doctors and historians of medicine.[3] There are also

3 Uteri are the other main category of internal organs that have (more recently) attracted the attention of doctors and historians of ancient medicine, see Charlier (2000); Dasen and Ducaté-Paarmann (2006); Ducaté-Paarmann (2007); Flemming (this volume). The (rarer) representations of bladders, testicles and hearts are still open to debate (Turfa, 1994, pp. 226–7).

reduced versions of this type of terracotta votive offering which represent the internal organs only rather than incorporating them into an anthropomorphic figure. These two different 'production lines' suggest that we should be cautious in considering the busts as exceptional and review all the attestations from the perspective of production and craftsmanship in order to shed light on both the anatomical knowledge of the craftsmen and the religious motivations of the worshippers. This chapter assesses the evidence for open bust votives, as well as highlighting the extent to which the interpretations placed on these objects must be connected with the circumstances of their discovery and collection.

History of the discoveries

Terracotta votives, especially anatomical *ex-votos*, have long been known and are attested fairly early in several (especially Italian) archaeological collections (see Tabanelli, 1962, p. 4; Bartoloni, 1970; Bartoloni and Bocci Pacini, 1996). However, it was chiefly in the nineteenth century, with the development of excavations in Italy, that objects of this type first entered the major European and then American museums. The smaller pieces in particular were found frequently near excavation sites or on the Roman and Neapolitan antiquities markets where they were often purchased by foreign travellers, being plentiful, inexpensive and easy to transport. Consequently, many of the nineteenth-century European collections founded on core collections assembled by private individuals feature feet, legs, hands, eyes, ears and so on that were brought back from Italy. Apart from votive uteri, various models of which were found over a fairly wide area (see Flemming, this volume), very few depictions of internal organs are attested at that time. The most complex model – a few known examples of which were found in the first half of the nineteenth century – consists of a single elongated polychrome plaque bearing a depiction of the internal structure of the chest and abdomen from the oesophagus to the intestines (Figure 9.3).[4]

Open busts are even rarer, with only two in the principal antique collections assembled in the nineteenth century. The first belonged to the collection of Edme-Antoine Durand, purchased in its entirety for the Musée du Louvre by Charles X in 1825. This rich collection of artefacts from ancient Italy contained only about 20 anatomical terracotta votives, to which the Chevalier Durand does not seem to have attached particular importance; rather, their presence reflects the relatively systematic and encyclopaedic nature of the collection,

---

4 A fragmentary specimen from the Campanari collection was purchased in 1839 by the British Museum (inv. 1839,0214.52–53; Turfa, 1986, p. 208, no. 1). Another was acquired by the Antikensammlung in Berlin in the first half of the nineteenth century (inv. TC 1333; Holländer, 1912, pp. 207–8, fig. 120; Decouflé, 1964, p. 27, pl. XI–XII; Berlin exhibition, 1988, p. 296, no. D 3.37; King and Dasen, 2008, p. 85, fig. 2.3; Kästner, 2010, p. 73, fig. 6.7). A third specimen (Figure 9.3) entered the Louvre with the Campana collection (Cp 9633; Rouquette, 1911, pp. 516–19, fig. 7; Tabanelli, 1962, pp. 58–9, fig. 28). The provenance of these fragments is uncertain, but similar fragments from Cerveteri (Caere) may suggest the same origin (Turfa, 1994, p. 226, fig. 20.1A).

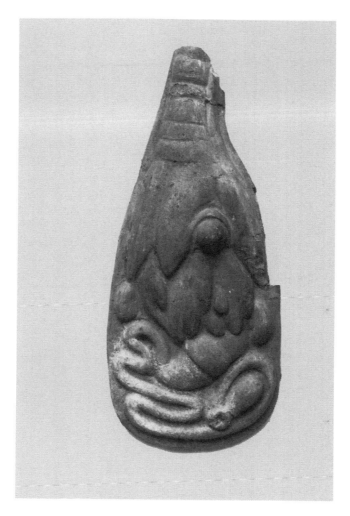

Figure 9.3 Plaque from the Campana collection. Musée du Louvre, Paris, inv. Cp 9633.
Source: Musée du Louvre, Dist. RMN-Grand Palais / image Musée du Louvre.

which comprised the main categories of ancient artefacts known at the time. Most of the votives in question are feet and male and female genitalia. In his catalogue Durand groups 'Votive monuments displaying a depiction of different ent parts of the human body' under the same heading (Paris, Musée du Louvre, Department of Greek, Etruscan and Roman Antiquities, inv. ED 2098–2117) but there is a separate entry for one small bust characterised by its open abdomen (Figure 9.4). The fact that the figure is female – as indicated by the breasts and a small incision for the vulva – led Durand to associate the votive dedication with a surgical intervention since he described the piece as a 'Votive

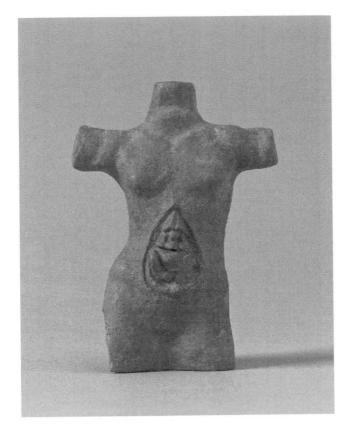

Figure 9.4 Bust from the Durand collection, h. 18.7 cm. Department of Greek, Etruscan and Roman Antiquities, Musée du Louvre, Paris, inv. ED 2097.

Source: RMN-Grand Palais (Musée du Louvre) / Stéphane Maréchalle.

torso dedicated to the caesarean operation' (Tabanelli, 1962, pp. 39–40, fig. 10; Haumesser, 2013, pp. 20–1, fig. 9–10). The second specimen, in Madrid's Museo Arqueológico Nacional, belonged to the collection of the Marquis of Salamanca.[5] Unfortunately, once again we have no precise information about the origin of this *ex-voto*, and there is no evidence for the claim that it comes from the vicinity of Capua (Holländer, 1912, p. 206; Tabanelli, 1962, pp. 41–2; Grmek and Gourevitch, 1998, p. 192; Bartoloni and Benedettini, 2011, p. 492) or, like most of the terracotta votives in the collection, from the excavations carried out by the Marquis at the Campanian sanctuary of Calvi (see Graells and Fabregat, 2011, pp. 8–15).

5 My thanks to Paloma Cabrera, director of the museum's Department of Greek and Roman Antiquities, for the indications she provided and for allowing me to examine the piece.

More and more discoveries were made in the late nineteenth century, with their number and quality sparking greater interest among scholars and collectors. This is why, despite fairly accurate information about the sites at which the votive deposits were found, many items were dispersed and have not all been located. An important find was made at Nemi in 1885: a draped female figurine whose torso is nonetheless open, exposing the internal organs (Nottingham Castle Museum, N 131, h. 26.5 cm; Blagg and MacCormick, 1983, p. 53; Moltesen, 1997, p. 161; Bartoloni and Benedettini, 2011, p. 494). A votive deposit found the same year at Civita Lavinia (Lanuvium) included two small male torsos with open abdomens (Museo Nazionale Etrusco di Villa Giulia inv. 42181 and 42182; Helbig, 1885, pp. 145–6; Moretti, 1967, p. 231; Coarelli and Rossi, 1980, fig. 79 mistakenly attribute it to Segni) (Figure 9.5).[6] However, in the late 1880s two sites in particular yielded a surprisingly rich

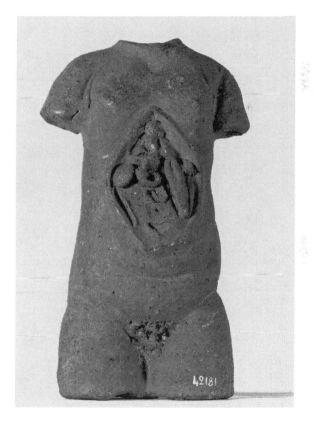

Figure 9.5 One of two busts from Lanuvium, h. 19.5 cm. Museo Nazionale Etrusco di Villa Giulia, Rome, inv. 42181.

Source: Museo Nazionale Etrusco di Villa Giulia.

6 My thanks to Maria Anna De Lucia for her help.

store of votive terracottas and especially of anatomical torsos and 'polyvisceral plaques'. First, several large deposits were found along the Tiber – especially in the vicinity of the Tiber Island – during work on the river banks (Pensabene et al., 1980, pp. 5–15). Most of these pieces entered the national collections and are now in the Museo Nazionale delle Terme. This is the case with the three torsos, or fragments of torso, that have illustrated many studies devoted to anatomical votive offerings (Figure 9.6). Other pieces were probably sold on the antiquities market, becoming part of private collections (Pensabene et al., 1980, pp. 5–6).

In 1889, shortly after these Roman finds, excavations conducted on behalf of the empress of Brazil by Rodolfo Lanciani unearthed some two thousand terracotta votives from a massive hoard in the Comunità area of Veii (Delpino, 1999, pp. 76–85; Liverani, 2004; Bartoloni, 2005; Bartoloni and Benedettini, 2011, pp. 11–19). Lanciani's report and the excavation drawings indicate that the

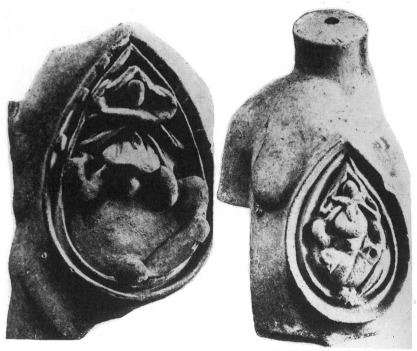

Figure 9.6 Left: Roman torso 2, Rome, h. 38 cm. Rome, Museo Nazionale delle Terme, inv. 14609. Right: Roman torso 1, Rome, h. 42 cm. Rome, Museo Nazionale delle Terme, inv. 14608.

Source: Wellcome Library, London.

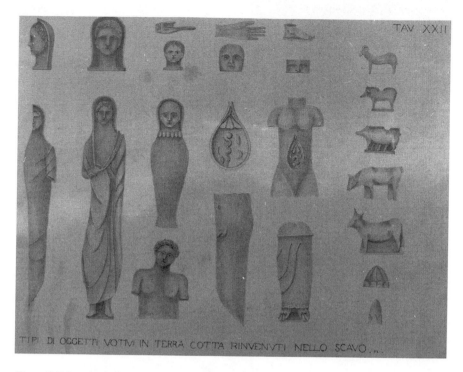

Figure 9.7 Lanciani, discoveries at Veii. Mss Lanciani 79.

Source: Biblioteca nazionale di Archeologia e Storia dell' Arte, Roma.

deposit contained several series of complex depictions of internal organs: various types of busts with exposed internal organs and reduced versions of anatomical plaques (Lanciani, 1889, p. 64).[7] Once again some of these *ex-votos* entered the national collections, whereas others found their way onto the antiquities market (Bartoloni and Benedettini, 2011, pp. 13–15) where they attracted the attention of a specific category of collectors: professors of medicine.[8]

7 Several plates in the Biblioteca di Archeologia e Storia dell'Arte in Rome document these excavations and the material found (Delpino, 1999). My thanks to Filippo Delpino for his help in finding these documents.

8 The institutions that recovered *ex-votos* from Veii (though their exact provenance cannot be determined) include the museum of Cluj Napoca in Romania where anatomical votives entered its collections in 1900, including a fragment of an open torso (Muzeul National de Istorie a Transilvaneiei, inv. V 19800; Crişan, 1970, p. 495, pl. II, 3). My thanks to Dr. Eugen Iaroslavschi for his information about this collection. The Pitt Rivers Museum, Oxford has a group of 27 terracottas donated in May 1896 by Robert William Theodore Gunther (inv. 1896.15.4–30; Kamash et al., 2013, pp. 351–2, fig. 16.8).

Doctors and collectors

Between the late nineteenth and early twentieth centuries, several European doctors compiled collections of terracotta votive offerings or added archaeological artefacts to collections devoted to the history of medicine (see chapters by Adams and Grove, this volume). Most of the votives they purchased came from Veii and Rome, although some were from other sites in Etruria and Latium. This information, gleaned from the few available documents, was usually contributed by the collectors themselves who often wrote about the works in their possession. This was the case with Ludwig Stieda, a German professor of medicine in Königsberg whose interest was aroused by a lecture delivered by archaeologist Alfred Körte in Düsseldorf in 1898 and who purchased a large group of votives at Isola Farnese in 1899 (objects therefore found at Veii, most of which probably came from the deposit at Comunità) and published two studies on the anatomical *ex-votos* (Stieda, 1899; 1901; Recke and Wamser-Krasznai, 2008, pp. 15–28). Stieda's terracottas are now in the Antikensammlung der Justus-Liebig-Universität (Giessen). Many of these doctors' collections followed a similar path: although some were dispersed or are untraceable, others were added to national collections which due to the collectors' academic careers tended to be located in university institutes devoted to the history of medicine rather than in archaeological museums. The famous Wellcome Collection in London is a case in point (Grove, this volume).

In 1894 on the occasion of the 11th International Congress of Medicine in Rome the English-Italian doctor Luigi Sambon presented a series of several dozen votive terracottas from the collection he had built up around objects found during the recent excavations in Rome and Veii, but which also included pieces from Bolsena and especially from Praeneste (modern Palestrina), another major production centre for votive terracottas which supplied an active market from the nineteenth century onwards. The following year Sambon published an overview of these terracotta pieces with references to collections compiled by colleagues, especially one belonging to a certain Dr Charles in Rome (Sambon, 1895a, p. 148; apart from a mention in Tabanelli, 1962, p. 9 we have no further information about Dr. Charles's Roman collection). The exhibition of 1894 so impressed William Oppenheimer, director of the eponymous pharmaceutical company, that he purchased the entire collection, exhibiting it the same year at the annual meeting of the British Medical Association in Bristol.

In 1910 the entire Oppenheimer collection – almost 1,300 objects including over five hundred terracotta votives – was purchased on behalf of Henry Wellcome, the wealthy owner of another pharmaceutical firm who had begun to amass a vast collection devoted to the history of medicine (Wellcome Library WA/HMM/CM/Col/87 'Sambon'; Grove, this volume). After this purchase a selection from the Oppenheimer collection was exhibited at the 17th International Congress of Medicine before this exhibition was transferred to the museum that was created shortly afterwards to house the Wellcome Collection in Wigmore Street, London (Handbook, 1913; Lawrence, 2003). The *ex-votos* were displayed in a small temple modelled on the Erechtheion (Grove, this volume, fig. 11.7). The most spectacular piece, which had already been given

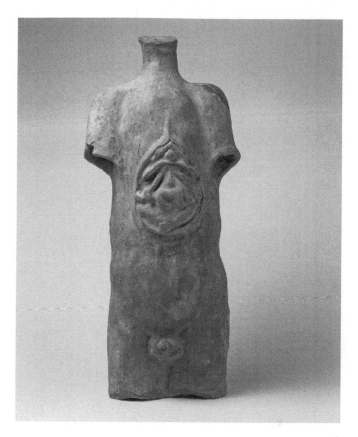

Figure 9.8 Bust from the Sambon collection, h. 70 cm. Science Museum, London, inv. A634998.
Source: Science Museum / Science & Society Picture Library.

pride of place in Bristol, stood in the centre: a headless bust some 70 cm high representing the internal organs. This piece, most probably found at Veii, is now on display at the Science Museum in London (Figure 9.8).[9]

Henry Wellcome's outstanding collection included some very rich series of anatomical votives, but these are largely unpublished and unfortunately rather poorly documented (Arnold and Olsen, 2003). The rhythm and number of acquisitions (sometimes complete collections) made it difficult to keep a precise and regular inventory. The dispersion of the collection from the 1930s onwards

9 The catalogue of the Wellcome Collection (Handbook, 1920, p. 33) and Thompson's (1922, pp. 2–3) study of the *ex-votos* it contained, give Isola Farnese as the place of discovery. Sambon (1895a, caption to fig. 5) says 'found near Rome'. Mention of 'Rome' in the typewritten inventory of the Sambon-Oppenheimer collection may correspond to a misunderstanding of the caption in Sambon's article (Wellcome Library, WA/HMM/CM/Col/87, 'Sambon').

further hindered the identification of the pieces and the reconstruction of the various series. A selection of objects is still on display today at the Wellcome Institute (Arnold and Olsen, 2003, pp. 388–9) but many items are now in the Science Museum, which acquired a large part of the collection (Richardson, 2003, pp. 330–2), and many other pieces were distributed (particularly in the early 1980s) to the major British museums (Russell, 1987). Nonetheless, the information contained in the archives is sufficient to identify the principal acquisitions and assess the number of ancient votives within the collection. In addition to the bust in the Oppenheimer collection Wellcome had acquired several particularly original *ex-votos* during the course of his search for artefacts, purchasing them at auctions or from collectors themselves. One such example is a small female bust acquired at an auction in 1918 on which the internal organs are indicated in slight relief (Figure 9.9).[10] Wellcome, like other collectors before him (including Sambon whose collection featured several copies of pieces in Roman collections), willingly included replicas in his collection, which he saw as essentially didactic. The cast that is most interesting from our perspective came from Germany: Johann Veit, a professor from Halle specialising in gynaecology, had seen the Wellcome Collection (the terracottas in particular)

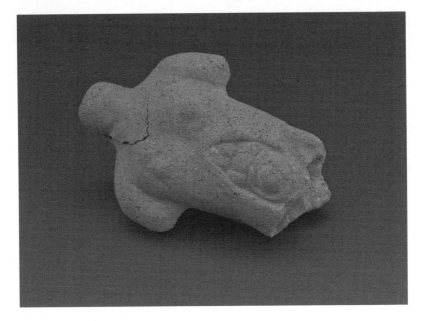

Figure 9.9 Female bust from the Wellcome Collection, h. 11.5 cm. Science Museum, London, inv. A 623134.

Source: Science Museum / Science & Society Picture Library.

10   The sales catalogue (London Catalogue, 1918, p. 19, no. 280A: 'A lot of Roman pottery, including a votive torso of a woman displaying the inner anatomy of the abdomen') gives no indication as to the provenance; it was part of a rather heterogeneous private collection.

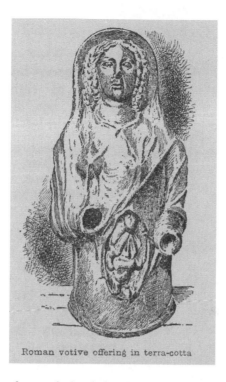

Figure 9.10 Illustration of a cast of a female bust formerly of the Wellcome Collection, h. 70 cm. Wellcome Collection, London, inv. R 4592/1936.

Source: Handbook (1920, p. 33).

at the 1913 International Congress of Medicine in London. Having indicated that he himself owned a large *ex-voto* from Veii he was immediately solicited by Wellcome.[11] Although Veit was unwilling to sell the piece, he agreed to the cast, which arrived in London in the spring of 1914 and became part of the museum display (Handbook, 1920, p. 33; Recke and Wamser-Krasznai, 2008, p. 69, n. 134) (Figure 9.10).[12]

11 The bust was already mentioned by Holländer (1912, p. 202; Thompson, 1922, p. 2). Evidently in this case the collector's clinical specialty was the reason for the acquisition. On Veit see Pickel et al. (2009). For the correspondence between Veit and Wellcome which allows us to trace the history of the piece, see the archive file Wellcome Library, WA/HMM/CO/Ear/998.

12 Unfortunately we have not yet been able to find this cast which features in the list of pieces transferred to British institutions by the Wellcome Trust in the 1980s (Wellcome Library, WA/HMM/TR/Abc/C.4/6 ('Classical Bronzes'): 'Replica of votive offering, Roman, terra cotta, showing internal organs'). Nor do we know whether the original in Halle was preserved. My thanks to Catherine Walker of the Wellcome Trust and Henryk Löhr of the University of Halle for their help with this research.

Unfortunately the provenance of other remarkable pieces – such as fragments of polyvisceral plaques – is still uncertain. In some cases there may be a connection with another significant acquisition dating from the same period: the part of the Gorga collection devoted to medicine. Wealthy Italian collector Evan Gorga had compiled a vast collection, the extraordinary variety of which has been highlighted by recent publications (Sannibale, 1998; Barbera, 1999a; 1999b; Cionci, 2004; Benedettini, 2012; Capodiferro, 2013; Ambrosini, 2013; on the votive terracottas see Roghi, 1999; Cenci, 2013 who both note the small number of such pieces in the Museo Nazionale Romano, a lack mistakenly associated with the attribution of a large series to the Museum of the History of Medicine at the Sapienza University in Rome). Negotiations with Gorga got under way in 1915, particularly through the intermediary of Arthur Amoruso, a lieutenant in the 31st Infantry Regiment. In December 1915 Amoruso, who was based in Naples at that time, sent C. J.S. Thompson (head curator of the Wellcome Collection) a report that provides an interesting account of the state of the collection. According to Amoruso, Gorga took him to a warehouse

> consisting of about 20 medium to small sized rooms *full* of boxes and trays each of which proved to be also full of specimens. In fact the first impression is that of the greatness of the collection. With the exception of a corridor full of Renaissance bas-reliefs, statuettes and ornaments, the remainder was chiefly of Roman origin. Naturally, but a fraction is of Medical interest, yet even that portion is very considerable. Unfortunately enough, it contains too many similar items.
>
> (Wellcome Library, WA/HMM/CM/Col/47 'Gorga')

Photos of the Gorga collection in situ confirm Amoruso's account (Cagiano de Azevedo, 2013, pp. 28–43, fig. 5–8). Among the 'very extensive collection of votive offerings' Amoruso saw

> all the usual limbs, a few internal organs (intestines and thoracic organs) of common type, heads and a couple of larger figures. The number of these objects must be really very large, since I have seen packing cases in several rooms full either of heads, hands, feet or genitals. A more careful and longer inspection might reveal some good specimens. I noticed particularly one uncommon representation of a womb. There are no end of small terracotta representations of animals, fruits etc.

The transaction was not completed until after the war in 1924; several hundred ancient and modern pieces including dozens of anatomical terracottas – notably 'internal organs' – thus arrived in London.

The importance accorded to ancient Italian votives in medical history collections is also reflected in the collection of Doctor Pierre Decouflé which was obviously on a smaller scale than that of Wellcome, bearing more resemblance to Stieda's collection. Around 1960 Decouflé purchased from a Paris dealer a large

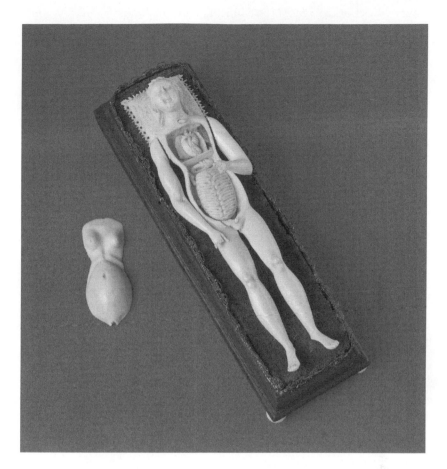

Figure 9.11 Anatomical model, Science Museum, London, inv. A 79643.

Source: Science Museum / Science & Society Picture Library.

Etruscan bust said to come from Canino which can be dated to the third century BC (Figure 9.2). Decouflé placed this votive bust (nicknamed 'Tarquin' by the children of the house) in the drawing room of his residence in Dakar (where he was practising at that time). It was displayed against a red velvet background between two seventeenth-century ivory anatomical models, probably similar to the model in Figure 9.11).

Other ancient medicine-related objects completed the Decouflé collection and the decoration of the doctor's home, of which unfortunately we have no photographs (Haumesser, 2013, p. 19).[13] This juxtaposition helps us understand

13 I am indebted for this information to Mme Decouflé, the collector's daughter, to whom I express my grateful thanks.

Decouflé's view of the *ex-voto*. Decouflé, like his predecessors, did not content himself with compiling a collection, he also devoted assiduous research to the objects it contained, gathering a wealth of documentation which served as material for his various publications on the bust, including the 1964 monograph in which he stressed its exceptional nature (also Decouflé, 1960; 1961). Distinguishing it from the plethora of simpler more repetitive representations of internal organs, Decouflé regarded the bust as an 'anatomical manikin' that reflected the importance of certain Etruscan sanctuaries as places where medical knowledge was transmitted. His published studies explicitly relate ancient open busts to the plates in Renaissance anatomical treatises and to the ivory models of the modern era (Decouflé, 1964, pp. 32–3). He even saw a form of continuity between Etruscan and Latin representations and Renaissance accounts (except for the 'period of regression, or at least of stagnation' in the Middle Ages) and suggested that ancient models may have been known during the Renaissance (Decouflé, 1964, p. 33). Whatever the truth of these hypotheses, the tradition of modern anatomical studies undeniably contributed to shaping the perceptions of Decouflé and the other doctor collectors, prompting them to investigate the accuracy of these ancient *ex-votos* and their place in the history of anatomical knowledge.

The doctors' view

Doctors' interest in anatomical terracotta votives stemmed first and foremost from personal inclination but can also be interpreted from a sociological perspective. Professors of medicine could afford to purchase relatively large collections, all the more so as the pieces (or at least the humblest among them) were inexpensive. Moreover, the doctors' medical training – still based on classical instruction in which the ancient world played a considerable role – enabled them to study these artefacts. Such interaction between the history of medicine and archaeology became fairly frequent from the late nineteenth century (as explored by Adams, this volume). This was not only the case with regard to terracotta votives: the few specimens of dental prostheses found in Etruscan tombs prompted many studies on Etruscan odontology (Naso, 2011), and the skulls themselves were also examined, particularly in the hope (typical of the attitude of the time) of identifying a specific feature of Etruscan skulls in comparison with Roman ones and thereby establishing the origin of the Etruscans. This, for example, was the aim of the work of Georges Cantacuzène who donated a series of skulls found at Tarquinia to the Muséum National d'Histoire Naturelle in Paris (Cantacuzène, 1909; Haumesser, 2013, p. 18).

Discounting a few pioneering studies on marble busts discovered long before in Rome by archaeologists such as Braun (1844) and by doctors (Charcot and Dechambre, 1857), the first diagnosis of the anatomical *ex-votos* was drawn up on the inspired initiative of Wolfgang Helbig. When examining two small busts found in 1885 at Civita Lavinia he asked the opinion of a doctor,

Corrado Tommasi-Crudeli (Helbig, 1885).[14] Although the doctor considered these pieces to have no anatomical accuracy, the debate on the scientific and clinical value of the various representations of organs was launched. In the following years, especially in the early twentieth century, several doctors (who had either collected such items themselves or were simply interested in the subject) devoted studies to Etruscan and Roman votive terracottas as well as those of other ancient Mediterranean regions (Holländer, 1912; the terracottas of Smyrna: Regnault, 1900; 1909a; Greek *ex-votos*: Meyer-Steineg, 1912).[15] After the previously mentioned article by Luigi Sambon (1895a), German doctor Ludwig Stieda published two successive studies based on his personal collection which represented an important stage in the research. Although fairly similar, the first of these studies was geared towards archaeologists and philologists, the second towards specialists in the history of medicine (Stieda, 1899, p. 230). Stieda's work was followed up in the German academic world in particular by Ludwig Aschoff (1903) synthesising the works of Sambon and Stieda, Gustav Alexander (1905) and a more general study by Eugen Holländer (1912, pp. 190–213). The French medical milieu also followed the trend. Particularly noteworthy are the works of Paul Rouquette (1911; 1912a; 1912b) – the first to publish several anatomical *ex-votos* belonging to the Musée du Louvre – and those of Félix Regnault who published certain terracotta votives from the museum of Madrid (Regnault, 1909b) and devoted a general study to the representations of internal organs in 1926. In Italy, Pietro Capparoni (1927) published a study of ancient anatomical *ex-votos* and the persistence of the phenomenon in the modern era, and his richly illustrated study features many pieces from the author's personal collection.[16] The trend was maintained in the early 1960s when doctors devoted major studies to the votive offerings of central Italy. The first was Mario Tabanelli (1960; 1962; 1963) with works on Etruscan medicine, particularly on anatomical representations. It was during this same period that Pierre Decouflé bought the large bust now in the Louvre and began to take an interest in ancient *ex-votos*. Indeed, the interest of historians of medicine has continued ever since: in addition to more specialist articles, reviews of ancient medicine and its representations continue to accord particular attention to the Etruscan and Latin *ex-votos* (Grmek and Gourevitch, 1998; King and Dasen, 2008, pp. 94–6).

---

14 This Italian professor of medicine, who also held political positions (he was a senator for life), was Professor of Pathological Anatomy at the University of Rome at the time and had just published a treatise on anatomy (Tommasi-Crudeli, 1882–84).

15 This type of research was not devoted exclusively to the ancient world; see, for example, Edgar Bérillon's (1911) work on Aztec *ex-votos*.

16 Judging by the illustrations, in addition to modern *ex-votos* from Greece, the collection included a relatively complete typology of Etruscan and Roman *ex-votos*: a head, eyes, an ear, a heart, arms, hands and feet but also a swaddled infant, another category often represented in these doctors' collections. Capparoni (1927, p. 55, no. 1) donated his collection to the Museo Storico della Medicina dell'Istituto Storico Italiano dell'Arte Sanitaria.

Most of the doctors who analysed the open busts concur that there was at least an intention to represent the internal organs of the human body. In several cases, basing their arguments both on *ex-votos* representing individual organs and on the overall arrangement of the organs on the open busts (Regnault, 1926, pp. 141–2; Tabanelli, 1962, pp. 77–8), the authors proposed some relatively complex interpretations, sometimes in the form of annotated diagrams (Regnault, 1926, p. 137, no. 2, figs. 1–4 and 6–7; Decouflé, 1964, figs. 11, 12, 15 and 21). Opinions diverged, however, as to the accuracy of these representations and the degree of anatomical knowledge they represented (Regnault, 1926, pp. 136–7; Tabanelli, 1962, pp. 19–21). Tommasi-Crudeli, the first 'professional analyst,' had concluded that the craftsmen of Civita Lavinia had no form of anatomical knowledge (Helbig, 1885, pp. 146–9), and Regnault (1926, p. 137) even claimed that it was 'easy to prove that the coroplasts who made these *ex-votos* had less anatomical knowledge than a butcher'. Decouflé (1964, pp. 20–9), on the other hand, noted a concern for precision and subtleties of presentation in the most accomplished *ex-votos* which he saw as an expression of precise medical knowledge – even as educational objects or 'anatomical manikins': 'We are convinced, for our part, that the scientific intention inherent in these manikins is evident, and equally sure that they may have been used for teaching' (Decouflé, 1964, p. 37).

The conclusions of Tabanelli (1962, pp. 85–91), who gathered the most abundant material and proposed an overview of the various prior interpretations, were more nuanced. The *ex-votos* sometimes showed an accuracy in the representation of isolated organs, but only rarely depicted the true arrangement of the different organs in the body (Tabanelli, 1962, pp. 77–83). These conclusions seem to accord with the measured opinion expressed by Rouquette (1911, p. 508, quoted in Regnault, 1926, p. 137) with which we fully agree: 'The arrangement of these anatomical plates was not simply due to the modeller's imagination, but expressed contemporary knowledge and commonly held medical beliefs'.

Craft traditions and production centres

The relative coherence of the various large *ex-votos* reflects a shared view of the anatomy of the thorax, visible, for example, in the central position of the heart which protrudes between the lungs on most of the terracottas (Tabanelli, 1962, p. 78). However, the treatment of the anatomical opening itself (its position, shape and dimensions) and the arrangement of the organs vary considerably from one piece to another and can be explained by the importance of local craft traditions. In his anatomical interpretation, Decouflé (1964, p. 32) reached the same conclusion: 'the manikins were produced by *schools of manikins*, as each reflects a personality and a greater or lesser degree of knowledge, with the result that they can be naturally divided into families'. More than a century after the first studies and 50 years after Decouflé's publication the increase in archaeological documentation has confirmed the importance of these craft traditions. Unfortunately, as is only too often the case, we have no precise information about the places of discovery of pieces that turned up on the antiquities market. This is the case, for example, with the large *ex-voto* from the Berman collection in the museum of Civita Castellana (Museo Archeologico dell'Agro Falisco, inv. 137222, h. 53 cm; Moretti Sgubini, 2004, p. 232) and of the bust now in the museum of Ingolstadt (Deutsches Medizinhistorisches Museum, inv. AB/720; Recke, 2013, pp. 1078–9). However, several votives that were discovered during excavations have allowed us to map the circulation of these anatomical models in central Italy with greater precision and in certain cases to attribute former finds of unknown provenance to these various centres.

One of the most important production centres – or at least the best documented – is undoubtedly Veii. Thanks to the concentration of anatomical *ex-votos* in the sanctuary of Comunità, especially representations of open busts and polyvisceral plaques (without equivalent in the Campetti sanctuary which is also well documented), this votive deposit is the best source of material for assessing the specificity of these representations. Lanciani (1889, p. 64) himself proposed a first typology of the votives found at Comunità. This can now be completed thanks to the recent publication of this assemblage (see Bartoloni and Benedettini, 2011, pp. 493–8 for the analysis of the types represented).[17] Six of the various types of *ex-voto* mentioned by Lanciani correspond to complex representations of internal organs, the first four of which are:

- '19. *Dischi ovoidali con visceri*': these are small plaques, the upper section of which represents the heart and three-lobed liver, while the lower section most probably depicts the stomach and intestines. The many recorded examples testify to mass production from a single model (Bartoloni and Benedettini, 2011, pp. 497–8 type H_{15}I–II and pp. 575–9, pl. LXXVIII f–g). Nonetheless, a number of variations can be distinguished, particularly a far simpler version drawn by Lanciani which can be compared with an *ex-voto* in the Wellcome Collection that is almost certainly attributable to Veii (Science Museum, inv. A636803. For similar examples from Veii: Recke and Wamser-Krasznai, 2008, pp. 114–17, no. 22a–23b).
- '9. *Busti dal seno all'ombelico, con ampio squarcio sul petto, dal quale pendono (all'esterno) gli intestini*': this category of smaller bust is well represented in the material from Comunità (Bartoloni and Benedettini, 2011, p. 496, types H_{14}IV–VI and pp. 573–4, pl. LXXVIII b–d).
- '11. *Busti con i seni femminili, e squarcio ovoidale sul petto, in capo al quale è rappresentato il membro virile, e sotto l'utero con altri intestini. Sotto lo squarcio, panneggio che vela il nascimento delle gambe*': the fragment of a large bust in the Stieda collection (Recke and Wamser-Krasznai, 2008, pp. 120–2, no. 25)

17 These types are catalogued as H_{14} and H_{15}. The various series from Veii provide further illustration, especially the pieces acquired in the years following the discovery, which can be attributed with relative certainty to Comunità, although Bartoloni and Benedettini (2011, pp. 13–16) are rightly cautious about the delimitation of the corpus and the attribution of other terracottas to this deposit.

helps us understand Lanciani's description. The chest and the vertical folds in the lower part of the drapery are represented in a distinctive manner. The '*membro virile*' in the upper part actually corresponds to the heart, which is often depicted as a cone protruding between the lungs in the different types of anatomical representation.

- '5. *Busti acefali grandi al vero, con membro virile, seni assai pronunciati, e squarcio sul petto che mostra gli intestini*': the female bust in Lanciani's drawing is a perfect illustration of this type, and the best example is now in Modena (Museo Civico, inv. unknown, h. 61 cm; Tabanelli, 1962, pp. 40–1, fig. 11; Bartoloni and Benedettini, 2011, pp. 494–5, type $H_{14}I$ and pp. 571–2, pl. LXXVII a).

These four types described by Lanciani are well documented, but the other two are still difficult to identify (as stressed by Bartoloni and Benedettini, 2011, p. 493, n. 203). The recent publication of the material from Comunità makes no mention of any pieces corresponding to Lanciani's type 34 '*Figurine muliebri, col ventre aperto che mostra gli intestini*'. It is tempting to think of a fragment of statuette from Veii now in Bonn (Bentz, 2008, pp. 116–17, no. 157) (Figure 9.12). However, it seems possible that Lanciani was referring to the type

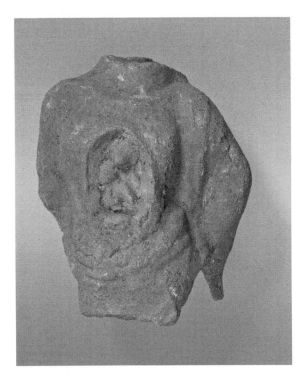

Figure 9.12 Fragment of statuette from Veii, h. 15 cm. Akademisches Kunstmuseum, Antikensammlung der Universität Bonn, inv. D 79.

Source: Akademisches Kunstmuseum – Antikensammlung der Universität Bonn (H. G. Oed).

of small female bust that includes the top of the legs, a smaller version of type 5 (Tabanelli, 1962, fig. 11; Bartoloni and Benedettini, 2011, p. 495, type H_{14}II and p. 572 with a bibliography that mistakenly refers to Lanciani's type 5, pl. LXXVII b–c). This type does not appear to be mentioned elsewhere by Lanciani. The second problematic type is number 18 '*Spine dorsali coi visceri appesi*'. This could refer to the complex form of representation in which the organs are arranged around the axis of the trachea either on plaques (see Figure 9.3) or sculpted in clusters (corresponding to the '*ex-voto animali*' well attested in several Etruscan sanctuaries: Regnault, 1926, pp. 137–9; Tabanelli, 1962, pp. 45–59).

On the other hand, Lanciani makes no mention of other types attested in the deposit. In addition to the small votive busts to which we have just referred (hypothetically identified with type 34) large female, and perhaps also male, busts are attested wearing tunics on which the anatomical plaques stand out. The best example is probably the large bust from the Veit collection (Figure 9.10) known to come from Veii (without further precision), but this type is also attested at Comunità (Bartoloni and Benedettini, 2011, pp. 494–5, type H_{14}III and pp. 572–3, pl. LXXVIII a). In this particularly interesting type of representation, the opening exposing the organs is contained within the clothing (Bartoloni and Benedettini, 2011, p. 495), which Decouflé (1961, pp. 3611–12) compared to certain anatomical plates in Renaissance treatises. Other votives displaying this feature include the female figure from Bonn, Decouflé's bust (Figure 9.2), that of the Berman collection from museum of Civita Castellana and statuettes from Nemi and Fregellae.

The multiplicity of models helps us understand how the craftsmen of Veii worked and to restore these votive offerings to their primary status as artefacts. It is evident that, as with the Comunità deposit, the craftsmen often reused models of simple busts into which they inserted plaques depicting the organs (Bartoloni and Benedettini, 2011, pp. 494–5).[18] This technique is the reason why the various types of busts feature an almost identical arrangement of the organs that is so characteristic of this site. This overall arrangement recurs in a simpler (sometimes almost diagrammatic) form on the separate plaques, which correspond to a different production line. So the differences between the latter and the large busts, rather than reflecting more accurate anatomical knowledge, probably represent greater investment on the part of the craftsmen who proposed various fairly standardised models. It is interesting to note that the most original representations of busts – those that differ the most from the standard model – are also the least sophisticated (Lanciani's class 9) and in a sense occupy an intermediary status between the separate plaques and the busts to which polyvisceral plaques were added.

18 The female bust in the Veit collection corresponds to the model of a bust from Veii now in the Medici collection (Bartoloni and Bocci Pacini, 1996, p. 453, fig. 11b). Another example is perhaps the large bust in the Sambon collection. However, although the attached plaque is of a type that was common in Veii, the other comparable busts are relatively different, perhaps suggesting that the bust came from another deposit at Veii.

The significance of this diversity in commissions from worshippers and in modes of craft production can also be observed at Rome in deposits found along the Tiber, particularly near Tiber Island. The many votives found in the late nineteenth century bring to light a local form of production consisting of fragments of torsos (Figure 9.6) distinguished by a relatively detailed treatment of the various organs: double lining around the almond-shaped section containing the organs, indication of the ribs, location of the heart in the upper part, development of the stomach and twisted shape of the intestines (Pensabene et al., 1980, pp. 235–6). The characteristics of these Roman artefacts distinguish them fairly clearly from the models found at Veii and reflect a separate tradition. They can also be seen on fragments of torso in the Wellcome Collection (Figure 9.13).

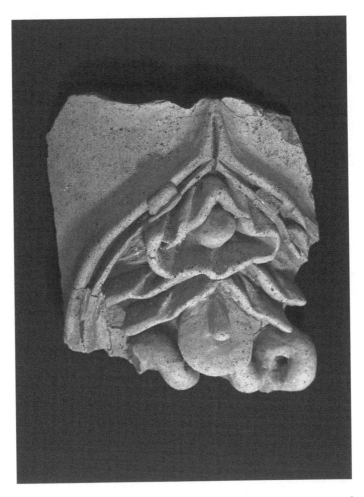

Figure 9.13 a) Fragment of torso, Science Museum, inv. A 634939; b) Fragment of torso, Science Museum, inv. A 635526.

Source: Science Museum / Science & Society Picture Library.

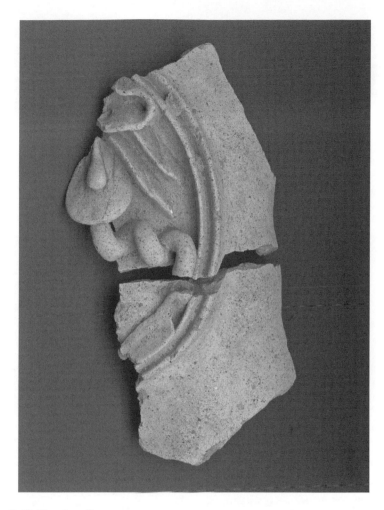

Figure 9.13 (Continued)

Although we lack documentation for these pieces, there is little doubt that they come from Rome and were probably among the late nineteenth-century discoveries. The Roman deposits, like those at Veii, contained isolated polyvisceral plaques which reproduce the model of the open torsos, sometimes in simplified form. Here again the characteristic treatment of the organs makes it possible to attribute a plaque in the Wellcome Collection, of uncertain provenance, to a Roman workshop (Figure 9.14). Other isolated Roman plaques follow the model of Veii, testifying to the circulation of models – and probably of craftsmen too – from one site to the other.

It is less easy to characterise the craft traditions of the other production centres in Latium (see sites listed in Fenelli, 1975; Comella, 1981; Bouma, 1996).

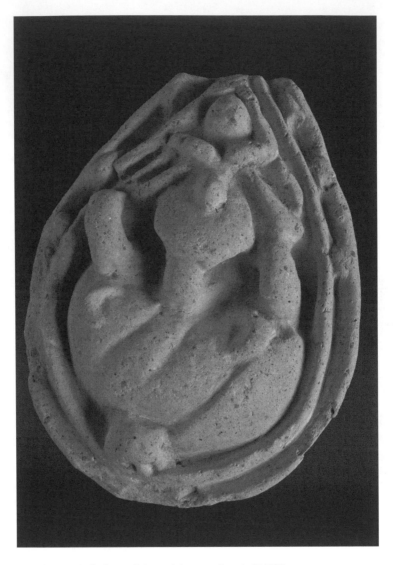

Figure 9.14 Anatomical plaque, Science Museum, inv. A 636802.

Source: Science Museum/Science & Society Picture Library.

The site of Lanuvium is remarkable for the number and concentration of attestations: in addition to the two torsos discovered in 1885 other specimens were found in 2012 in the Pantanacci votive deposit, including 11 small and medium-sized torsos whose publication is awaited for further information about the characteristics of the treatment of the organs (Attenni and Ghini, 2014, p. 159). A similar small torso found in a votive deposit at Aprilia probably belongs to the same craft tradition (inv. SBAL 146824, h. 11 cm; Pannella, 2013, p. 87, no. 114).[19] The small torso in the Wellcome Collection (Figure 9.9) strongly resembles the latter and probably comes from the same area. Praeneste seems to have been another important centre. A small female bust found out of context and attributed to the sanctuary of Hercules (Museo Archeologico Nazionale Prenestino, inv. 13732, h. 18.5 cm: Quilici, 1983, pp. 88–103 and p. 96; Baggieri, 1999, p. 56; Pensabene, 2001, p. 114; Demma, 2002, p. 91; Fabbri, 2010, p. 23) is very similar to two torsos of unknown provenance: the female torso in the Louvre (Figure 9.4) and a male torso in the Getty (inv. 73.ad.83, h. 21.6 cm; Smithers, 1993, pp. 13–32; Recke and Wamser-Krasznai, 2008, p. 137) for which I have also suggested an attribution to Praeneste, although we cannot exclude the possibility that the model circulated (Haumesser, 2013, pp. 20–1). The diversity of traditions at Praeneste is attested by two other examples: an atypical statuette in the Museo Nazionale Romano (inv. 50150, h. 19.5 cm; Regnault, 1926, p. 140; Pensabene, 2001, pp. 367–8, no. 331) and a recently discovered fragment of a male torso (Gatti and Demma, 2012, p. 360). Apart from these two centres the anatomical busts attested in the various sanctuaries of Latium are usually isolated and correspond probably to private commissions made by local craftsmen. Although the overall layout and disposition of the organs are relatively similar and testify to a fairly homogeneous level of anatomical knowledge, the formal approaches are generally different. We also know of a fragment of a life-size bust at Fidenae (Barbina et al., 2009, p. 342; di Gennaro and Ceccarelli, 2012, p. 221) and a small bust at Velletri which disappeared during the Second World War (Melis and Quilici Gigli, 1983, p. 12, no. 366). Other centres in Latium probably produced similar *ex-votos*.[20] The statuettes found at Nemi and Fregellae (the latter during scientific excavations: Coarelli, 1986a) should also be considered.

The example of Veii shows that this type of votive offering also circulated in Etruria. Several other Etruscan sanctuaries have yielded complex representations of organs but few open busts, which, to date, evidence suggests was a primarily Latin type. It also seems likely that the specimens found at the other Etruscan sites should be dated from the period of Romanisation, as was the case with Veii which had long been Romanised by the time the anatomical *ex-votos*,

19 The link between the two sites was confirmed by the discovery of an *ex-voto* in the form of a mouth characteristic of the Pantanacci deposit (Pannella, 2013, p. 87, no. 113; Attenni and Ghini, 2014, p. 156, fig. 7 ('*cavi orali*'), no. 9).

20 Holländer (1912, p. 202) mentions an *ex-voto* of this type supposedly found in a votive deposit at the temple of Jupiter at Terracina and now in the Museo Nazionale Romano. As the museum administrators kindly informed me, such a piece does not appear to belong to the museum's collection. According to Holländer's brief indications, it is a statue with a very large polyvisceral plaque ('*das Medaillon für die Statue viel zu groß ist*'). This could be the statuette published by Pensabene (2001) with all the groups of terracotta votives from Palestrina in the Museo Nazionale Romano. Holländer may have confused Terracina and Palestrina, or was the provenance from Terracina lost and the piece added to a group from Palestrina?

dated generically between the fourth and second century BC, were probably produced. This would explain why the models from Veii tended to travel to Rome rather than to Etruria (Bartoloni and Benedettini, 2011, pp. 789–90). The representations of organs from the trachea to the intestines are in the form of plaques like the previously mentioned examples from Cerveteri (Caere), but also of 'clusters' modelled in the round attested especially at Tarquinia (Ara della Regina: Comella, 1982, pp. 154–7), Bolsena (Pozzarello: Acconcia, 2000, pp. 49–52) and Vulci (Tessennano: Tabanelli, 1960; Costantini, 1995, pp. 76–8 and pp. 100–103). However, the latter site also yielded a fragment of open torso. Here again the arrangement of the organs corresponds to that attested on the isolated polyvisceral plaques from the same site, thereby confirming the use of the techniques employed in Veii or Rome (Tabanelli, 1962, p. 53; Costantini, 1995, p. 103). The bust in the Decouflé collection probably also belonged to the sanctuary of Tessennano. Although it is supposed to come from the nearby town of Camino (Haumesser, 2013, p. 22), the head is very similar to votive heads from the Tessennano deposit (Söderlind, 2002). Likewise, the treatment of the organs, although more meticulous on the large bust, is suggestive of the previously mentioned fragment and the isolated plaques, especially with regard to the representation of the stomach as a round ball sitting above the indistinct tangle of the intestines.

Anatomy and devotional practices: an open question

The attribution of the open busts to a site or even to a sanctuary is insufficient to determine their role within a particular cult. Even in the case of the best-documented deposits, such as those at Veii or Tessennano, it is difficult to identify precisely the deities to whom these offerings were addressed. We have very few examples of inscriptions accompanying an *ex-voto* (de Cazanove, 2009). In most cases the open torso, which accompanied other types of anatomical votive, is certainly related to healing cults. The spread of the cult of Asclepius comes naturally to mind, particularly for the votive deposits surrounding the Tiber Island and for the sanctuary at Fregellae (Comella, 1982–83; Coarelli, 1986a), as do aspects of the Etruscan cult of Apollo (Costantini, 1995, pp. 147–53; Haack, 2007b). However, other more specific practices cannot be excluded as it has been (cautiously) suggested for the sanctuary related to the Comunità votive deposit at Veii (Bartoloni and Benedettini, 2011, p. 494 and p. 788). Interesting information will doubtless emerge from the excavation of the votive deposit at Pantanacci where a large group of open torsos was found in context. As the presence of many other types of anatomical *ex-voto* suggests, a healing cult must have been practised here (Attenni and Ghini, 2014, p. 156 and p. 160). Interestingly, these open torsos, placed near a very particular type of terracotta representation of the oral cavity (if this interpretation is correct), were themselves placed in a cave, an opening in the rock.

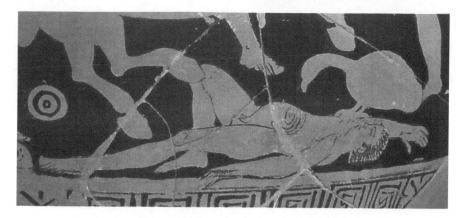

Figure 9.15 Faliscan vase with a dead warrior, fourth century BC. Akademische Kunstmuseum, Bonn, inv. 1569.

Source: After Beazley (1947).

In the absence of precise data concerning their cult value, the appreciation
of anatomical votive busts is centred on their 'artefact' dimension.[21] They were
costly offerings, bearing the same relation to polyvisceral plaques and other
anatomical votives as that of statues and busts to simple votive heads. The
quality of the anatomical representations on the busts therefore depended first
and foremost on the dedicator's spending power and cultural imperatives. The
polyvisceral votives probably reflect a form of general knowledge in Etruscan and Latin societies also apparent in a representation on a fourth century
BC Faliscan vase of a dead warrior whose roughly depicted entrails are being
devoured by a scavenger (Beazley, 1947, pp. 96–7; Bentz, 2008, pp. 32–3; for
the motif see Scheffer, 2006, pp. 507–8 and p. 511) (Figure 9.15). Like the
vase painter, the worshippers and makers of the votive offerings knew that the
belly contained rolls of intestines and bundles of organs. However, the more
detailed and anatomically more ambitious depictions on the large votives reflect
a greater awareness of the different organs which is unlikely to be attributable
to the craftsmen alone. Decouflé (1964, p. 36) suggests that the doctor must
have 'guided the craftsman's hand'. Others see the influence of an awareness of
animal anatomy which was presumably more widespread due to ritual sacrifice
and the observation of the organs (Regnault, 1926, p. 140). The craftsmen who

21 Although the open busts do indeed have equivalents in the modern age, these are more likely to be
found in *ex-votos* and popular devotional practices than in scholarly representations in treatises and
anatomical models. On the persistence of forms of worship between antiquity and the modern age
and the recurrence of forms, see especially Regnault (1926, pp. 148–9), Capparoni (1927) and (with
a Warburgian analysis) Didi-Huberman (1998).

created these high-quality votives probably endeavoured to depict the organs in the greatest possible detail, basing their depictions on common knowledge and perhaps on information gleaned from holders of anatomical and medical knowledge in order to offer (to the dedicator at least, and perhaps to the deity) a precise presentation of the anatomical facts of the dedicator's ailment (Tabanelli, 1962, pp. 86–7). The resulting votive busts must have contributed in their turn to forming a picture of the internal organs in the imagination of visitors to the sanctuaries, and it is essentially (and perhaps only) in this respect that they can legitimately be regarded as anatomical models.

10 Fragmentation and the body's boundaries

Reassessing the body in parts

Ellen Adams

Introduction

This chapter explores the potential range of functions and meanings of anatomical votives by drawing together a number of interrelated themes.[1] The first of three sections contrasts ancient and modern attitudes to the normal and disabled body. It charts the shift from the classical ideal to today's desirable norm. It also considers cultural views towards the more complicated issue of the 'abnormal' disabled body as fundamental background to anatomical votives. The second section considers approaches to healing the body and the role of prostheses as a coping or 'normalising' mechanism. It is argued that ancient anatomical votives served as a form of ritual prostheses, incorporating modern case studies for additional insights into how an individual may react to such aids. These votives are then set against modern Anatomy, which developed during the Enlightenment era, involving a complex dialogue with antiquity. First, this was when British collectors became aware of both ancient and modern anatomical votives from areas of the classical world, and they often formed part of collections of more prestigious antiquities, including classical sculpture. Second, studies of the human body (such as écorchés and anatomical publications) were often framed around the growing corpus of known (and generally fragmentary) classical sculpture.

The concluding section of this chapter examines more closely the relation between the parts of the physical body and the whole, extending to the wider concept of personhood. It develops the contrast made in the previous section between anatomical models and fragmentary sculpture in two ways: the role the latter has had in explorations of disability in modern art, and whether these representations of the ideal should be rendered complete through reconstructions. The term 'anatomical' itself is dissected, as there are many ways to break down the body. A final related theme explores how the body can be moulded into material culture just as objects, like anatomical votives, may represent the body.

1 I am grateful to the organisers of the conference for the invitation and the hospitality enjoyed while in Rome. The paper benefited from the responses of the two anonymous readers and also from comments by Alexia Petsalis-Diomidis.

Exploring the body in parts requires a range of considerations and themes and, in this case, different time periods need to be explored.

Other chapters in this volume have focused on the classical context of anatomical votives, so that outline is only sketched here. However, a form of chronological triangulation is required whereby *antiquity* and its influence on the *modern* are viewed through the lens of the *Enlightenment* period of the discovery and collection of classical anatomical votives alongside other kinds of bodily fragments. During the 'long' eighteenth century of the Enlightenment, notions of the 'normal' body moved away from the classical ideal. This period also witnessed the shift from aesthetic to didactic or 'professional' collections, which drove disciplines in certain directions (for example, sculptural art history, with its fascination with the classical ideal, and surgery, which involves dissection and the construction of anatomical specimens and models). We shall also explore recent developments in Disability Studies to explore notions of the 'complete' body and the relationship between the part and the whole. It is argued that anatomical votives served as a kind of ritual prosthesis; as such, they shed light on notions of the broken body and completeness.

Changing perceptions of the body, normality and disability

Classical ideal to average norms

This section compares ancient and modern concepts of the body in the light of crucial developments since the Enlightenment. The malfunctioning or impaired body is inevitably set against an idea of the able-bodied whole, so fragmentary bodies in material culture, whether anatomical votives or ancient marble sculptures, need to be considered against this framework. Anthropological studies indicate that 'most cultures have notions of a "normal" or "ideal" body-mind', but 'the specific character of those norms and the extent to which they are negotiable varies considerably across and within societies' (Oliver and Barnes, 2012, p. 33). Both antiquity and modernity share an aesthetic engagement with the ideal body form, although these have changed greatly. However, there has been a shift in modern medicine towards an appreciation of the *typical* body grounded in statistics: this is a parallel type of ideal. It has been argued that 'normal', used as a concept of able-bodied or complete body, has been used as such only since around 1840 (Davis, 1995, p. 24). As a concept, it is closely linked to the rise of statistics. The General Register Office was established in 1837 to generate data for the changes in policies resulting from legislation such as the Reform Act (1832) and Poor Law (1834). The *average norm* was the desired goal of study rather than an unattainable aspiration such as the celebrated classical ideal (certain characteristics were ranked, such as intelligence, but the main aim was to blend in; Davis, 1995, p. 27). This quantitative, data-based practice has increased, so that today's medical trials with statistically meaningful numbers of volunteers are a vital part of scientific advancement.

This notion of the norm enshrined in statistics relies on measurement, which was also a concern in antiquity, but we can perhaps note a general shift from art to science. During the Enlightenment, collectors such as Payne Knight recognised that measurement and proportion were key concepts to classical approaches to the body: 'When we speak of the *beauty of the human form*, we mean the pleasing result of well-balanced and duly proportioned limbs and features' (Payne Knight, 1805, p. 12).[2] Polyclitus's *Canon* 'represented the body as a measure of beauty and perfection that was available to all, not only kings and heroes' (Vlahogiannis, 1998, p. 21), but the focus remained on the ideal rather than the normal. The Renaissance sculptor Leon Battista Alberti (*De Statua, c.*1464) was inspired by the classical account of Zeuxis, who attempted to depict the perfect Helen by assembling the best parts of several women (Mansfield, 2007; see also Angelica Kauffman's 1778 painting *Zeuxis selecting models for his painting of Helen of Troy*). However, Alberti's approach was based on measuring the finest women available to him and establishing the 'perfect' average from them all, looking towards the statistical model. Against this backdrop we can discern other similarities and differences between attitudes to disability as well.

Disabled bodies

In all societies, what happens when the body goes wrong is a fundamental concern, and the body in fragments, such as anatomical ritual votives or medical specimens, is a clear nod to that anxiety. The issue of whether a body should strive to be an unachievable ideal or average norm marks an important distinction between antiquity and modernity, but there are also many similarities regarding attitudes to health and disability. This section aims to explore attitudes to disability over time, incorporating modern social theory, ultimately to see how anatomical votives may be reevaluated.

Rose (2003), Garland (2010) and Laes et al. (2013) offer very useful surveys of the evidence for disabilities in the ancient world, but pain, sometimes associated with illness, has generated much more interest overall (for example, Brilliant, 2000; King, 2002; Hughes, 2008; also pertinent here is the reception of classical treatments of pain, for example, Budelmann, 2007). The social standing of disabled people in the ancient world is unclear, and it would be misleading to generalise across time and space. For example, the Spartans checked the 'viability' of newborns, but the Athenians did not prescribe that deformed babies be killed (Garland, 2010). But what if you should encounter deformity and disease later

---

2 The artist Hogarth (1753, p. 13 and p. 21) comments that it is the *relation* between parts that 'is of the greateſt conſequence to the beauty of the whole', criticising the Laocoön for the 'abſurdity of making the fons of half the father's ſize' but with the proportions of grown men. Leonardo's 'Vitruvian Man' would have been a well-known image at the time. The regular rhythms of the body (a palm is four fingers, a foot is four palms, a cubit is six palms, four cubits make a man, a pace is four cubits, a man is twenty-four palms . . .) can be matched in architectural measurements, man's ultimate outer covering and protection against the elements.

on in life? Illness and disability may hit those in their prime, in addition to the degenerating process of ageing, although discussions about the elderly are not necessarily couched in terms of disability (but see Appleby, 2010, p. 52).

The bodily ideals of the Greco-Roman world generated prejudice, and it is widely held that such views form the roots of disablism today (Oliver and Barnes, 2012, p. 56), not least in the idea that the problem is due to the fault or sin of the individual. From literary accounts 'physical disability was a metaphor for punishment' (Vlahogiannis, 1998, p. 14; Vlahogiannis, 2005). In certain cases a ritual confession was made when stricken by illness or accident (van Straten, 1981, p. 101; Potts, this volume). In societies where disabilities are not understood in medical terms, they may be ascribed to witchcraft or a semi-human state and status (Oliver and Barnes, 2012). This places the responsibility for dealing with the disability squarely on the individual; this was their personal tragedy/lot/fault and not society's problem to deal with.[3] However, help could be sought both from doctors and the gods, and the Athenians bestowed limited financial support on those unable to work (for example, Lysias 24.6, cited in Vlahogiannis, 1998, p. 15). Offering anatomical parts at open sanctuaries does not suggest the attempt to cover up the problem, but is a public declaration in order to help resolve the issue.

Hephaestus is one of the few disabled figures of Greek mythology, and he was thrown out of Olympus by Zeus (the myths vary: in some he is thrown out because of his form, in others his limp is caused by the fall; Ebenstein, 2006). Hephaestus is therefore a victim, provoking pity, laughter and awkwardness. Disabled or disfigured people could also incite disgust (for example, Thersites in Homer, *Iliad* 2) and be considered less than human; in modern terms they may be a target of abuse and perceived as a drain on resources if in receipt of extra support. In contrast, Socrates may have been notoriously ugly (arguably an impairment in the Greek world), but his intellect marked him out for special status; he was superhuman, like the Paralympians. At both extremes, subhuman and superhuman, disabled people are neither normal nor ideal in both antiquity and modernity.[4] In terms of considering what a 'complete' person may entail, these extremes stand below or beyond this.

Disabilities have social implications as well as medical, and attitudes to impairments and the associated terminology are culturally specific. There is no single and general Greek word for 'disabled' (Rose, 2003, p. 11), nor did they have our

---

3 Some inscribed dedications may have been made by other family members rather than the afflicted individual, but this was not seen as a social problem.

4 An exception is the disabled hero. For example, E.H. Baily's statue of Lord Nelson in Trafalgar Square portrays him with only one arm and his empty sleeve pinned to his chest. The loss of his arm was a war wound, and the disability is therefore presented as heroic and also minimised by his sleeve being shown pinned to his chest (but with no prosthesis; see also Richard Westmacott's statue of Nelson in the Bull Ring, Birmingham). Baily does not show his other disability, the blindness of his right eye. John Flaxman's portrayal of the hero in St Paul's Cathedral disguises his missing arm and does not depict his blind eye.

specific medical terminology. The Enlightenment was the age of taxonomy: if one could classify the world, one could understand and control it, and medicine and disease was a part of this process. There remains, however, a tendency to speak of 'disability' as a simple category without making even simple distinctions between physical, communicative and mental impairments and also types of illnesses.[5] One might, for example, distinguish between impairments (deafness) and disease and/or pain (earache). Furthermore, it is significant whether the problem is temporary or permanent; in the latter case, the compensatory strategies adopted are likely to have a long-term impact on personality and behaviour. Conventionalised gestures, for example, appear to have been developed for deaf mutes in the ancient world (Plato, *Cratylus* 422e). It is possible to be a perfectly healthy but impaired person who requires certain supports and strategies if they are not to be disabled from participating in society.[6]

This chapter attempts to introduce these issues into classical reception studies while recognising that modern ideas and terminology should not be projected back: crucial differences between the classical and modern worlds exist as well. On the one hand, the modern West is more progressive than the ancient world, and there is a strong sense of the social, shared responsibility in terms of an individual's impairments. However, this is a very recent development, enshrined in Britain in the 2010 Equality Act. On the other hand, it has also been argued that the rise of capitalism and industrialism brought with it increasing segregation of the 'defectives', since there was little apparent room for disabled people in this new way of working (Oliver and Barnes, 2012). 'Able-bodied' refers mainly to being able to work, so how the concept is framed will be closely linked to modes of production. Combined with the impact of industrialism and the increasing separation of work and home, the physical as well as social segregation of 'defectives', particularly in the nineteenth century, may be a historical anomaly.

Disability Studies is a very young discipline in modern sociology (Oliver and Barnes, 2012, pp. 11–12), especially in comparison with studies of gender and race. One recent work, *The Body: Key Concepts*, does not deal with disability or impairment, despite the presence of a chapter entitled 'Bodies and difference', which considers 'the body as central in understanding how social differences, such as race, class, sexuality and gender, pass into our very being and becoming' (Blackman, 2008, p. 59). Disability has yet to be recognised as an inherent and unavoidable (albeit often hidden) aspect of social life, generally leading to socio-political disadvantages. Health and illness are covered briefly (Blackman, 2008, pp. 98–101), but the people who have malfunctioning or absent parts are also

---

5 This chapter focuses on physical rather than mental impairments in line with the physicality of the objects under discussion.

6 The terminology is problematic. It may be useful to distinguish between medical *impairments* and the *disabilities* that may result if sufficient technological supports and/or social adaptation are not provided, which lead to social segregation.

completely missing from such studies. Around 15 per cent of the world's current population is classified as disabled according to the WHO (2011) *World Report on Disability*. This depends on the criteria set (the dialogue is framed within Western views of 'disability' and 'normality'), but it is clear that this group comprises a significant minority in all societies. Each society needs to outline expectations concerning the extent to which these individuals are expected to integrate and participate, and how this is to be achieved. The relevance here for anatomical votives is how these parts are framed within the setting of the complete body, and how they may have served as compensatory strategies or 'ritual prostheses'.

Changing approaches to healing the body

Ancient medicine and anatomical votives

The ancients deployed a wide range of healing strategies. A crude distinction can be made between scientific approaches and those that engaged the gods. Case 3 in the Greek and Roman Life room (69) at the British Museum sets out this contrast well: familiar medical tools are laid out on the left side and the right exhibits votives, including anatomical parts. Despite the use of surgical tools, ancient medicine was framed around the concept of the humours, where health was achieved with a holistic balance of these essences.[7] For example, Galen recommended blood letting in order to mend injured limbs (Rose, 2003, p. 18). Anatomy had been studied in the ancient world – Galen himself dissected monkeys. On the whole, however, the dissection of human corpses was not considered acceptable, with the exception of the work of Herophilus and Erasistratus in the third century BC (von Staden, 1992). The right side of the British Museum exhibit is much less familiar to those visiting the museum today, even though such dedications have been made in Italy in modern times. It is generally agreed that classical anatomical votives signify either requests for healing or gratitude for health (van Straten, 1981; see also the introduction to this volume).[8] They are representations, serving as substitutes for body parts that require special attention. They are also dedications, deposited in the ritual sphere and reaching out to realms beyond the body's experience. It follows from this that a part of the body is singled out because of a disease or impairment, so the object becomes a symbol for that predicament rather than associated with the dedicator's entire body and person.

7 The four humours each had certain characteristics: blood was cheerful, fire and hot; phlegm was slow-moving, air and cold; yellow bile was quick tempered, water and moist; and black bile was melancholic, earth and dry.

8 Hughes (2008, p. 222) points out that this was not the only way a particular part of the body could be signified, as demonstrated by the figurines from Sardinia where the figure points to the affected part with an expression of pain: no fragmentation occurs here. It has been suggested in the Minoan context that a representation of the entire body may also be linked to ritual healing (Peatfield and Morris, 2012, p. 239).

The sanctuaries of the healing god Asclepius were clearly amongst the most popular choice for the deposition of anatomical votives, especially in Greece, and it has been suggested that some sanctuaries specialised in particular diseases (Oberhelman, 2014). So, the Athenian Asclepieion focused on ocular diseases, and the healing sanctuary at Ponte di Nona in Italy paid particular attention to legs, feet and head pains. Turfa (1986, p. 205) points out that the presence of these anatomical votives does not reveal much about the cult practice associated with their deposition (see Roebuck, 1951, p. 116 on Corinth). They were initially displayed on shelves or walls and then buried in trenches or more permanently displayed in other contexts.

The practice of dedicating anatomical votives is particularly common in Etruria and Italy more widely where around 150 relevant sanctuaries have been discovered. In most of these, healing rites and dedications were incorporated and added to other practices, whereas a few sanctuaries appear to have focused on healing (Turfa, 1994, p. 224). Terracotta anatomical votives were particularly common from the fourth to first centuries BC (Turfa, 1994, pp. 224–5). Etruscan and Latin votive assemblages include more examples of internal organs than are found in Greece, including uteri (van Straten, 1981, p. 111; Flemming, this volume). Greek Hippocratic practice included the instruction not to cut into the body, which would discourage any such inner exploration. These representations were in any case stylised rather than realistic – these are far from the teaching tools of the Enlightenment and beyond.[9]

Anatomical votives as ritual prostheses

This chapter suggests that ancient anatomical votives served as ritual prostheses, deployed to render the body whole and healthy again. Because ancient attitudes towards prostheses are so poorly known, we turn to modern case studies in order to gain insights. A prosthesis is a replacement of a missing bodily part, such as a limb or tooth, with an artificial substitute. It may be functional, enabling mobility and walking, for example, or it may be cosmetic such as a glass eye. The latter would support social functionality given the common cultural aversion to physical deformity or abnormality. There is considerable evidence for dental prostheses in the ancient world but much less for 'extremity prosthetics' (Bliquez, 1996). There are literary sources such as Herodotus's (*Histories* 9.37) reference to a wooden foot that Hegesistratus had made following a self-amputation of part of his own (see also Draycott, 2014 for reference to a manufacturer of artificial limbs). Physical evidence is weak, and there is no convincing visual evidence of their use in the iconography (Bliquez, 1996). There is a replacement right leg from Capua made of wood with bronze sheeting which dates to around

---

9 This is not to say that body parts are not ritualised in the modern era as well. Dissection 'was a ritual act, a performance staged for particular audiences within carefully monitored frameworks of legal and religious regulation' (Kemp and Wallace, 2000, p. 23; Bleeker, 2008).

300 BC. Bliquez (1996, p. 2670) concludes that this device did not have a foot attached and could not have performed particularly well as a replacement leg (most similarly afflicted people probably had peg legs). Although this evidence is limited, there may be more indications that the ritual sphere was called upon to provide a different kind of prosthetic device.

While the request/gratitude for healing has long been recognised as the key function of anatomical votives, Hughes (2008, p. 226) has explored how they may also indicate ancient concerns about the metaphorical fragmentation of the body and the relationship between the part and the whole, pointing out that modern patients often describe their bodies in terms of disintegration, not just 'broken' but also 'shattered'. A slightly different way of viewing this is to consider these votives as ritual prostheses and to explore the cultural norms associated with the use of such aids. Ancient Greek votives were nearly always depictions of the healthy body part; in other words the desired 'normal' fragment is depicted with no sign of the 'problem' (Petsalis-Diomidis, 2006, p. 210 and p. 220). In this case, the object is not a representation or likeness of the damaged part, but a replacement with a healthy part. Some of these anatomical votives may serve as a memory aid for a lost part, such as an amputated leg (van Straten, 1981, p. 76).[10] The healed, or to-be-healed, votive might also embody divine favour and presence, becoming the miraculous part (Petsalis-Diomidis, 2006, p. 211; 2010, p. 238 and p. 262). Anatomical votives could offer pilgrims a sense of regaining control over their bodies (Petsalis-Diomidis, 2010, p. 260); they can therefore be viewed as a psychological prosthesis or an aid to feeling whole. In this case they should be viewed as an aid to the healing process, not as an aid to compensate for a disability such as modern limb prostheses. But in both cases the aim is to 'make whole again', to achieve the elusive and culturally specific 'normality'.

Aids serve as a material acknowledgment of illness and disability, issues that often cause social embarrassment and are therefore ignored and brushed out of sight. A prosthesis is both an extension of the body and a replacement or sub-stitute of a part of an 'incomplete' person; at least, the latter is in the view of the etic observer. The emic, experienced view is more variable. Ideally, prostheses are enablers but inert and controlled by the user (setting aside the very modern development of cyborgs). It may be the case that if the aid is successful the user's attention is only drawn to it when it goes wrong or becomes 'disabled' itself: the aid is incorporated into a 'natural', 'normal' whole (Sobchack, 2006, p. 22, where users of such objects are described as 'posthuman'). Or it may be the case that, if

---

10   In contrast, 'the anatomical votives of antiquity could be seen to represent the disaggregation of the dedicant's whole body (rather than the amputation of a single part of it)' (Hughes, 2008, p. 225). Rose (2003, p. 20) suggests that preventative amputation was not conducted at all in the Classical Greek world, but a range of medical approaches were available, and she points out literary references to this procedure (for example, Plato, *Symposium* 205e). The Roman Celsus (7.33.1–2; quoted in Garland, 2010, pp. 134–5) describes the technique in some detail.

an individual is denied the right to feel normal as a disabled person, the pressure to normalise has other damaging consequences.

Modern prostheses add insights into the attempt to 'normalise', whether to the classical ideal or average norm discussed earlier. Although the sophisticated and personalised prostheses built today were not available in antiquity, the responses of two successful, outspoken and, in different ways, integrationist modern individuals shed light on such 'normalisation' aids for disabled people. Both Alison Lapper and Oscar Pistorius were born disabled, with the latter undergoing below-the-knee amputation before learning how to walk. Lapper (2005, p. 32) describes her visits as a child for fittings for prostheses in a lukewarm manner, stating: 'they wanted to normalize us. I can see that from an able-bodied person's point of view that is the logical thing to do'. Oscar Pistorius (2012, p. 119), the 'fastest man on no legs', stated that he would not necessarily desire 'normal' legs if they could be magically applied; the disability, or rather the manner in which one responds to it, becomes too engrained in the personality, lifestyle and worldview to be so suddenly dismissed. In an apparently effortless 'normalisation' process, he relates childhood routines with his brother: 'every morning while Carl put on his shoes, I would slip on my prostheses; it was all the same to me' (Pistorius, 2012, pp. 22–3). He would then go and play rugby. Since the events of Valentine's Day 2013, when the golden boy of the Paralympics killed his girlfriend Reeva Steenkamp, the world has been quick to judge the possible strain that this lifelong normalisation programme inflicted. In other words, if success is measured by the extent to which one may appear normal, thereby denying both the disability and actual body in question, this may in itself be unhealthy.

The hypothesis here is that dedication of anatomical votives is also an attempt to achieve the ideal of 'normality', albeit with an appeal to other worlds rather than the attempt to integrate and be integrated into the surrounding society, by adapting the body to become normal. Anatomical votives may be seen as ritual prostheses, the material manifestation of the divine support mechanism. Although it is true that 'a basic, unchallenged assumption is that they [anatomical votives] are petitions or thank-offerings for healing or fecundity' (Turfa, 1994, p. 224), this does not exclude further meanings involving personal identity and attitudes towards disability. This approach may indeed be less blunt and traumatic than the physical and literal process of normalisation as practiced in modern medicine. Further considerations of the discovery of these objects and how they are perceived in the modern world are important, precisely in order to avoid projecting back modern values.

The emergence of modern anatomy and the ancient world: a dialogue

Many accounts have charted the link between ancient and modern medicine, particularly with reference to the humours, but the issue of anatomical votives is less well explored. Here we return to the Enlightenment. Early collectors were aware of classical healing votives from ancient literature (for example,

Livy 45.28.3, mentioned by Middleton, 1733, p. 24).[11] Middleton (1733, p. 23) explored the apparent continuities between classical paganism and popery, including the dedication of anatomical votives: '*Legs, Arms*, and other *Parts of the Body*, which had formerly been hung up in their *Temples* in Teftimony of fome divine Favour or Cure effected by their *tutelary Deity* in that particular Member [original emphasis]'.[12] Half a century later, Sir William Hamilton, the great collector of Greek vases, published an account of rituals performed by Italian peasants at Isernia, suggesting that the practice was a continuation of ancient ones (Hamilton, 1786[1894]; Davis, 2008).[13] This continuity may have caused chronological confusion: Sigmund Freud, who possessed phallic amulets, apparently believed that they were ancient, but they were probably modern (Davis, 2008, pp. 107–8). In a discussion of amulets of genitalia worn by women in Herculaneum and Pompeii, Payne Knight (1894[1865], p. 28) states that: 'The female organs of generation were revered as fymbols of the generative powers of nature or matter, as the male were of the generative powers of God'. The idea of a single deity or 'Creator' is projected back, apparently justified by the explicit link with eighteenth-century practices. It is therefore imperative to consider these objects in the light of how and when they were discovered, as contemporary values may have been projected back on account of this apparent continuity.

Hamilton's collection of modern wax phalli, which was placed in the British Museum in 1785 (Jenkins and Sloan, 1996; Grove, this volume), also possesses classical anatomical votives such as terracotta uteri from Charles Townley's collection (acquired in 1814) and a marble votive relief with eyes from Lord Elgin's collection (acquired in 1816) (see Turfa, 1986). These were incidental artefacts in the major collections based on 'higher' forms of art. Hamilton's main focus was Greek vases, whereas Townley's was free-standing sculpture and Elgin's was architectural sculpture. The market and aesthetic value of anatomical votives were far beneath these classes of material. Rouse, in 1902, stated of the votives: 'this custom shows how low the artistic taste of the Greeks had already fallen, but it is not without its moral interest' (Rouse, 1902, pp. 210–1). In Britain, this great age of collecting classical antiquities coincided with the period when anatomy, enabled by dissection, became a recognised and respected discipline in its own right. It has even been suggested that sculptural fragments 'implicitly legitimated the collecting practices of anatomists' (Alberti, 2011, p. 72). The relationship between classical art and anatomy is traditionally close (Adams, 2009, pp. 84–7).[14] For example, both professions are as much tactile as visual, although

---

11 There are more references to votive tablets recording treatments, for example, at Epidaurus (Strabo, *Geography* 8.6.15; Pausanias, *Description of Greece* 2.27.3) and also dedicating locks of hair (for example Pausanias, *Description of Greece* 2.11.6; see Draycott, this volume).

12 The dedication of anatomical votives was later discovered to go back to the Minoan peak sanctuaries of the second millennium BC (for example Myres, 1902–03).

13 Recently Carabelli (1996, p. 48) described Hamilton's Isernian phalli as survivals, 'residues of a senseless, archaic and taboo custom: anatomical fragments in a landscape without figures'.

14 Hume (1758, p. 285) argued that the 'anatomist presents to the eye the most hideous and disagreeable objects; but his science is useful to the painter in delineating even a Venus or a Helen . . . Accuracy is, in every case, advantageous to beauty . . . .'

it is not now allowed in either art or anatomy museums to touch exhibits. In an early display Quatremère 'compared the Elgin Room of the British Museum to the sculptor's workshop, where it was possible to lay hands on the sculptures' (Jenkins, 1992, p. 27). The practice of dissection is one that offers the opportunity to learn how to feel around the body. Both disciplines also explore the body through its parts, and in both questions of how to restore or preserve the 'complete' body are raised.

Anatomy attempts to understand how the body works and its pathology by cutting into it, separating the parts from the whole and analysing them in turn. Not striving for beauty (regarding the discussion on measurement and proportion earlier) the value of this process was to understand the workings of the parts of the body and the diseases that targeted particular areas. From the seventeenth century onwards, the body was perceived as a machine (Tarlow, 2011, p. 71). Particular areas were seen and treated as distinct working parts serving the whole (Bell, 1797, pp. 1–2; Sawday, 1995, p. 32). This is completely different from the traditional classical idea of humours with their view of holistic health. During the Enlightenment, Anatomy was therefore one rare profession that was engaged with breaking away from the classical tradition, particularly with protagonists such as John Hunter, who reacted bitterly against the stranglehold that Classics had over education in the Eighteenth century (Adams, 2013).

His brother, William Hunter, was also a surgeon and was more receptive to the Classics. Once, for example, when he received the body of an executed criminal, instead of performing a full dissection where the bodily parts would be separated, he flayed the cadaver to reveal the muscles and tendons, and set the body in the pose of the Dying Gaul. Smugglerius is the name given to the original 1776 écorché and the copies made of it (the sculptor Agosino Carline made the initial bronze cast to preserve this figure, although only plaster casts of this survive today; Edinburgh Cast Collection, n.d.) (Figure 10.1). The

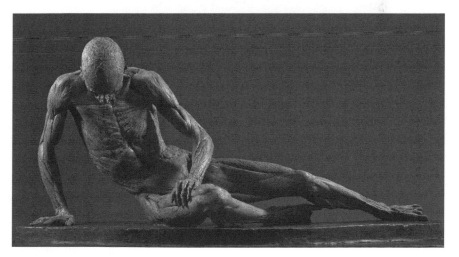

Figure 10.1 Smugglerius, artists William Pink and Agostino Carlini, plaster cast, *c.*1834.
Source: Royal Academy of Arts, London.

Dying Gaul, now in the Capitoline Museum at Rome, was first recorded in 1623 and became one of the most famous images of classical sculpture. The majesty of the piece is little diminished by the fact that the left leg is pieced together from shattered remains or that the right arm is reconstructed. The cool gleam of the polished marble hints at the body within, with muscles and veins running beneath the surface, while the wound in his side offers a more direct, literal window into it. Lifelike, but with his life ebbing away, the sculpture inspired the immortalisation of a man of uncertain identity (probably a highway robber named James Langar) and his transformation into material culture, a work of art and a training tool for future artists.[15]

Similarly, Cheselden's *Osteographia* included a plate of a skeleton with the same proportions and attitude as the Belvedere Apollo (Figure 10.2), the sculpture

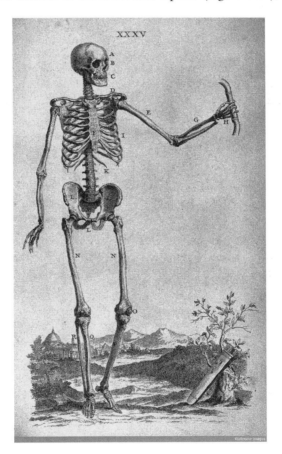

Figure 10.2 William Cheselden, *Osteographia* (1733).
Source: Wellcome Library, London.

15 While the classical statue provides 'a paradigm of physical and aesthetic perfection', écorchés reveal 'myological insights which were otherwise available only to the professional anatomist and student

championed by Winckelmann as the best example of the classical ideal. Cheselden's *Osteographia* was published in 1733, the same year that Middleton composed his letter regarding ritual continuity in Italy. Cheselden's skeleton is 'reconstructed', complete with left hand (here holding part of a bow) and right lower arm, which are missing from the sculpture (these were restored by Giovanni Angelo Montorsoli, a pupil of Michelangelo, and later removed). A tree stump supports a quiver to the side of Cheselden's skeleton echoing the larger tree trunk (a kind of prosthesis?) needed to support the sculpture. The Apollo is nude apart from sandals, *strophium* and cloak, but Cheselden's skeleton, stripped to the bone, offers a new interpretation of 'nude'. Since the Renaissance, the autonomous individual has been defined as 'a bounded corporeality that is assumed to "end" with the skin' (Fraser and Greco, 2005, p. 12), but more detailed explorations of the body challenged this view. The boundaries of the body are fluid at various different times of the life/death cycle, and this is highlighted when the body is placed under the spotlight and studied in the context of an anatomical collection. Like a surgeon, the art critic has a tendency to zoom in on the body, appreciating parts before reconstructing and reevaluating the whole (Davis, 2005). Barrell (1989) has discussed this concerning the early eighteenth century; still in the twentieth Bernard Ashmole (1929) was advocating an approach to sculpture that began from multiple photographic close-ups: 'The value of the photography of details was that, like the child's telescope of a plain cardboard tube, it helped them to see things more clearly because it cut out the objects around'.

The history of the body has very much been couched in the history of ideas. For example, Descartes's earlier ideas of the self-contained, clearly bounded and presumably able-bodied individual (with a distinct mind) gained universal acceptance during the Enlightenment. Anthropological work on partible and permeable bodies has more recently sought to challenge this view of bounded agents, notably with the use of non-Western examples (Strathern, 1988; Busby, 1997; Graham, this volume). But we can also locate non-Cartesian attitudes to the body within the Western sphere. Since the Enlightenment the presentation, display and viewing of various kinds of body fragments have also helped to form modern perceptions and in just as important ways. Attitudes to the body are also processed when constructing representations and models, such as anatomical votives, and building collections, such as antiquities or anatomical specimens. This side of the story requires as equal weight as the abstract theorising (Adams, 2009). These collections challenge the perception of the distinct, bounded and 'complete' individual by constantly renegotiating the boundaries between parts and the whole. Classical antiquities, from the high sculpture to the lowly anatomical votives, have helped to shape this process. Issues surrounding the fragmentary body will be considered further in the following section.

---

of medicine' (Postle, 2004, p. 55). In real life William Hamilton inverted the Pygmalion myth by presenting his wife Emma as a painting or sculpture during her 'Attitudes' (Coltman, 2006, p. 66).

The fragmentary body

Much scholarship has concentrated on the decomposed, fragmented dead and their relationship with objects (Chapman, 2000), but here we consider anatomical objects that concern the disabled living. It is argued that we need to move beyond a focus on the body part and pay attention to the implications for a person's impaired body having to deal with a malfunctioning or absent part. We consider not just the relationship between the sum and the parts, but also whether all parts are working; this is a much more subtle yet everyday consideration than the ultimate life/death dichotomy. It has been suggested that the ancients were unaware of the idea of literary fragments. Their texts survive as fragments, but they themselves do not appear to have 'thought of *making* fragments or to have thought about the fragment as a possible form' (Wanning Harries, 1994, p. 12). This is not completely true, and certainly not so concerning material culture. The idea of busts representing important individuals was very much present in the ancient world, and anatomical votives are clearly constructed *as* fragments. Indeed, one aspect of the classical legacy is the idea of the intended fragment as well as the accidental, broken one (Petsalis-Diomidis, 2010, pp. 260–1 refers to novels and medical and physiognomical writings that work on the theme of the fragmented body).

The use of busts, one of the most familiar forms of intended fragment, in Enlightenment collections and libraries is worthy of note. Busts tend to provide commentary on inspirational accomplishments (Baker, 2003, pp. 145–6; Opper, 2003), standing for achievements beyond the specific individual. For example, in the Hunterian and Soane Museums today you can see busts of the two protagonists (John Hunter and John Soane) surveying their kingdoms. As a way of achieving immortality the busts stand for their contributions to surgery and architecture, respectively. This is more or less the opposite of our main focus: the intended fragment of the anatomical votive presented with reference to underachieving/damaged parts. Anatomical votives are one kind of body part; by setting them against other ways in which the body has been fragmented, we may explore the complex relations between the parts and the whole and the body's boundaries. Both art and anatomy explore the body through its parts. If sculptural fragments are synecdochic for individuals, then medical museums accommodate body parts that become metonymic for particular areas or diseases.

Fragments of antiquity: classical sculpture

Over time, the collections of the British Museum were set within a hierarchy of cultures: classical sculpture is at the top, with the Parthenon marbles taking pride of place.[16] The modern perception of classical sculptures as 'art' can veil

---

16 This is perhaps most strikingly seen in James Stephanoff's (1848) vision 'An Assemblage of Works of Art, from the Earliest Period to the Time of Phydias'. Payne Knight (1805, p. 5) commented on 'the precious remains of Grecian sculpture, which afford standards of real beauty, grace, and elegance in the human form, and the modes of adorning it'.

their original, ritual context as votives. In the case of sculpture the 'beautiful fragment becomes a place where pagan worship is turned into the religion of art' (Barkan, 1999, p. 123). More importantly this medium is notably fragmentary. The main survivals are broken marble sculptures, because the vast majority of bronze sculptures have been deliberately broken/melted down and recycled. These marble remains did not need to be complete in order to be considered perfect. Art students studied as standard the Belvedere Torso, one of the most famous sculptural fragments (Petherbridge, 1997, p. 69; John Flaxman, the neo-classical sculptor, turned a copy of the Torso Belvedere into a 'complete' Hercules and Hebe, but overall the piece was admired and copied as a fragment). Fuseli's image of 'the Artist moved to despair by Roman ruins' of 1778 is a famous comment on the awe that ancient sculptural fragments could inspire (Nochlin, 1994). Besides the great works of art with missing limbs, such as the Belvedere Torso, a single foot and hand can be enough to send the wretched imitator into a state of depression: these past achievements are irreplaceable and unrepeatable. This section considers this response to broken classical sculpture in contrast to attitudes to the disabled.

One of the most famous examples of a fragmented statue is the Venus de Milo. A recent discussion of the statue outlines how her distinctive silhouette resonated with Romantic sensitivities (Prettejohn, 2012, p. 82). To discount the fact that her disability is interwoven with our aesthetic enjoyment is both common and worrisome. Rarely is it pointed out that the lack of arms renders the woman 'a symbol of sexual allure without the ability to resist' (Davis, 2005, p. 172, who notes that a replica of the statue in the film *Boxing Helena* highlights the theme of sexualised powerlessness). Art historians such as Kenneth Clark (1956) hardly discuss absent limbs, and phantom limbs pervade the literature; it is supposed that the viewer somehow normalises the object in their mind. As Barkan (1999, p. 207) notes,

> If the *Torso Belvedere* is the paradigm of ancient sculpture and Michelangelo is the tragic hero of the fragment, that is because he based his career in part on what could be imagined and not seen or because he appeared so often to be unable to produce statues more complete than the fragments that inspired him.

Moreover, 'one is dealing not simply with art history but with the reception of disability, the way that the "normal" observer compensates or defends against the presence of difference' (Davis, 1995, p. 133). This unspoken practice is perhaps akin to that of dedicating healthy votives of damaged body parts, willing the body to the ideal complete form – a form of restoration.

It has been artists, not academics, who have really engaged with the fragmentary nature of classical sculpture, although references to these creative responses have appeared in scholarly publications. Nead (1992, pp. 77–9) refers to Mary Duffy's work *Cutting the Ties that Bind*, and Squire (2011, pp. 27–8) cites Mark Quinn's *Alison Lapper Pregnant* (Figure 10.3): the latter 'looks to the Venus de

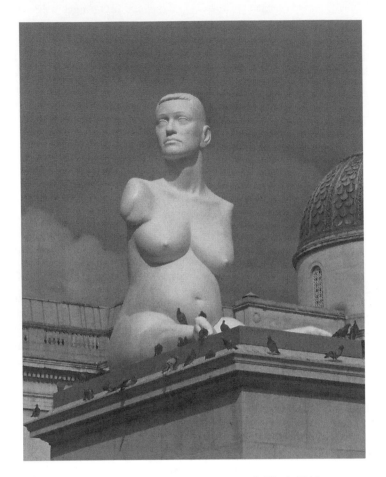

Figure 10.3 Alison Lapper Pregnant by Marc Quinn, Fourth Plinth 2005.

Source: Photograph by Michael Squire.

Milo in an effort to champion a wholly *non*-canonical image of beauty (or indeed disability)' (see also Lapper, 2005, p. 186; Quinn, 2006). Millett-Gallant (2000, p. 66) takes a wide range of examples in some depth, comparing these artworks to modern approaches in medicine including anatomical displays. Beyond these contrasting values of beauty and (dis)ability, these modern artworks challenge the notion of 'wholeness' as being a person equipped with all limbs and faculties (they are nude to reinforce this). Duffy deliberately sets her own armless body in contrast to the 'amputated' Venus de Milo, but it is Duffy's body that is 'whole, complete and self-bounded' (Nead, 1992, p. 79): in modern terms it is offensive to describe her as 'less' of a person because of these missing parts. Duffy and Lapper are complete, albeit disabled, in a way that the Venus is not; this is the reversal of the perception of disabled people as partial and classical sculpture as the perfect ideal. Mark Quinn's series *The Complete Marbles* is a direct reference to the fluid nature of the body's boundaries with respect to personhood: these disabled individuals are strong, not broken.

One dilemma that faced collectors was whether to reconstruct antiquities and make them whole again. The Enlightenment was the golden age of restoration, although there was less enthusiasm for this in Britain than the Continent. For example, Haskell and Penny (1981, p. 103) describe how in 1809 Edward Daniel Clarke celebrated the fact that the caryatid he acquired from Eleusis would not be 'degraded by spurious addition' as had commonly occurred in France, although Antoine-Chrysostôme Quatremère de Quincy's recommendation that the Venus de Milo's arms not be restored was followed (Prettejohn, 2012, p. 81). Antonio Canova declined to restore the Parthenon marbles brought to London by Elgin, unlike Bertel Thorvaldsen who extensively restored the Aegina marbles. Indeed, the Parthenon marbles' fragmentary state, unattractive to a private collector, 'became the proof of their superiority to the merely commercialized objects traded on the art market for purposes of interior decoration' (Prettejohn, 2012, p. 58). Likewise, Payne Knight was careful to make sculptural additions clear in his illustrations, separating the ancient and the modern.[17] Authenticity is valued over completeness, whereas the anatomical votives strove to restore full health.

Anatomy and the relationship between the part and the whole

The question of restoration or the need to preserve human remains add further depth to what we might mean by a complete, perfect, natural or even normal body: 'All the fragments on display together make up a multi-authored, diseased body . . . no longer an individual . . . but rather a *dividual* body, that is, composed of different separated parts from different sources' (Alberti, 2011, p. 8). Preserving anatomical specimens and attempting to avert the natural process of decomposition and fragmentation is the opposite of sculptural reconstruction; both negotiate the question of the body in parts from different angles. Anatomical votives can either be of body parts with external boundaries such as legs and ears or of internal organs such as intestines or uteri. Bare skin is the body unclothed, but skin also serves to veil the body, and dissection could be a 'form of unveiling' (Jordanova, 1989, p. 99). The Hunterian Museum has examples of the human body in various stages of undress, indicating that the term 'anatomical part' is also rather fluid. Anatomical representations can strip layers of the body as well as divide the body into distinct parts. The Evelyn tables represent a different form of delayering: the mapping of veins on the wooden slab, for example, is one type of body part. Sculpture may depict veins, tense muscles and flesh but it is

---

17 He states, for example, with reference to Townley's Discobolus, that 'our duty to the public obliges us to acknowledge that the head appears to us to have belonged to a totally different figure' (Payne Knight, 1809, p. OIV). There is an irony here since the Roman marble sculptures Payne Knight was discussing were so often copies – a different kind of artistic restoration and representation.

essentially recording the body's surface. However, 'when the artist represents the surface of the body he or she is engaging, consciously or unconsciously, with questions about the body's borders, and the relations between its interior and the exterior' (Fend, 2005, p. 311).

The 56 plates in Cheselden's *Osteographia* (1733) depict life-size examples of each bone with how they are assembled together in smaller scale. Cheselden was not only interested in the relationship of the part to the whole but also provided illustrations of diseased bones and the growth of bones.[18] This logic extended to medical collections: 'curators re-compose these partible bodies as encyclopaedias of disease – not the partible living persons anthropologists observe, but like them multi-authored dividuals composed of relations, with different parts from different places' (Alberti, 2011, p. 71). Modern anatomical collections strive to illustrate the typical body but need also to explore the abnormal, diseased or impaired parts as well (for example, Joseph Merrick, 'the Elephant Man', was measured and recorded for use by the medical community and to stimulate interest for those viewing him as freak: Petsalis-Diomidis, 2010, pp. 114–15). This focus on the diseased part has a considerable overlap with anatomical votives and contrasts, or even contradicts, the holistic Hippocratic approach to health. There is therefore a specific focus on a particular part of the body, as with anatomical votives. Figure 10.4 inverts this tendency for comic effect. Set

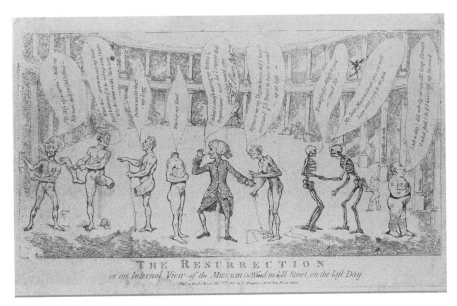

Figure 10.4 Thomas Rowlandson, 'The resurrection or an internal view of the museum in W-d-m-ll Street, on the last day' (1782).

Source: Wellcome Library, London.

18 In the house-museum of John Hunter the theme of the 'growth of bones' juxtaposed embryos with the colossal skeleton of the Irish Giant, or Charles Byrne (Chaplin, 2009, p. 375).

in the anatomical collection of the physician and dissector William Hunter, it depicts the people missing parts rather than the parts themselves. 'Where's my head?', asks one bemused subject.

But the relationship between the part and the whole and what it means to be a 'complete person' is medically very complicated. The skin will grow over amputated limbs so that person will become a disabled individual but is still 'complete' if differently so, and the complete embryo also forms part of its mother. William Hunter's *The Anatomy of the Human Gravid Uterus* (1774) explores the lives of embryos and the relationship between baby and mother (Figure 10.5). Increasing understandings of how pregnancies work contributed

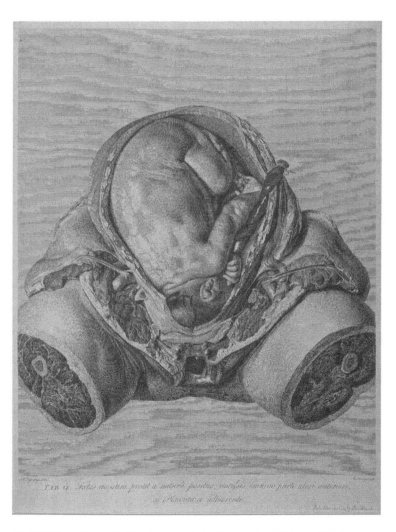

Figure 10.5 William Hunter's *The Anatomy of the Human Gravid Uterus* (1774).

Source: Wellcome Library, London.

not only to notions of personhood and when life begins, but also to whether the baby is viewed as part of the woman or a complete, separate person with associated human rights. Votives depicting uteri and swaddled babies – the helpless newborn – suggest that the point at which children become recognised as 'fully human' may have also been a consideration in antiquity (Graham, 2013; chapters by Flemming and Glinister, this volume). The relationship between the body part and the whole was a concern in antiquity as well as modernity, even if it was articulated differently.

Naming the body

In terms of the 'complete person', a sense of identity is vital, and this extends well beyond the physical body. Names are a central part of personal identity, and collectors attempt to identify both sculpture and body parts. Classical fragments may become more complete if they can be named – and they were valued more; for example Payne Knight (1809, Pl. VII) commented on a marble suspected to be of Venus, 'though it has nothing of the exquisite and voluptuous beauty, which later artists, in ages of greater refinement, attributed to the goddess of love' – the main desire is actually to name these figures.[19] This approach can still be seen today. The *Spinario*, or boy with the thorn in his foot, is a complete bronze sculpture but 'what renders it fragmentary is rather the mystery of the boy's identity' (Barkan, 1999, p. 150). Pliny identified art on the basis of concrete evidence, such as signatures rather than artistic style or special characteristics, as became more common in the modern era (Isager, 1991, p. 156). Naming sculptures also affected the theatricality of the collectors' house-museums, since the sculptures were turned from anonymous props into named actors, forming part of the assembly (Adams, 2009).

We attempt to breathe life into sculptures by naming them, while body parts may be easier to cope with if presented as anonymous material culture rather than the butchered remains of an individual. This objectification and materialisation of disease is paralleled in the anatomical votives, both ancient and modern. Over time, and especially with the introduction of the Anatomy Act (1832), the use of the poor (who could not afford burials) for dissections as well as criminals encouraged general anonymity (Tarlow, 2011, p. 90). Pathologists 'dismembered the dead body and preserved the fragments, whether by injection or by storage in fluid, *fashioning them into material culture*' (Alberti, 2011, p. 3; my emphasis). Anonymity facilitated the objectification and commercialism of body parts, although if patient details and case history were known then specimens could reach a better price (Alberti, 2011, p. 93). Body parts provoke even more fascination when a name can be attached to them, whether religious

---

19 Payne Knight (Pl. VIII) also refers to the common confusion between Bacchus/Plato and Socrates/Silenus in sculpture, revealing the frustration felt by art historians as they attempted to identify artworks.

relics, famous individuals or infamous criminals. One example is the skeleton of Charles Byrne, the Irish Giant. It is documented that he explicitly did not want to be paraded in death as he was in life, a professional freak, but John Hunter thwarted his attempt to be buried at sea. Most anatomical votives are nameless, but some provide an example of an associated inscription that names the dedicator. Petsalis-Diomidis (2010, p. 265) argues that the visual votives contained the identity of the dedicant. They certainly serve as a part of them but alone are unable to signify the individual too specifically. Naming provides a bridge between the body and the person as a whole and is therefore the final layer when thinking about the relationship between parts and the complete individual.

Conclusion

Hughes (2008) is right to look for further meanings of anatomical votives beyond the request or desire for healing. But in order to do so, we need to dissect modern uses of the terms we now labour under, and the cultural conditions under which these objects were found. Ideas of what comprises a 'complete' body may be culturally specific, but we can gain insights from the recent growing body of theory in Disability Studies and art that explores this explicitly. The notion of disability implies that a function is missing, but there is a contradiction in that the individual's experience is not necessarily less 'full', with a truncated identity. However, compensatory strategies are often deployed in order to reach or imitate the perceived norm, and it is argued here that anatomical votives have this role as ritual prostheses, attempting to achieve 'normality' through the healing process.

It has also been argued that the relationship between the part and the whole can be fruitfully explored through a comparison of art and anatomy. Art represents the human, while dissection transformed human remains into material culture through the process of preservation; the two disciplines seem to approach the same themes from different angles. Both the artist (or craftsman) and the surgeon engage with questions about the body's boundaries; these are many and fluid depending on context. The debates about whether to reconstruct sculpture highlight the importance of authenticity over completeness and different values of perfection. This paper has drawn a contrast between the average norm as processed by the rise of statistics and the unattainable classical ideal. Disabled people are not literally partial in personhood, but neither are they seen as normal or ideal. The focus on a body part, such as an anatomical votive, reveals the full complexities of this issue.

11 Votive genitalia in the Wellcome collection

Modern receptions of ancient sexual anatomy

Jen Grove

In West London, in what was once a Post Office headquarters and is now a vast storage facility for the capital's biggest museums, lies what remains of a collection put together by the American-born pharmaceutical millionaire Sir Henry Wellcome. Wellcome opened his 'Historical Medical Museum' in 1913, and his vast collection is famed for its extraordinary quantity of medical memorabilia. The objects now in storage attest to a collector with exceedingly wide-ranging interests who ran a 30-year campaign to gather material from across the world and throughout history relating broadly to the history of medicine and far beyond (Turner, 1980; Arnold and Olsen, 2003; Hill, 2004; Larson, 2009). At times topping the British Museum's annual expenditure on acquisitions, Wellcome acquired around one million items by the time of his death in 1936 (Skinner, 1986, p. 383).[1] In the stores we find historical contraceptives, eighteenth-century European 'parturition chairs', medieval torture equipment, Middle Eastern smoking pipes and Victorian bedpans painted with amusing poems to entertain the user. One large room is dominated by a collection of around six hundred Roman and Etruscan anatomical votives in terracotta, clay and marble. At the time of writing a fraction of these objects are on display at the galleries of the Wellcome Collection in London within a small exhibition which showcases a selection of the 'vast stockpile of evidence about our universal interest in health and the body' which Wellcome acquired (Wellcome Collection, n.d.). These votives appear in the shape of body parts such as heads, hands, feet, legs, mouths and eyes, as well as more unusual forms such as hair, tongues and torsos opened up to reveal internal organs (for discussions of hair and of open torsos see chapters by Draycott and Haumesser, this volume). The focus of this chapter,

---

1 An edited version of this article by Skinner appeared under the name Lawrence in Arnold and Olsen (2003). At the time of writing there is no definitive published catalogue of Wellcome's collection as it existed in the early twentieth century. That which was not dispersed after Wellcome's death is now on permanent loan to the Science Museum London and listed online at http://collectionsonline.nmsi. ac.uk/ [Accessed 13 February 2015]. Unless otherwise stated, material described in this chapter is part of this latter collection and is referenced with a museum number beginning with the letter A or R.

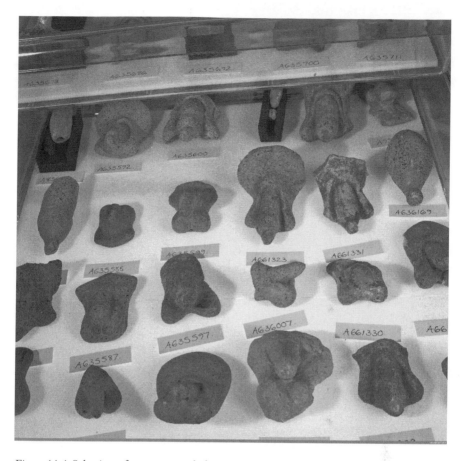

Figure 11.1 Selection of terracotta and clay Etrusco-Roman votive male genitals.
Source: Wellcome Library, London.

however, is the collection of 65 penis-shaped votives – either a dismembered organ or attached to a groin with hair and testicles – (Figure 11.1) as well as a group of six simple triangle-shaped vulvae (Figure 11.2). Wellcome's collection is used as a case study to examine the modern reception of ancient votive genitalia. Wellcome's story introduces a new dimension for understanding modern responses to such sexually explicit remains of the ancient past, challenging prevailing historiographies focused on censorship and suppression. His deliberate engagement with such material within a context which posed itself as genuinely scientific in outlook prompts us to explore the intersections between material culture, the classical past and modern debates around medicine, sexuality, religion and wider human culture.

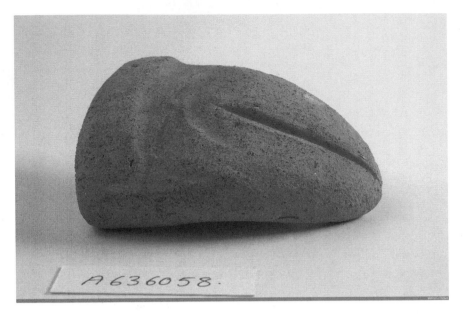

Figure 11.2 Terracotta Roman votive vulva, 200 BC–AD 200. Science Museum/Wellcome Collection, A636058.

Source: Wellcome Library, London.

Challenging the 'secret cabinet' model

Where collection histories of Roman and Etruscan votive genitalia in modern times exist they have tended to focus on their censorship and suppression, in particular their appearance within the so-called 'secret cabinets' of European museums (Johns, 1982, p. 59; de Caro, 2000a, p. 17). The most famous of such cabinets is the 'Gabinetto Segreto' of the National Archaeological Museum, Naples. Since the late eighteenth century this special collection, or its forerunners, has housed classical antiquities featuring sexual imagery from the excavations of the nearby ancient cities of Pompeii and Herculaneum and has been subject to various levels of restricted access (for a history of the *Gabinetto Segreto* and the politics surrounding its opening and closing see de Caro, 2000b; Fisher and Langlands, 2011; Beard, 2012). A number of votive genitalia (as well as votive breasts and uteri – types also collected by Wellcome: Figures 6.6 and 11.3) were brought into the collection in the 1860s from an excavation at the ancient city of Cales, north of Naples (de Caro, 2000a, p. 17). Votive genitalia have also been identified as one of the features of the British Museum's own 'secret' collection (Johns, 1982, p. 59). Sexually themed material from across this institution was kept together from at least the 1830s in a segregated area with restricted access that came to be known as the 'Secretum' (Johns, 1982, pp. 29–30; Gaimster, 2000).

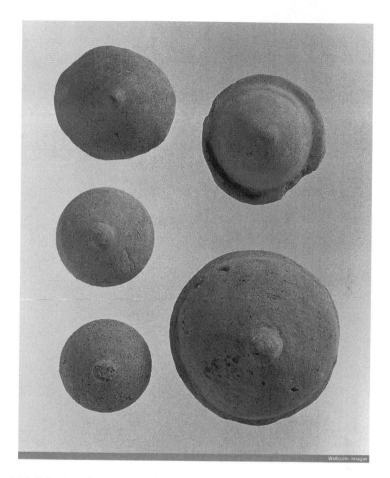

Figure 11.3 Selection of terracotta and clay Etrusco-Roman votive breasts. Science Museum/ Wellcome Collection, A2502/1936, A2502/1936, A2529/1936, A2531/1936 A10945.

Source: Wellcome Library, London.

The enduring notion of these clandestine repositories set up to deal with supposedly 'difficult or troublesome artefacts' (Frost, 2008, p. 31) from the ancient world has led to perceptions of the modern treatment of ancient sexual imagery being dominated by notions of censorship and repression (Johns, 1982, pp. 29–30; Kendrick, 1987; Gaimster, 2000; Varone, 2001, p. 15; Clarke and Larvey, 2003, p. 28; Frost, 2007; 2008; 2010). Recent research, however, has begun to problematise this historiography. In 2011, Fisher and Langlands challenged the 'censorship myth' which has developed around the Naples *Gabinetto Segreto*, demonstrating that it was not created initially to lock out of sight permanently the great numbers of offensive objects as soon as they were found at Pompeii and Herculaneum. Rather, restricted access to certain objects began on an ad hoc basis, and once an official 'secret' collection had been created it was accessed regularly, widely known about and deliberately added to, sometimes for the purposes of creating a scholarship about sex (Fisher and Langlands, 2011). As we have seen with the example of the votive genitalia, material was added piecemeal to the collection, perhaps to create a more comprehensive picture of ancient attitudes to sexuality. The appearance in Wellcome's collection of votive genitalia as well as a large number of phallic figures and amulets (Figure 11.4) and other sexually themed antiquities of the type found in these 'secret' collections

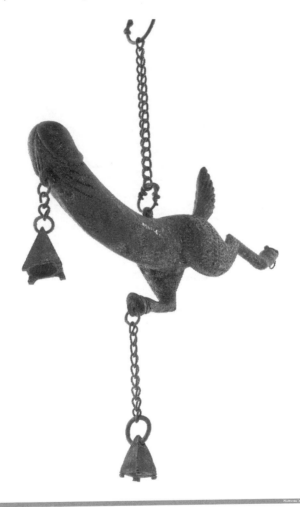

Figure 11.4 Solid bronze *tintinnabulum* in the form of a phallus with hindquarters of a horse, suspended by a chain, with pendants attached at base, Italy, 100 BC–AD 100. Science Museum/Wellcome Collection, A154056.

Source: Wellcome Library, London.

(for example, a ceramic oil lamp decorated with an image of a man and woman having acrobatic sexual intercourse: Museum No. A665703) also suggests a different model of treatment. They were deliberately and systematically sought out as important specimens for a project which ambitiously attempted to re-create the history of human health through the display of objects (Skinner, 1986, p. 399; Larson, 2009, pp. 88–90).

Despite Wellcome's reputation as a 'magpie' collector, records show that there was a clear collecting policy which included the acquisition of votive genitalia. The Wellcome Historical Medical Museum (WHMM) opened its doors in London's Wigmore Street in 1913 with the aim of presenting 'the history of medicine and allied sciences throughout the world from prehistoric times' (WHMM Handbook, 1927, p. 1, WA/HMM/PB/Han/20).[2] Items from Wellcome's collection which it displayed included medical apparatus through the ages, such as birthing forceps and the surgical saw; material relating to central figures in the development of medical science, including antiseptic pioneer Joseph Lister; reconstructions of historical workshops of 'quacks', chemists and apothecaries across the world; and a large 'ethnographical' display reflecting the medical practices of so-called 'primitive' cultures, both historical and contemporary, with which the British empire was increasingly connecting (Turner, 1980; Larson, 2009). Wellcome's collection has frequently attracted attention for its seemingly endless variety of material, which often appears to go beyond the remit of the historical-medical. Joan Braunholtz, who worked at the museum between 1928 and 1932, recalled later that 'Sir Henry was . . . buying through his agent anything and everything, almost regardless of its connection with the history of medicine – coaches, carriages, prams, African spears, skeletons, porcelain, Japanese netsuke all arrived almost daily in huge consignments' (Braunholtz to H.J.M. Symons, 29 July 1985: WA/HMM/ST/LAT/A.29). As comments from L.G. Matthews, the director of the Wellcome Foundation from 1944–1960, suggest, there is a notion that Wellcome 'had started as a genuine collector but it had become a magpie collection. . . . He lost the medical and historical science theme and would collect anything' (quoted in Gould, 2007, p. 14). Together with such accounts of indiscriminate collecting there is an oft-repeated story of shrewd dealers who would offload unwanted material onto Wellcome by combining it in group lots at auction with items they knew he could not resist (Turner, 1980, p. 37 and p. 42; Russell, 1987, p. 21; Larson, 2009, p. 83). If the Roman and Etruscan votive genitalia had been brought into the collection by these incidental methods this would present no challenge to prevailing notions about the modern reception of sexually themed antiquities. Other collection histories have described their discovery by horrified archaeologists, reluctant acceptance by museums and hurried removal by anxious curators into special locked rooms (Johns, 1982, pp. 20–32; Kendrick, 1987, p. 6; Carabelli, 1996, p. 1

2 All references beginning with 'WA/HMM' refer to archival material relating to the WHMM held by the Wellcome Library.

and p. 129; Gaimster, 2000). In this atmosphere the idea of deliberate acquisition of such material seems incongruous. This squeamish response to ancient sexual imagery is often identified with the height of European 'Victorianism' in the 1860s (Johns, 1982, pp. 28–31; Gaimster, 2000) but is thought to have continued until at least the mid-twentieth century if not beyond (Johns, 1982, p. 32; Gaimster, 2000; Frost, 2010, pp. 140–1). In fact, the reverberations of previous generations' supposed prudishness in dealing with ancient sexuality is thought to obscure our proper understanding of ancient depictions of sexuality even in the modern day (Johns, 1982, p. 35). My research in the archival records of Wellcome's museum (now accessible in the Wellcome Library) reveals, however, that votive genitalia together with a vast range of other sexually themed artefacts were not treated as embarrassing acquisitions to be secreted away, but rather were acquired deliberately and systematically to be studied and displayed prominently in the museum. As Gislaine Skinner has argued, there is evidence that despite his enthusiasm Wellcome in fact had a distinguishable collecting policy and kept close control over what was acquired: 'the enormous (but not limitless) diversity of items was certainly intentional' writes Skinner (1986, p. 395, n. 79; see also Engineer, 2000, p. 396). It is very clear that this applied to the acquisition of the votive genitalia.

'Stalking' the votive genitalia

Before even opening his museum Wellcome had already acquired a good number of ancient penis and vulva-shaped votives. Several of these were purchased along with dozens of other anatomical shapes as part of a collection of Italian medical antiquities. This collection had been put together in the late nineteenth century by another London-based producer of pharmaceuticals-turned-collector, Oppenheimer Son and Co Ltd. Much of Wellcome's wider collection is frustratingly lacking in provenance; however, the records show that many of Oppenheimer's votives had been gathered from an ancient deposit found in 1887 on the Via Carlo Botta in Rome, possibly the site of the temple of Minerva Medica mentioned by Cicero and other authors of the Republic (Sambon, 1895b; for the votive deposit see Gatti Lo Guzzo, 1978). Other Oppenheimer votives came from the Temple of Maternity near Capua as well as the former Etruscan sites of Tarquinia, Civitavecchia, Lavinium and Veii (Sambon, 1895b; WHMM Handbook, 1920, p. 33: WA/HMM/PB/Han/17; some votive genitalia later acquired by Wellcome came from Tiber Island, Rome: WHMM Handbook, 1920, p. 33).

The acquisition of the Oppenheimer collection in 1910 was a great coup for Wellcome. The WHMM's first employee and conservator Dr Charles John Samuel Thompson declared that he had been 'stalking this collection' for some years (Thompson report, 18 November 1910, 'Sambon Collection': WA/HMM/CM/COL/87). It was already known to the medical community and coveted by other historical medical collectors, having been displayed previously at the British Medical Association annual meeting in Bristol in 1894, where the votives were declared to be the highlight of the collection along with a group of Roman surgical instruments, and it was reportedly of interest to the Royal College of Surgeons who were to become one of Wellcome's biggest rivals in historical-medical collecting (Sambon, 1895a; Larson, 2009, p. 103). A report by Thompson to Wellcome explains that a representative from the Oppenheimer firm approached him 'in a mysterious way' and asked him if he were interested in buying the collection (Thompson report, 18 November 1910, 'Sambon Collection': WA/HMM/CM/COL/87). It was requested that Thompson should pretend to be a private collector, as Messrs Oppenheimer had expressly stated that the collection should not go to Wellcome. The report does not explain why but it may have been prejudice against an American collecting in Europe or a dislike of the multimillionaire's already zealous collecting tactics (Larson, 2009, p. 97). The two carried out an elaborately clandestine operation in which Thompson played nonchalant so as not to let on how much he wanted the purchase and, true to reputation, as he boasted to Wellcome in his report, Thompson managed to secure the collection at two-thirds of what he considered its true value and a third of the price which Cambridge University had previously offered (Thompson report, 18 November 1910, 'Sambon Collection': WA/HMM/CM/COL/87). Wellcome declared that he was 'very thankful' to have it and that it filled a 'very important place' within the collection (Wellcome's handwritten notes on Thompson report, 18 November 1910, 'Sambon Collection': WA/HMM/CM/COL/87). This document is typical of the type of detailed report which Wellcome insisted on from his growing staff of collectors (see Engineer, 2000, p. 396; Larson, 2009, p. 72 and p. 116). These reports, together with Wellcome's responses to them (which appear mostly as scribbled notes in the margins), provide clear evidence that he kept a close eye on acquisitions, ensuring that his collectors were seeking out material that he especially wanted and that this included votive genitalia.

The group of votive genitalia from Oppenheimer, while substantial, had been acquired by Wellcome within a larger group of other votives and as part of an even wider collection of Italian medical antiquities. As proof of Wellcome's particular interest in sexually themed ancient material archival records show that he and his collectors went on to deliberately add to the collection of penis and vulva-shaped votives (as well as breasts and uteri) by purchasing them individually from auctions and private collectors. Like much of the classical material in Welcome's collection, a large number of the votive genitalia were acquired at the turn of the 1930s as part of Wellcome's newly developed 'international policy' which saw him investing serious money and energy into collecting abroad (Larson, 2009, pp. 232–3; on the wider classical collection see de Peyer and Johnston, 1986: much of the material arguably goes beyond what I have established as Wellcome's extremely wide definition of the 'medical-historical'). Wellcome employed a dedicated overseas collector, Peter Johnston-Saint, a well-connected ex–Indian Army General who used adept networking and shrewd collecting skills to acquire thousands of items for Wellcome in Europe and the Middle East (Engineer, 2000, p. 396; Arnold and Olsen, 2003, p. 108–10; Larson, 2009, pp. 232–3). Johnston-Saint's meticulous report writing, which had secured him his role as 'foreign-secretary', as Wellcome jokingly referred to him (Arnold and Olsen, 2003, p. 109), provides an invaluable record of visits to foreign collectors, dealers and markets and of the sort of material which he had been instructed to seek out. Johnston-Saint purchased dozens of penis-shaped votives as well as a number of vulvae, breasts and uteri in Rome and Florence, as well as acquiring hundreds of other ancient objects featuring sexual imagery in both Europe and the Middle East. For example, in 1929 Johnston-Saint visited the 'wonderful private collection' of a 'Signor Cafiero' in Florence. Johnston-Saint describes 'an old gentleman who was very fussy about having his things moved or handled and consequently was very difficult to deal with' (Johnston-Saint Travel Diaries, January–April 1929, entry 23 March 1929: WA/HMM/RP/JST/B.3). Despite these difficulties he managed to secure some 'very important material' for the museum, which included two terracotta models of male genitals along with several Roman surgical instruments, 12 bronze phallic amulets, some 'instruments for flagellation', an artificial hand, a 'curious African figure' and a speculum (Johnston-Saint Travel Diaries, January–April 1929, entry 23 March 1929: WA/HMM/RP/JST/B.3). On the same trip Johnston-Saint visited several of his regular dealers in Rome and reported to Wellcome the purchase of another votive marble penis together with a pottery breast and a uterus (WHMM accession notebooks '1–1362', entries A292, A295, A519: WA/HMM/CM/NOT/1).

This deliberate and prolonged acquisition of votive genitalia challenges not only Wellcome's reputation as a haphazard collector, but more importantly, the paradigm of censorship and repression currently associated with the modern reception of sexually themed antiquities. In fact, the archival material shows that Wellcome saw the *Gabinetto Segreto* in Naples in particular not as a solution for dealing with difficult archaeological material once reluctantly accepted into a collection but as a model for building a world-class collection of sexual antiquities. Johnston-Saint's reports tell us that he visited and studied the material in this 'secret' collection and then used this knowledge in putting together a collection for Wellcome to match – or even to better – its contents (Johnston-Saint Travel Diaries, January–April 1929, pp. 19–20: WA/HMM/RP/JST/B.3; February–April 1930, p. 41 and p. 55: WA/HMM/RP/Jst/A.7; for the *Gabinetto Segreto* as a desirable museological asset see Blanshard, 2010, p. 32). The Wellcome museum did not accidentally acquire votives shaped as sexual parts of the body and then deliberately suppress them; rather it invested significant monies and energy into actively seeking them out.

The 'scientific museum' and the 'science of sex'

The context in which such material was deliberately gathered for the WHMM encourages a new model for thinking about the display and discussion of sexually related ancient material in museums in this period, looking beyond suppressive and repressive responses towards engagement with it for the purposes of serious research. From the beginning Wellcome declared his project to be 'strictly professional and scientific in character' ('Historical Medical Exhibition

London', 1903, p. 1: WA/HMM/PB/HAN/1). At the opening of the museum he announced: 'In organising this Museum my purpose has not been simply to bring together a lot of 'curios' for amusement. This collection is intended to be useful to students and useful to all those engaged in research' ('XVIIth International Congress of Medicine, London, 1913. Historical Medicine Museum of the Section of the History of Medicine', p. 23: WA/HMM/PB/Han/13). Here Wellcome employs the language of the 'scientific institution', a museological model developed in the late nineteenth century in which the systematic categorisation and display of material culture came to be viewed as vital data for understanding the world and especially the history of human culture (Murray, 1904, p. v; Skinner, 1986, pp. 389–90). This was positioned as the antithesis of an older method of organising collections, the so-called 'cabinet of curiosities', perceived by these later curators as a ragbag of disparate artefacts which were displayed without any order and meant simply to amuse and entertain visitors (Murray, 1904, p. 226; Hooper-Greenhill, 1992, p. 7 and p. 79). The best known proponent of the 'scientific museum' is the nineteenth-century archaeologist, ethnologist and collector Augustus Pitt Rivers, who insisted on the importance of gathering together, classifying and comparing large amounts of material culture to demonstrate his theories about the cultural evolution of humanity (Chapman, 1985; Bowden, 1991). In the early twentieth century Wellcome named the Pitt Rivers museum at Oxford University his 'closest counterpart' and emulated its mission to treat collections of museum objects on 'scientific' lines ('Oral evidence, memoranda and appendices to the final report', 1929, p. 39: WA/HSW/OR/L.5; Skinner, 1986, p. 391–3 and p. 399; James, 1994, p. 335; Larson, 2009, p. 67, p. 76 and pp. 88–90). Wellcome insisted that the WHMM was not meant for 'popular entertainment, to gratify those who wish to view strange and curious objects' ('Oral evidence, memoranda and appendices to the final report', 1929, p. 107: WA/HSW/OR/L.5). It is likely that he felt defensive about his huge and varied collection, much of which could arguably have found a place in an old 'cabinet of curiosities' including such gruesome items as tattooed human skin (Object No. A530, probably dated 1899, France) and shrunken heads (Object No. A642477, acquired in Venezuela in 1936). Ancient anatomical votives had featured in 'cabinets of curiosities' too. There is a reference to them in this context from 1729 by man-of-letters Conyers Middleton (1729, p. 23). As we have seen, these objects also appeared in the 'secret' collections of European museums from the mid-nineteenth century. The 'secret cabinet' model has much in common with the 'cabinet of curiosities' in the way it has been critiqued by later commentators. Like late nineteenth century curators' disapproval of what they perceived as the unscientific 'cabinet of curiosities' model, in recent times curators have criticised the 'secret cabinet' for diminishing the academic value of the material housed within it. Stuart Frost (2008, p. 31) of the British Museum argues: 'By segregating material either formally or informally nineteenth and twentieth century museums supported the notion that there was something wrong, unnatural, or "pornographic" about this material and stifled research'. Catherine Johns, then of the British Museum, suggests in her seminal book of 1982 on ancient sexual imagery that 'it would have been impossible until quite recently to display or discuss an *ex voto* in the form of a penis in the same way as one in the form of a foot. Such a distinction is academically invalid' (Johns, 1982, p. 59). In the Wellcome museum votive genitalia were not segregated within special collections but discussed and displayed openly alongside nonsexual votives (including feet).

The 'secret cabinet', like the 'cabinet of curiosities', has also been perceived as having more to do with 'gratifying' the visitor and providing them with a voyeuristic peek at extraordinary artefacts than any serious research purpose. Historical claims of erudition by visitors to restricted collections have been viewed with scepticism by later observers. There is an enduring image of the nineteenth-century elite gentleman 'pornophile' who claimed to be able to respond in a detached scholarly way to sexual imagery but who was really covering up his lascivious interest in viewing naughty pictures (Funnell, 1982, p. 58; Johns, 1982, p. 28; Godwin, 1994, p. 22; Carabelli, 1996, pp. 10–11 and p. 112; Gaimster, 2000; Lyons and Lyons, 2004, p. 59; Janes, 2009, p. 122; for a critique of this characterisation see Fisher and Langlands, 2011, p. 310). While it is impossible, and actually quite unhelpful, to try to distinguish between intellectual and emotional responses to museum material, Wellcome's museum – which set itself up as an antidote to any and all unscholarly 'gratification' in engaging with material culture – helps us to think beyond clandestine titillation and toward other motivations in the modern interest in sexual antiquities. Although some research has drawn attention to serious academic study of sexual antiquities from at least the time of their mass modern discovery in the eighteenth century (Carabelli, 1996; Davis, 2010; Fisher and Langlands, 2011), Wellcome's interest should be seen as part of the developing specialised and increasingly 'scientific' study of sexuality developing in the late nineteenth century. It is increasingly being recognised that this new 'sexual science' or 'Sexology', although known for its 'medicalisation' of sex embraced the methodologies and evidence of history, archaeology and anthropology (Fisher and Funke, 2015). The collection and study of sexual antiquities by these sex researchers for the purpose of better understanding human sexuality is only just beginning to be researched (see Funke, 2015 on Magnus Hirschfeld; the majority of research has focused on Freud's ancient collection: Davis, 2001, pp. 249–50; 2008; Armstrong, 2005, p. 20; Burke, 2007, p. 36–7.

This new 'scientific' study of sexuality gave researchers licence to deal with certain subjects and material in a more frank way than would be possible in a public forum. Wellcome's museum was officially closed to the public, believing as he did that 'most people visit museums simply as "stragglers"' ('Oral evidence, memoranda and appendices to the final report', 1929, p. 107: WA/ HSW/OR/L.5). In this way it did create certain restrictions on viewing the sexual material which it displayed. It did not allow the kind of free, public access to view sexuality of the past that has been called for in recent museological discourses. However, Wellcome's motivation was not to censor the material out of a prudish response to its sexual content but rather to enhance the scholarly credentials of his collection. Furthermore, despite his mandate that only researchers and medical students should be allowed entry, the records show that a wide range of visitors came to the museum, including parties of schoolchildren and the then Queen Mother ('WHMM Reports to WBSR': WA/HMM/RP/HMM/1 and WA/HMM/RP/HMM/2). Although these visitors may have received directed tours, they could hardly have missed the model penises and vulvae which, as we will see, were displayed in the centre of the main hall of the museum. Neither a seedy private collection nor a 'secret cabinet' within a public museum, Wellcome suggests an alternative model for the modern museological treatment of sexual artefacts.

'Interesting and dependable pathological data'

The votive genitalia were deliberately acquired as important evidence in debates around humanity's wide-ranging response to health. They are crucial to our understanding of Wellcome's broad definition of 'medical history', which incorporated both the biomedical and the anthropological. Firstly, these objects were valued as evidence of ancient pathological and anatomical knowledge. In the late nineteenth century anatomical votives had begun to be 'diagnosed' by medical historians, believed to depict the particular disorder that the dedicant had been suffering from (see Haumesser, this volume). The Oppenheimer collection of anatomical votives which Wellcome acquired had been important in this development: the agent whom Oppenheimer had employed to collect for him was Louis (Luigi) Sambon, an Italian medic who later became well known for his work for the London School of Tropical Medicine (Larson, 2009, p. 103).[3] After collecting them Sambon had published an article on the ancient anatomical models in 1895 in the *British Medical Journal*. 'From the vast quantities of anatomical terra-cottas bought and dedicated by patients of all classes,' he writes, 'we can surmise that gross anatomy was thus far better known to the general public [in the ancient world] than it is at the present day' (Sambon, 1895a, p. 148). Of the votive vulvae, Sambon suggests that many show the 'characteristics of childhood, at other times, those of puberty' (Sambon, 1895a, p. 149). The study of votives, he later wrote, also reveals far more 'interesting and dependable pathological data of antiquity than could be gathered from the written records' (quoted in Haddow, 1936, p. 25). Many of the models of male genitals he collected show a 'long foreskin completely covering the glans penis' which indicate 'phimosis from venereal disease' (Sambon, 1895a, p. 148). This condition whereby the foreskin cannot be retracted (the name of which

---

3 In 1903 Wellcome purchased a personal collection from Sambon which contained 24 votive offerings in terracotta, bronze and marble featuring a particularly 'unique' votive vulva: 'Sambon, Louis', 1913–21: WA/HMM/CO/EAR/845.

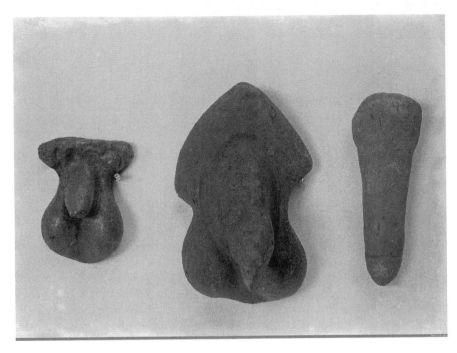

Figure 11.5 Selection of terracotta and clay Etrusco-Roman votive male genitals, the middle possibly depicting the condition phimosis.

Source: Wellcome Library, London.

derives from the Greek word meaning 'muzzled') is no longer associated with sexually transmitted infections. An elongated foreskin appears often in Roman and Etruscan votive male genitalia as well as on ancient phallic figures (Figure 11.5). Wellcome's museum clearly adopted this biomedical understanding of the votive genitalia, especially after Sambon himself came to work there in 1919 ('Sambon, Louis', 1913–21: WA/HMM/CO/EAR/845). The WHMM handbook of 1920 (WA/HMM/PB/Han/17, p. 20) highlights a display of 'rarer Roman votive offerings of anatomical, pathological and obstetrical interest' and draws the visitor's attention to numerous examples of 'pudenda' and male genitals. These latter are identified in the handbook as showing a 'long, swollen prepuce' suggesting phimosis from sexually transmitted infections (WA/HMM/PB/Han/17, p. 20). In criticising the supposed prudish responses to ancient votive genitalia of previous generations, Johns (1982, p. 59) has insisted that these objects should be considered 'no more obscene than . . . a diagram in a medical textbook'. Taking its lead from Sambon's scholarship the Wellcome museum treated sexual votives in precisely the way Johns prescribes – not as 'pornography' but as illustrations of ancient medical knowledge.

The 'religio-medico'

Whereas Sambon and Oppenheimer had approached these objects from an almost exclusively biomedical perspective, Wellcome's extremely broad definition of the 'historical-medical' meant that he also valued them as cultural records of an ancient religious practice. This was part of his wider interest in the way humanity has historically turned to the supernatural in order to solve health problems (Mack, 2003). In this Wellcome and his museum were influenced by contemporary anthropological theory such as the work of physiologist and psychologist W.H.R. Rivers, under whom the museum's second conservator, Louis Malcolm, had studied at Cambridge. Rivers identified a conflation of religious and medical practice in many cultures (Rivers, 1924; see also Mack, 2003, pp. 220–21). The masses of objects classified as 'Religio-Medico' material made up a substantial part of Wellcome's collection and included, for instance, wooden African and Native American masks labelled as used in 'shamanic' healing (for example Object No. A645087), Buddhist and Shinto shrines of deities associated with curing disease (for example Object No. A199221) and thousands of 'amulets, charms and talismans' from ancient Egypt to contemporary London (for example Object No. A666092). This collection was an essential part of Wellcome's presentation of the cultural history of health outside of the Western so-called 'rational' biomedical tradition. He explained: 'in all the ages the preservation of life and health has been uppermost in the minds of living beings, hence the omnipresent medicine man and the religio-medico or priest-physician' ('Oral evidence, memoranda and appendices to the final report', 1929, p. 108: WA/HSW/OR/L.5). The Roman and Etruscan votives were classified within the 'Religio-Medico' collection and were joined by other objects which demonstrated the universal practice of dedicating something to a deity in thanks or in appeal for an issue relating to health or the body. For instance the collection of *retablo*, nineteenth- and early twentieth-century tin roof tiles from Mexico and Italy dedicated in thanks to the Catholic Saints and painted with images of accidents which the dedicant had survived (for example Wellcome Library no. 44885i). Wellcome's interest in the classical version of this ritual practice is evidenced in his acquisition of fourth century BC Greek plaques showing Athenians bringing anatomical votives to healing shrines on the Acropolis (object nos. A3526 and R7451/1936; on the healing shrines see Aleshire, 1989) (Figure 11.6).

In modern scholarship which aims to 'correct' the supposed damage done by our 'irresponsible predecessors' (Johns, 1982, p. 10) a key idea is that the act of censoring sexual artefacts obscured their 'original' ancient meaning: grouping material together purely on the basis of its sexually explicit appearance (that is, treating it as 'pornography' for sexual titillation in one definition of this term) detracts from the variety of functions such material appears to have had in daily life in the ancient world, including in religious contexts (Johns, 1982, pp. 10–11; Gaimster, 2000; Varone, 2001, p. 15; Clarke and Larvey, 2003, p. 28; Frost, 2007, p. 69; 2010, p. 144). In categorising objects shaped as the penis and vulva as 'votives' and part of a 'Religio-Medico' collection, Wellcome clearly understood

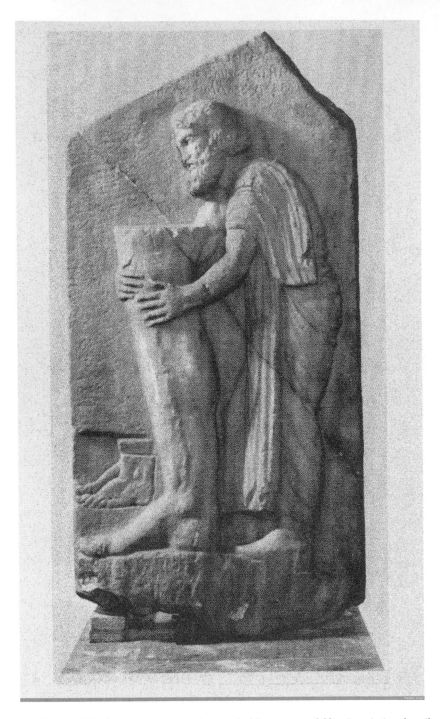

Figure 11.6 Marble plaque showing bearded man holding up a model leg. Inscription describing offering of Lysiamachides, son of Lysimachos the Acharian, Greek, fourth century BC. Found on the west slopes of the Acropolis. Original museum no. 3526 (current location not known).

Source: Wellcome Library, London.

them to have been connected with faith in their historical setting. They were exhibited with other anatomical votives in the centre of the WHMM in a 'model of a Greek shrine after the temple of Erechtheion', a display case with a plain pediment and ionic columns like the eastern portico of the temple on the Acropolis in Athens upon which it was apparently modelled (Figure 11.7). In the museum this 'temple', had spacious room around it and four glass sides such that the objects could be viewed all the way round, giving them maximum impact. This must have created the very opposite effect to that supposedly produced by the dark and secluded 'secret cabinets' of other museums. Not only did this allow excellent viewing of these objects, but also demonstrates an attempt by Wellcome at re-creating the 'original' religious context in which these objects featured. Despite the historical inaccuracies – the Erechtheion has never been associated with votive giving – Wellcome's display was designed to suggest to the visitor something of the ritual setting in which these objects are thought to have been 'displayed' in antiquity, that is hung up or placed around an altar in healing shrines. In a comparable display the museum constructed a Catholic 'chapel' to replicate the modern setting in which its Mexican *ex-voto* painted roof tiles were hung. Wellcome did not segregate the votive genitalia from the other anatomical models and treat them as obscenities to be hidden away in a special collection, but displayed

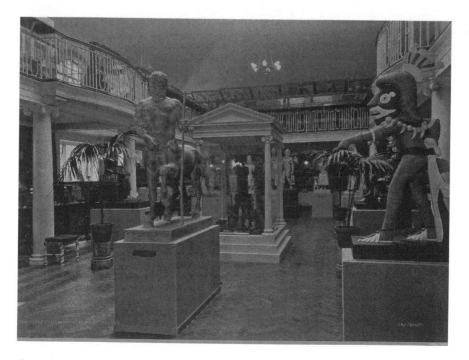

Figure 11.7 'Hall of Statuary', Wellcome Historical Medical Museum, 1913, Wellcome Library archives (WA/PHO/Hmm/1).

Source: Wellcome Library, London.

all votive types together, thus demonstrating the idea that in the ancient world objects featuring sexual imagery had appeared in public spaces alongside other nonsexual objects of the same function. Walter Kendrick's (1987) book *The Secret Museum* did much to promulgate ideas of censorship and pornography in connection with the modern reception of sexual antiquities and particularly the story of the removal of objects from Pompeii and Herculaneum to the Naples *Gabinetto Segreto*, lamenting that 'modern classifiers had to rip them from their Roman street corners and entrance halls and group them under a single heading' (Kendrick, 1987, p. 32). If this demonstrates the disembodiment of ancient sexual material from its 'original' context, Wellcome's display of votive genitalia attempted to put it back into its ancient context.

'Illustrative of phallic worship'

In addition to their role as records of pathological knowledge and ancient healing cults, the ancient votives shaped as human genitals were also viewed by Wellcome as evidence of the specific connection between sex and religion in antiquity. This was part of Wellcome's interest in the long-standing anthropological theory on the universal origins of all religious belief in the worship of procreation (for the most thorough account of this intellectual tradition see Carabelli, 1996). Investigations of 'phallic worship' had risen in the Enlightenment when antiquarians were struck by the ubiquitous image of the erect penis and other sexual imagery across ancient cultures, especially that found at the recently excavated cities of Pompeii and Herculaneum, as well as the newly 'discovered' Hindu temples of India (Funnell, 1982, pp. 52–3; Haskell, 1984, p. 187; Rousseau, 1988, pp. 116–17; Godwin, 1994, p. 9; Carabelli, 1996, pp. 26–8 and p. 66). The centrality of Roman material culture in this developing discourse is evidenced in the enduring use of the phrase 'The Worship of Priapus' (a reference to the Greco-Roman fertility god depicted with an oversized erect penis) to refer to cross-cultural fertility cults. This appeared in the title of the first and still best-known full-length treatise analysing sexual imagery from across cultures for its religious significance. *A Discourse on the Worship of Priapus, and Its Connection with the Mystic Theology of the Ancients* by collector Richard Payne Knight was published privately in 1786 by the Society of Dilettanti, of which Payne Knight was a member, together with letters on the subject by fellow member Sir William Hamilton, Britain's Extraordinary Envoy to Naples (on this work and its debt to classical sexual imagery see Funnell, 1982; Johns, 1982, pp. 22–8; Davis, 2008, pp. 109–30; 2010, pp. 51–82). This work and its many derivatives throughout the nineteenth and early twentieth century present evidence of a supposed primeval cult of fertility in the universal use of particular symbols across ancient art, not least the image of the phallus (see Carabelli, 1996; also Johns, 1982, pp. 26–8; Godwin, 1994, pp. 22–4; Lyons and Lyons, 2004, pp. 57–9). Roman culture provided not only representations of the god Priapus but a cavalcade of phallic figures associated with fertility, such as the half-goat, half-man figure of Pan and his companions the satyrs, as well as the widespread production of the ubiquitous amulet shaped as the *fascinum* – the divine phallus worn in particular by Roman boys and soldiers to provide protection from danger (Johns, 1982, especially chapters 2–4).

Like these theorists before him Wellcome was especially drawn to such phallic imagery from antiquity, collecting over three hundred ancient Roman phallic objects alone. But he also sought out material from across cultures which would prove the theory that the worship of fertility was a universal phenomenon. His 'phallic worship' collection was especially wide ranging, including artefacts from ancient Egypt (Object No. A87303: Ptolemaic stone figure of phallic god Harpocrates, 390–100 BC), pre-colonised Peru (AA153142: pottery jug in form of man clutching his erect penis) and contemporary Japan (Object No. A641145: bamboo and paper model of a house with model phallus inside, late nineteenth century). The Roman and Etruscan votive genitalia were included in this collection in addition to the 'votives' section so that their entry in the museum accession registers reads 'VO/PHA' (for example WHMM Index Cards No. A113296: WA/HMM/CM/INV/A.144). However, unlike most other artefacts in the 'phallic worship' collection that featured the phallus (that is, the erect penis) Wellcome's votive objects from ancient healing shrines almost exclusively represent a flaccid organ. Arguably these objects are meant to represent fragments of the ancient human body for the purpose of communicating with the divine as opposed to the divine phallus, itself imbued with some supernatural power to provide fertility and protection. This rule regarding the erect versus flaccid penis does not always apply for ancient materials as we will see later. This singling out of penis-shaped votives from other anatomical types and equating them with the worship of fertility gods (in addition to regular healing cults) can be traced to the Enlightenment and the beginnings of the theory of universal fertility cults. One of the most important and now well-known collections of artefacts to inspire the theory of 'phallic worship' was a set of modern Italian wax penises which William Hamilton acquired and presented to the British Museum in 1784, where they can still be seen (Museum no. M.560–4; Hamilton, 1894, p. 6; Carabelli, 1996; Jenkins and Sloan, 1996, p. 142 and pp. 238–9). These objects were illustrated in the engraved frontispiece of the original 1786 publication of *Worship of Priapus*. In addition to the objects themselves Hamilton (1894, p. 6) had obtained a first-hand account of a festival in which these *'ex-voti* of wax, representing the male parts of generation' were dedicated at the shrine of St Cosmos and St Damian by sterile women or the wives of sterile men in Isernia, Naples. Hamilton (quoted in Carabelli, 1996, p. 2) declared: 'I have actually discovered the Cult of Priapus in its full vigour, as in the days of the Greeks and Romans'. He believed these wax models of male genitalia to be the modern survivors of the numerous specimens of Greek and Roman phallic deities which he and his colleagues were then acquiring and depositing in the British Museum. However, as they are most likely wax representations of the genitals of actual members of the Isernian community, it could be suggested their more logical ancient parallel are the votive genitalia – representations of ancient human organs used to communicate with the divine (and which Hamilton and

Payne Knight themselves acquired). Most of the wax models, like the ancient votives, are flaccid penises, although some do depict erections. Whitney Davis (2008, p. 115) insists Hamilton's 'determination to construe an ordinary healing cult as a cult of priapic worship' is evidence of his derisory commentary on the Catholic Church's sacred ceremonies. The Society of Dilettanti's anticlerical mission was to expose not only a surviving paganism but also a prudish hypocrisy at the core of Catholicism (Turner, 1981, pp. 1–2; Godwin, 1994, pp. 1–4; Carabelli, 1996, p. 25, pp. 35–7). Hamilton (1894, p. 3) made clear that his research was intended to provide 'fresh proof' to support the earlier treatise of Conyers Middleton on the 'exact conformity between Popery and Paganism'. However, Hamilton seemingly ignored the reference from Middleton (1729, p. 23) on the practice of dedicating votive body parts (although not specifically genitalia) in both ancient and modern Italy. Hamilton (1894, p. 6) acknowledged that other parts of the body were offered in wax to the saints Cosmos and Damian; however, the greater number of male genitalia dedicated at the festival allowed him to propagate the more damaging idea of Catholic women worshipping the very image of the penis itself rather than simply using effigies of their husbands' penises to communicate with the healing saints. Payne Knight (1894, p. 16) in his essay goes onto equate the women's actions with the highly eroticised ancient female Bacchic ceremonies (Davis, 2008, p. 117). Hamilton and Payne Knight's associate Pierre-François Hughes, the French writer, pseudo-aristocrat and self-styled 'Baron d'Hancarville', had already published several volumes of purportedly ancient gems with depictions of women performing ceremonies around the phallic statue of Priapus (d'Hancarville, 1771; 1782). If this 'confusion' between religious practices was indeed intentional by Hamilton and Payne Knight, it was nevertheless taken up by their many followers throughout the nineteenth and twentieth century who repeated the idea that the modern Italian wax models of the penis were clear evidence of trans-historical 'phallic worship'. Crucially, those influenced by these Enlightenment theories, of which Wellcome was one, also set apart ancient votive genitalia from other anatomical votives, not for reasons of prudery but as extra evidence of the special connection between religion and sexuality.[4]

Classical 'primitivism'

The heterogeneous treatment of ancient votive genitalia by Wellcome is bound up with a key premise in late nineteenth- and early twentieth-century understanding of human culture and a related ambiguity in modern perceptions of classical cultures. As anthropological theorising developed in this period, a pertinent question arose as to whether the Greeks and Romans should be viewed as 'primitive' or 'civilised' cultures from a modern viewpoint (Orrells et al.,

---

4 Images of votive genitalia appeared in nineteenth- and twentieth-century publications as evidence of 'phallic worship', see Davenport (1869, pl. vi) and Licht (1925, v. 3 p.8).

2011, p. 4). While some of Wellcome's wider collection of classical material was relevant to this question, votive genitalia in particular troubled the distinction between these two definitions of human culture and the place of antiquity within them. Popularised by Edward Tylor's 1871 *Primitive Culture,* the nineteenth century had seen the rise of a cultural evolutionary theory which proposed a steady progression of humanity from 'primitivism' to 'civilisation' as 'man transcended, by means of his rationality and inventiveness, enslavement to his basic animal needs' (Skinner, 1986, p. 390; Stocking, 1987). But in many ways classical culture did not fit neatly into these newly consolidated specifications, presenting both 'primitive' and 'civilised' cultural characteristics. As Sebastian Matzner (2010, p. 60) has recently suggested:

> Throughout Europe's cultural history, the reception of Classical antiquity is marked first and foremost by the intrinsic ambivalence of it being at the same time the foundation and the Other of contemporary cultural identity. It is, as it were, the resident alien at the core of Western civilisation (see also Armstrong, 2005, p. 5)

The 'alterity and identity', as Matzner puts it, in modernity's relationship with the classical past is embodied in Wellcome's dual approach – both biomedical and cultural – to his ancient anatomical votives. Classical antiquity could be viewed in this one object type as both the father of Western observatory medicine (found also in Wellcome's displays of manuscripts of Hippocrates and Galen, WHMM Handbook 1914, p. 65: WA/HMM/PB/Han/15) and a group of societies which routinely turned to the supernatural as part of their approach to healthcare. This seemingly twofold superstitious and sophisticated approach to health in antiquity is also embodied in a plaque (Museum no. A3369) acquired by Wellcome which had been found at the sanctuary to the mythical hero Amphiaraos at Oropos in Greece where he was worshipped as a healing god (Figure 11.8). It shows him as a doctor tending to the shoulder of a man while in the background the same man is shown practicing incubation whereby a sick person slept in a healing shrine in the hope of being cured by the deity overnight. Pausanias (*Description of Greece* 1.34.4–5) writes about incubation at the Amphiareion (for interest in healing at this sanctuary and the practice of incubation at the time Wellcome was collecting, see Jayne, 1925, p. 305). Wellcome's anthropological approach to medical history, which saw such 'primitive' and 'folk' medicine as worthy subjects, was regarded by other medical historians with suspicion and derision at a time when twentieth-century medical museums usually featured alternatives to biomedical history only as a warning of their dangers and to establish the superiority of orthodox medicine (Skinner, 1986, p. 414; Larson, 2009, p. 145).

The strict division between the anthropological and biomedical history of medicine found elsewhere in medical history exhibits was challenged by Wellcome in the importance he placed on the role of religion in ancient healthcare

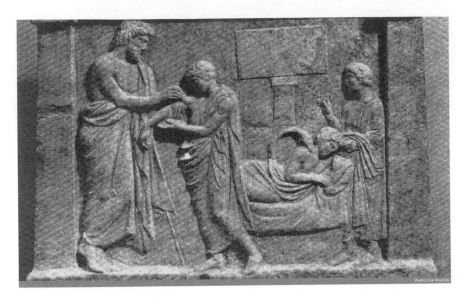

Figure 11.8 Marble plaque showing a shrine. The inscription described the offering of Archinos to Amphiaraos. Greek, fourth century BC. Found at Oropos. Science Museum/Wellcome Collection, A3369.

Source: Wellcome Library, London.

together with the 'primitive' practices of other cultures in their attempt to preserve healthy communities. At the opening ceremony of Wellcome's museum in 1913 Norman Moore, the future president of the Royal College of Physicians, identified the material around him as representing 'two great branches of medicine': one concerning 'local superstitions, with charms and amulets and incantations' which was represented by the 'primitive figure' of Ixtlilton, the god of medicine of the Aztecs, the other 'the control and causation of disease' represented by a plaster copy of the Apollo Belvedere – as the father of Asclepius – who embodied 'the true ancestors, the true observing predecessors of Hippocrates and Galen' (WHMM Handbook 1927, pp. 26–7: WA/HMM/PB/Han/19). For Moore antiquity properly belonged to only the second 'true' branch of the history of medicine. For Wellcome it belonged to both, a concept embodied in the ancient anatomical votive.

The votive genitalia in particular, as we have seen, also embodied an aspect of antiquity which was seen in Wellcome's time as indicative of 'primitivism': the idea that sex and religion did not necessarily need to be hostile concepts. These objects reflected for Wellcome a preoccupation with reproduction and sexuality – a greater acknowledgement of humanity's 'basic animal needs' – in classical cultures. During the mass excavation of ancient sexual imagery at Pompeii and Herculaneum in the eighteenth century, this material had been compared to that used in the ritual practices of modern 'savages', such as the

Pacific Islanders 'discovered' by explorer James Cook (Jenkins and Sloan, 1996, p. 241; Coltman, 2006, p. 107). The recognition of the similarities between classical and modern 'primitive' culture has been characterised by later commentators in terms of a 'trauma' for Western culture, as ancient sexuality threatened the place of antiquity as the founder of civilisation itself (Johns, 1982, p. 21; de Caro, 2000a, pp. 11–12; 2000b; Gaimster, 2000; Harris, 2007, p. 113; Frost, 2010, p. 140). As we have seen, the assumption is that previous generations simply removed the evidence which disturbed their image of antiquity. However, in the tradition of research into 'phallic worship' inspired by these finds, the 'primitivism' (and 'paganism') of antiquity had been embraced, even celebrated. Following this thinking Wellcome did not suppress ancient images of genitalia but instead deliberately sought out these objects, which acted for him as emblems of ambiguity in the cultural status of antiquity and its role in the history of healthcare.

Conclusion

Taking Henry Wellcome's early twentieth-century collection as a case study for the reception of one type of anatomical votive, I have shown that, contrary to previous assumptions, Roman and Etruscan models of genitalia at this time were not always anachronistically dismissed as 'pornographic' and therefore silenced from intellectual debates about ancient healthcare and culture. As museum artefacts they were not segregated in a special area with other sexually themed material, thereby obscuring their ancient context and meaning. They were instead deliberately and systematically sought out as important research data into human culture and displayed prominently alongside their nonsexual counterparts to convey an understanding that sexual imagery was not separated from daily life in antiquity. They were valued as records of ancient anatomical and pathological knowledge and simultaneously as evidence of cultural responses to human health, encouraging consideration of how humanity has thought about the healthy body and its functions by both 'rational' and 'nonrational' means. These objects therefore troubled the distinction between 'primitive' and 'Western' or 'civilised' medicine and wider culture present in the late nineteenth and early twentieth century and highlighted the complex position that the classical past held within this discourse.

What implications can be drawn from this case study? Wellcome's story illuminates the role of Roman and Etruscan votive genitalia and the anatomical votive more generally in modern debates around health, the body, sexuality, religion and the development of culture and highlights how interconnected these have been. While the role of classical literature for the modern negotiation of sexuality in particular has been mapped more comprehensively (Halperin, 1990; Dowling, 1994; Verstraete and Provencal, 2005; Orrells, 2011), the history of how interactions with ancient material culture have influenced our modern sexual knowledge is far from being fully understood. In particular, more research is needed on the collection of antiquities and the expanded discourses on human sexuality in the period Wellcome was active, as part of the increasing understanding of the importance of historical, archaeological, anthropological and artistic evidence and methods for sexologists and sex researchers in the late nineteenth and early twentieth century.

Wellcome's response to the sexual content of historical material, however, should not be seen simply as an indication of changing attitudes and a greater licence to scrutinise sex in this period; rather it should encourage us to look again at the treatment of sexually themed antiquities in even earlier collections and museums beyond the story of censorship and repression and perhaps towards that of serious intellectual interest in such material. Finally, given the difficultly of elucidating the meaning and intent behind the practice of ancient votive giving, the observation of modern responses to these objects is evidently worthwhile. The various modern labels given to ancient votive models of genitalia which we have seen throughout this chapter – from titillating 'pornography', sophisticated medical diagram and 'primitive' fertility object – can be useful benchmarks for the further understanding of their meaning to the people who dedicated them in antiquity.

12 Votive futures

An afterword

Jessica Hughes

In the last months of 2014 posters appeared around Paris urging the public to *Faites vos voeux! (Make your vows!)*. The central image showed a grimacing red devil sitting outside a hut in a desert landscape painted in the traditional style and colours of a Mexican votive *retablo*. The poster directed viewers not to any of the city's churches, but rather to an exhibition of 'votive art' inside the Musée de la Poste in Montparnasse where they could scribble down their vows, or even just their wishes, inside a makeshift chapel before moving on to contemplate a series of other works by artists who had been inspired by the concept of the votive offering.

Images of body parts were everywhere in the Paris show, from the tiny *milagros* in which disembodied heads were caressed by outstretched silver arms to the over–life-size anatomical photos arranged in fragmentary jigsaws on the gallery floor. The Armenian artist Sarkis had juxtaposed three hundred tarnished metal *ex-votos* – including many anatomicals and swaddled babies – with a triptych of bright pigments and a book entitled *Mnemosyne* (Memory). The Polish sculptor Xawery Wolski had contributed a series of clay *Organes* whose creamy-white colour evoked 'our first nutrition – the milk that heals and purifies whatever is contaminated, whose emptiness can put out fires' (Wolski, cited in Anon, 2014, p. 85) (Figure 12.1). One of the most striking uses of body parts was by the Parisian artist Coco Fronsac who had arranged assemblages of tiny votive-like objects in front of colourful portraits of 'canonised' celebrities, thereby using the relationship between mortal and divine as an evocative template for other forms of worship and dependence (Figure 12.2).

Faites vos Voeux confronted visitors with the extraordinary range of ways in which votive body parts might be given new life and made relevant to the modern world. And the artists in this show are far from the only ones to have been inspired by anatomical offerings in recent years. Hanging on a gallery wall in the Wellcome Collection, in close proximity to the ancient terracotta body parts discussed by Jen Grove earlier in this book, is a work by Julian Walker entitled *Acts of Faith*. It consists of hundreds of tiny body parts sculpted from nonprescription pills and communicates, amongst other things, the quasi-religious regard that patients have for their doctors, as well as the blind hope and trust inherent in the act of swallowing medicine (Figure 12.3). Across London,

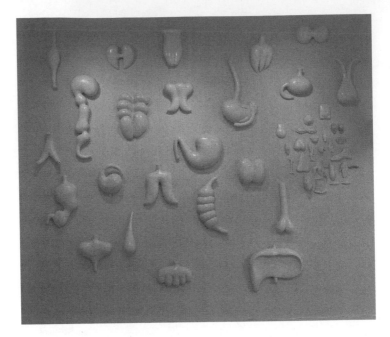

Figure 12.1 *Organes* by Xawery Wolski (2014).

Source: Courtesy of Xawery Wolski.

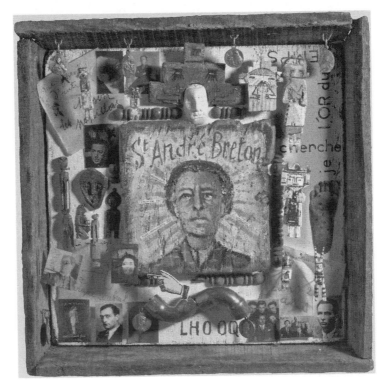

Figure 12.2 *St. Andre Breton*, Coco Fronsac (2014).

Source: Courtesy of Coco Fronsac.

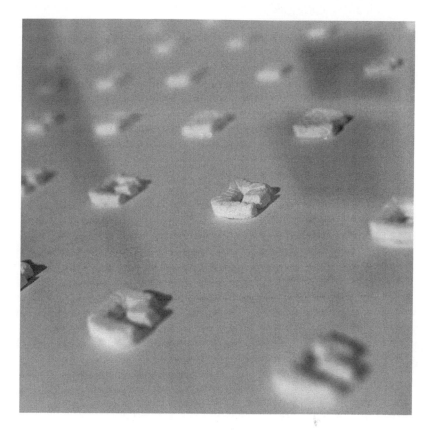

Figure 12.3 Acts of Faith (detail, stomach), Julian Walker (2003).
Source: Courtesy of Julian Walker.

the ceramicist Christie Brown experiments with anatomical votives as symbols of lost knowledge and as a way of exploring the relationships between archaeology, psychoanalysis and fragmentation. And many of the contemporary works on display in the 2014 exhibition 'Out of Body: Fragments in Art' held at the Israeli Museum in Jerusalem were clearly in dialogue with the ancient anatomical votives that were displayed alongside them.

All these contemporary artworks are profoundly interesting in their own right. However, they take on an extra level of significance when they are considered collectively. What might account for the apparent 'renaissance' of anatomical votive imagery in modern art? Can the rising numbers of *ex-votos* in our galleries be attributed in some part to the increasingly diverse attention paid to this type of object by academics and museum curators, as attested by the wide-range of starting points and approaches employed by the studies in this volume? Or do we need to see these scholarly works on votives in the same terms – that is, as reflecting a much broader cultural shift in ways of understanding the body and the sacred? Certainly the fragmentation of the body is something that is often in the news headlines, whether it takes the form of violent decapitation in the context of global religious conflict or the 'miraculous' disassembly enacted in new medical procedures such as organ transplants and gene therapy. Contemporary artworks such as those in the Paris exhibition sometimes respond quite explicitly to these modern practices, drawing on the ancient votive tradition to reassure, to reenchant or simply to reflect on the anxieties and hopes that these new ways of disassembling the body generate.

The cultural factors underlying the 'votive turn' in twentieth- and twenty-first-century art will no doubt become clearer with the passing of time. But these modern works can already help us deepen our understanding of the ancient objects studied in this book. In part this can be achieved by ringing the changes between old and new: How do modern artists fragment the body differently from their ancient counterparts, and what might this tell us about the broader sociocultural differences between the past and present? Contemporary artworks also raise new questions that we might ask in relation to the ancient votives – questions about the symbolism of the sculptural materials, for instance, or about the relationship between sacred and 'rational' medical healing. Some of the body parts used in the modern artworks actually have their origins in historical religious spheres, having passed from church to workshop via market stalls or online auctions on eBay. These 'liminal' objects remind us that all votives have biographies and demonstrate how far the changing context of a votive has the power to drastically alter its function, value and meaning.

The current book has, in fact, already started to articulate and explore many of these questions. The individual contributors have engaged closely with the form and materiality of votives from specific geographical areas, and the juxtaposition of all of these case studies has allowed us to begin dissecting the relationships between votives from different periods and places. Over the coming years the debates about votives will hopefully grow even louder and livelier, with many more voices being added to the conversation besides those of historians and contemporary artists. Some of these voices may belong to academics from disciplines beyond the humanities – psychologists, neuroscientists and behavioural economists among them. Some may belong to those who continue to make, dedicate and curate anatomical offerings within a religious context, whether this be a Catholic church, a Hindu temple or any of the other sacred spaces worldwide in which anatomical votives still form part of the material horizons. Ultimately, the future of the votive is not a singular one; instead, its various strands will unfold in different ways in the university, in the art gallery, in the church and on the Internet as well as in other yet-to-be-discovered places. Identifying how all these different trajectories are connected and mutually influential will be one of the most challenging aspects of future votive study but one which can only help to deepen our understanding of these powerful yet fragile 'bodies of evidence' which continue to be a source of fascination, inspiration and hope for so many people.

Bibliography

Acconcia, V., 2000. *Il santuario del Pozzarello a Bolsena. Scavi Gabrici 1904.* Corpus delle stipi votive in Italia X, Regio VII, 5. Rome: Giorgio Bretschneider Editore.

Adams, E., 2009. Defining and displaying the human body: Collectors and Classics during the British enlightenment. *Hermathena*, 187, pp. 65–97.

Adams, E., 2013. Shaping, collecting and displaying medicine and architecture: A comparison of the Hunterian and Soane museums. *Journal of the History of Collections*, 25(1), pp. 59–75.

Agelidis, Z., 2011. Kulte und Heiligtümer in Pergamon. In: R. Grüßinger, V. Kästner and A. Scholl, eds. *Pergamon: Panorama der Antiken Metropole: Begleitbuch zur Ausstellung: eine Ausstellung der Antikensammlung der Staatlichen Museen zu Berlin.* Berlin and Petersberg: Antikensammlung, Staatliche Museen zu Berlin and Michael Imhof Verlag, pp. 175–83.

Agostini, A., 2012. New perspectives on Minaean expiatory texts. *Proceedings of the Seminar for Arabian Studies*, 42, pp. 1–12.

Ahearne-Kroll, S.P., 2014. The afterlife of a dream and the ritual system of the Epidaurian Asklepieion. *Archiv für Religionsgeschichte*, 15(1), pp. 35–52.

Akıncı Öztürk, E. and Tanrıver, C., 2008. New katagraphai and dedications from the sanctuary of Apollon Lairbenos. *Epigraphica Anatolica*, 41, pp. 91–111.

Akıncı Öztürk, E. and Tanrıver, C., 2009. Some new finds from the sanctuary of Apollon Lairbenos. *Epigraphica Anatolica*, 42, pp. 87–97.

Akıncı Öztürk, E. and Tanrıver, C., 2010. New inscriptions from the sanctuary of Apollon Lairbenos. *Epigraphica Anatolica*, 43, pp. 43–9.

Alberti, S.J.M.M., 2011. *Morbid curiosities: Medical museums in nineteenth-century Britain.* Oxford and New York, NY: Oxford University Press.

Aldhouse-Green, M.J., 1999. *Pilgrims in stone: Stone images from the Gallo-Roman sanctuary of Fontes Sequanae.* Oxford: Archaeopress.

Aldhouse-Green, M.J., 2004a. Crowning glories: Languages of hair in later Prehistoric Europe. *Proceedings of the Prehistoric Society*, 70, pp. 299–325.

Aldhouse-Green, M.J., 2004b. Chaining and shaming: Images of defeat, from Llyn Cerrig Bach to Sarmitzegetusa. *Oxford Journal of Archaeology*, 23(3), pp. 319–40.

Aleshire, S.B., 1989. *The Athenian Asklepieion: The people, their dedications, and the inventories.* Amsterdam: J.C. Gieben.

Aleshire, S.B., 1991. *Asklepios at Athens: Epigraphic and prosopographic essays on the Athenian healing cults.* Amsterdam: J.C. Gieben.

Alexander, G., 1905. Zur Kenntnis der etruskischen Weihgeschenke nebst Bemerkungen über anatomischen Abbildungen im Altertum. *Anatomische Hefte*, 30(1), pp. 155–98.

Allason-Jones, L., 2005. *Women in Roman Britain.* 2nd ed. York: Council for British Archaeology.

Ambrosini, L., 2013. *Evan Gorga al CNR: Storia e immagini di una collezione*. Rome: CNR edizione, Consiglio Nazionale delle Ricerche.

Ammerman, R.M., 2002. *The sanctuary of Santa Venera at Paestum II: The votive terracottas*. Ann Arbor, MI: University of Michigan Press.

Ammerman, R.M., 2007. Children at risk: Votive terracottas and the welfare of infants at Paestum. In: A. Cohen and J. Rutter, eds. *Constructions of childhood in the ancient world*. Hesperia supplement 41. Princeton, NJ: American School of Classical Studies at Athens, pp. 131–51.

Anon., 1981. *Enea nel Lazio: archeologia e mito*. Rome: Fratelli Palombi.

Anon., 2014. *Faites vos vœux: ex-voto d'artistes contemporains*. Exposition, Paris, L'Adresse Musée de La Poste, 6 octobre 2014–3 janvier 2015. Gand: Snoeck.

Appleby, J., 2010. Aging as fragmentation and dis-integration. In: K. Rebay-Salisbury, M.L. Stig Sørensen and J. Hughes, eds. *Body parts and bodies whole*. Oxford: Oxbow Books, pp. 46–53.

Arbach, M. and Audouin, R., 2007. *Collection of epigraphic and archaeological artifacts from al-Jawf sites, San'â' National Museum. Part II*. San'â': UNESCO and Social Fund for Development.

Armstrong, R.H., 2005. *A compulsion for antiquity: Freud and the ancient world*. Ithaca, NY: Cornell University Press.

Arnold, C.E., 2005. 'I am astonished that you are so quickly turning away!' (Gal 1.6) Paul and Anatolian folk belief. *New Testament Studies*, 51(3), pp. 429–49.

Arnold, K. and Olsen, D., eds. 2003. *Medicine man: The forgotten museum of Henry Wellcome*. London: British Museum Press.

Aschoff, L., 1903. Die Sambon'sche Sammlung römischer Donaria (im Besitz der Firma Oppenheimer in London). *Mitteilungen zur Geschichte der Medizin und der Naturwissenschaften*, 2(1), pp. 1–8.

Ashmole, B., 1929. Study of ancient art: The value of casts. *The Times*, 24 October, p. 21.

Attenni, L. and Ghini, G., 2014. La stipe votiva in località Pantanacci (Genzano di Roma-Lanuvio, Roma). In: E. Calandra, G. Ghini and Z. Mari, eds. *Lazio e Sabina 10. (Atti del Convegno 'Decimo incontro di Studi sul Lazio e la Sabina', Roma, 4–6 giugno 2013)*. Rome: Lavori e Studi della Soprintendenza per i Beni Archeologici del Lazio, pp. 153–61.

Audollent, A., 1923. Les tombes gallo-romaines à inhumation des Martres-de-Veyre (Puy-de-Dôme). *Mémoires présentés par divers savants à l'Académie des inscriptions et belles-lettres (Paris)*, 13, pp. 275–328.

Baggieri, G., 1998. Etruscan wombs. *The Lancet*, 352, p. 790.

Baggieri, G., 1999. Archaeology, religion and medicine. In: G. Baggieri and M.L. Rinaldi Veloccia, eds. *L'antica anatomia nell'arte dei donaria (Ancient anatomy in the art of votive offerings)*. Rome: Ministero per i Beni e le Attività Culturali, pp. 80–6.

Baggieri, G., Margariti, P.A. and di Giacomo, M., 1999. Fertilità, virilità, maternità. In: G. Baggieri and M.L. Rinaldi Veloccia, eds. *L'antica anatomia nell'arte dei donaria (Ancient anatomy in the art of votive offerings)*. Rome: Ministero per i Beni e le Attività Culturali, pp. 22–7.

Baglione, M.P., 1976. *Il territorio di Bomarzo*. Rome: Consiglio Nazionale delle Ricerche.

Baglione, M.P., 2001. Le statue ed altri oggetti votivi. In: A.M. Moretti Sgubini, ed. *Veio, Cerveteri, Vulci: città d'Etruria a confronto*. Rome: 'L'Erma' di Bretschneider, pp. 69–78.

Baker, M., 2003. Bodies of enlightenment: Sculpture and the eighteenth-century museum. In: R.G.W. Anderson, M.L. Caygill, A.G. MacGregor and L. Syson, eds. *Enlightening the British: Knowledge, discovery and the museum in the eighteenth century*. London: British Museum, pp. 142–8.

Baker, P., 2013. *The archaeology of medicine in the Greco-Roman world*. Cambridge: Cambridge University Press.

Barbera, M., ed. 1999a. *Museo Nazionale Romano: la collezione Gorga*. Milan and Rome: Electa and Ministero per i beni e le attività culturali, Soprintedenza archeologica di Roma.

Barbera, M., 1999b. Gorga e il collezionismo antiquario a Roma fra Ottocento e Novecento. In: M. Barbera, ed. *Museo Nazionale Romano: la collezione Gorga*. Milan and Rome: Electa and Ministero per i beni e le attività culturali, Soprintendeza archeologica di Roma, pp. 3–13.

Barbina, P., Ceccarelli, L., Dell'Era, F. and Di Gennaro, F., 2009. Il territorio di Fidenae tra V e II secolo a.C. In: V. Jolivet, C. Pavolini, M.A. Tomei and R. Volpe, eds. *Suburbium II. Il suburbio di Roma dalla fine dell'età monarchica alla nascita del sistema delle ville (V–II secolo a.C.)*. Rome: École française de Rome, pp. 325–45.

Barkan, L., 1999. *Unearthing the past: Archaeology and aesthetics in the making of Renaissance Culture*. New Haven, CT and London: Yale University Press.

Barrell, J., 1989. 'The dangerous goddess': Masculinity, prestige, and the aesthetic in early eighteenth-century Britain. *Cultural Critique*, 12, pp. 101–31.

Bartman, E., 2001. Hair and the artifice of Roman female adornment. *American Journal of Archaeology*, 105(1), pp. 1–25.

Bartoloni, G., 1970. Alcune terrecotte votive delle collezioni medicee ora al Museo Archeologico di Firenze. *Studi Etruschi*, 38, pp. 257–70.

Bartoloni, G., 2005. Il deposito votivo rinvenuto a Veio negli scavi del 1889. In: A. Comella and S. Mele, eds. *Depositi votivi e culti dell'Italia antica dall'età arcaica a quella tardo-repubblicana: atti del convegno di studi, Perugia, 1–4 giugno 2000*. Bari: Edipuglia, pp. 171–8.

Bartoloni, G. and Benedettini, M.G., 2011. *Veio. Il deposito votivo di Comunità (scavi 1889–2005)*. Corpus delle stipi votive in Italia XXI, Regio VII, 3. Rome: Giorgio Bretschneider Editore.

Bartoloni, G. and Bocci Pacini, P., 1996. De 'donariis'. In: M.G. Picozzi and F. Carinci, eds. *Studi in memoria di Lucia Guerrini: Vicino Oriente, Egeo, Grecia, Roma e mondo romano. Tradizione dell'antico e collezionismo di antichità*. Studi Miscellanei, 30. Rome: 'L'Erma' di Bretschneider, pp. 439–56.

Βαβρίτσας, Α., 1973. Ἀνασκαφή Μεσημβρίας. Πρακτικά τῆς ἐν Ἀθήναις ἀρχαιολογικῆς ἑταιρείας. Athens.

Bataille, G., 2008. *Les Celtes: des mobiliers aux cultes*. Dijon: Éditions Universitaires de Dijon.

Battaglia, D., 1990. *On the bones of the serpent: Person, memory, and mortality in Sabarl Island society*. Chicago, IL and London: University of Chicago Press.

Beard, M., 2012. Dirty little secrets: Changing displays of Pompeian 'erotica'. In: V.C. Gardner Coates, K. Lapatin and J.L. Seydl, eds. *The last days of Pompeii: Decadence, apocalypse, resurrection*. Los Angeles, CA: J. Paul Getty Museum, pp. 60–9.

Beaumont, L.A., 2012. *Childhood in ancient Athens: Iconography and social history*. London and New York, NY: Routledge.

Beazley, J.D., 1947. *Etruscan vase-painting*. Oxford: Clarendon Press.

Becker, M.J. and Turfa, J.M., 2017. *Etruscan false teeth and the history of dentistry*. London and New York, NY: Routledge.

Belayche, N., 2008. Du texte à l'image: les reliefs sur les steles 'de confession' d'Anatolie. In: S. Estienne, ed. *Image et Religion dans l'antiquité gréco-romaine: actes du colloque de Rome, 11–13 décembre 2003 organisé par l'Ecole française de Rome, l'Ecole française d'Athènes*. Naples and Athens: Centre Jean Bérard and École française d'Athènes, pp. 181–94.

Bell, J., 1797. *The anatomy of the human body. Volume I. Containing the anatomy of the bones, muscles and joints*. 2nd ed. Edinburgh and London: G. Mudie and Son and Cadell and Davies.

Benedettini, M.G., ed. 2012. *Il Museo delle Antichità Etrusche e Italiche. III. I bronzi della collezione Gorga*. Rome: Casa editrice Università La Sapienza.

Benedum, C., 1986. Asklepios und Demeter: zur Bedeutung weiblicher Gottheiten für den frühen Asklepioskult. *Jahrbuch des Deutschen Archäologischen Instituts*, 101, pp. 137–57.

244   *Bibliography*

Bentz, M., ed. 2008. *Rasna, die Etrusker: eine Ausstellung im Akademischen Kunstmuseum, Antik-ensammlung der Universität Bonn, 15. Oktober 2008–15. Februar 2009.* Petersberg: M. Imhof.

Berger, J., 1972. *Ways of seeing.* London: British Broadcasting Company and Penguin Books.

Bérillon, E., 1911. *La pathologie précolombienne d'après les ex-voto aztèques.* Paris: Maloine.

Berlin exhibition, 1988. *Die Welt der Etrusker. Archäologische Dekmäler aus Museen der sozialist-ischen Länder (catalogue de l'exposition de Berlin, Altes Museum, 4 octobre – 30 décembre 1988).* Berlin: Staatliche Museen zu Berlin.

Bernabò Brea, L. and Cavalier, M., 2000. *Meligunis Lipara, 10: Scoperte e scavi archeologici nell'area suburbana di Lipari. Studi e documenti d'archivio.* Rome: 'L'Erma' di Bretschneider.

Biancifiori, E., 2012. I pendenti bivalve. In: M.G. Benedettini, ed. *Il Museo delle Antichità Etrusche e Italiche. III. I bronzi della collezione Gorga.* Rome: Casa editrice Università La Sapienza, pp. 338–52.

Blackman, L., 2008. *The body: The key concepts.* Oxford and New York, NY: Berg.

Blackman, W.S., 2000[1927]. *The Fellahin of Upper Egypt.* Cairo: American University in Cairo Press.

Blagg, T.F.C., 1985. Cult practice and its social context in the religious sanctuaries of Latium and Southern Etruria: The sanctuary of Diana at Nemi. In: C. Malone and S. Stoddart, eds. *Papers in Italian archaeology IV.* BAR International Series 246. Oxford: Archaeopress, pp. 33–50.

Blagg, T.F.C. and MacCormick, A.G., eds. 1983. *Mysteries of Diana: The antiquities from Nemi in Nottingham museums.* Nottingham: Nottingham Castle Museum.

Blanshard, A.J.L., 2010. *Sex:Vice and love from antiquity to modernity.* Chichester and Malden, MA: Wiley-Blackwell.

Bleeker, M., ed. 2008. *Anatomy live: Performance and the operating theatre.* Amsterdam: Amsterdam University Press.

Bliquez, L.J., 1996. Prosthetics in classical antiquity: Greek, Etruscan, and Roman pros-thetics. In: W. Haase, ed. *Aufsteig und Niedergang der römischen Welt: Geschichte und Kultur Roms im Spiegel der neueren Forschung. II Principat. 37, Philosophie, Wissenschaften, Technik. 3, Wissenschaften* (Medizin und Biologie). Berlin and New York: W. de Gruyter, pp. 2640–76.

Blundell, S., 2006. Beneath their shining feet: Shoes and sandals in Classical Greece. In: G. Riello and P. McNeil, eds. *Shoes: A history from sandals to sneakers.* Oxford and New York, NY: Berg, pp. 30–49.

Bodel, J., 2009. 'Sacred dedications': A problem of definition. In: J. Bodel and M. Kajava, eds. *Dediche sacre nel mondo Greco-Romano: diffusione, funzioni, tipologie. Religious dedica-tions in the Greco-Roman world: Distribution, typology, use. Institutum Romanum Finlandiae, American Academy in Rome 19–20 Aprile 2006.* Rome: Acta Instituti Romani Finlandiae 35, pp. 17–41.

Bohtz, C., 1981. *Das Demeter-Heiligtum. Altertümer von Pergamon 13.* Berlin: W. de Gruyter.

Boivin, N., 2009. Grasping the elusive and unknowable: Material culture in ritual practice. *Material Religion*, 5(3), pp. 266–87.

Bonfante, L., 1986. Votive terracotta figures of mothers and children. In: J. Swaddling, ed. *Italian Iron Age artefacts in the British Museum.* London: British Museum, pp. 195–203.

Bonfante, L., 1989. Iconografia delle madri: Etruria e Italia antica. In: A. Rallo, ed. *Le donne in Etruria.* Rome: 'L'Erma' di Bretschneider, pp. 85–106.

Bonfante, L., 1997. Nursing mothers in classical art. In: A.O. Koloski-Ostrow and C.L. Lyons, eds. *Naked truths: Women, sexuality, and gender in classical art and archaeology.* London and New York, NY: Routledge, pp. 174–96.

Bonghi Jovino, M., 1971. *Capua preromana. Terrecotte votive II (Le statue).* Florence: Sansoni.

Bord, J., 2004. *Footprints in stone: The significance of foot- and hand-prints and other imprints left by early men, giants, heroes, devils, saints, animals, ghosts, witches, fairies and monsters.* Wimeswold: Heart of Albion.

Bouma, J.W., 1996. *Religio votiva: The archaeology of Latial votive religion: The 5th–3rd centuries BC votive deposit south west of the main temple at Satricum-Borgo le Ferriere.* Three volumes. Groningen: Rijksuniversiteit Groningen.

Bowden, M., 1991. *Pitt Rivers: The life and archaeological work of Lieutenant-General Augustus Henry Lane Fox Pitt Rivers, DCL, FRS, FSA.* Cambridge: Cambridge University Press.

Braun, E., 1844. Studi anatomici degli Antichi. *Bullettino dell'Istituto di corrispondenza archeologica*, pp. 16–19.

Brelich, A., 1955–57. Les monosandales. *La nouvelle Clio*, 7–9, pp. 469–84.

Brilliant, R., 2000. *My Laocoön: Alternative claims in the interpretations of artworks.* Berkeley, CA: University of California Press.

Brunaux, J.-L., 2006. Religion et sanctuaires. In: C. Goudineau, ed. *Religion et société en Gaule.* Paris: Errance, pp. 95–116.

Bruneau, P., 1970. *Recherches sur les cultes de Délos à l'époque Hellénistique et à l'époque Impériale.* Paris: E. de Boccard.

Bruzza, L., 1861. Bassorilievo con epigrafe greca proveniente da Filippopoli. *Annali dell'Istituto di corrispondence archaeologica*, 33, pp. 380–88.

Bryson, N., 1988. The gaze in the expanded field. In: H. Foster, ed. *Vision and visuality.* New York: The New Press, pp. 86–113.

Buckler, H.W., 1914–16. Some Lydian propitiatory inscriptions. *Annual of the British School at Athens*, 21, pp. 169–83.

Budelmann, F., 2007. The reception of Sophocles' representation of physical pain. *American Journal of Philology*, 128(4), pp. 443–67.

Burke, J., 2007. *Sigmund Freud's collection: An archaeology of the mind.* Melbourne: Monash University Museum of Art, in association with the Nicholson Museum, University of Sydney.

Burkert, W., 1987. *Greek religion.* Cambridge, MA: Harvard University Press.

Busby, C., 1997. Permeable and partible persons: A comparative analysis of gender and body in South India and Melanesia. *Journal of the Royal Anthropological Institute*, 3(2), pp. 261–78.

Byl, S., 1993. Les pieds remarquables d'Oedipe. *Cuadernos de Filología Clásica*, 3, pp. 99–108.

Cagiano de Azevedo, E., 2013. Evan Gorga. Dalla collezione ai musei. In: A. Capodiferro, ed. *Museo Nazionale Romano: Evan Gorga: la collezione di archeologia.* Milan: Electa, pp. 28–43.

Cairoli, R., Cosentino, S., and Mieli, G., 2001. Le grotte. In: A. Campanelli, ed. *Il tesoro del lago: l'archeologia del Fucino e la collezione Torlonia.* Pescara: Carsa, pp. 130–7.

Cairoli, R., d'Alessandro, A., Grossi, G. and Papi, R., 2001. Luco dei Marsi. In: A. Campanelli, ed. *Il tesoro del lago: l'archeologia del Fucino e la collezione Torlonia.* Pescara: Carsa, pp. 254–79.

Canal, A., 1988. Découverte d'un sanctuaire rural à Viuz-Faverges. *Bulletin d'Histoire, édité par 'Les Amis de Viuz Faverges'*, 29, pp. 2–8.

Cantacuzène, G., 1909. Contribution à la crâniologie des Étrusques. *L'Anthropologie*, 20, pp. 329–52.

Canto, A.M., 1984. Les plaques votives avec 'plantae pedum' d'Italica: un essai d'interprétation. *Zeitschrift für Papyrologie und Epigraphik*, 54, pp. 183–94.

Capodiferro, A., ed. 2013. *Museo Nazionale Romano: Evan Gorga: la collezione di archeologia.* Milan: Electa.

Capparoni, P., 1927. La persistenza delle forme degli antichi 'donaria' anatomici negli ex-voto moderni. *Bollettino dell'Istituto Storico Italiano dell'Arte Sanitaria*, 7(2), pp. 39–57.

Carabelli, G., 1996. *In the image of Priapus.* London: Duckworth.

Cassell, A.K., 1991. Santa Lucia as patroness of sight: Hagiography, iconography, and Dante. *Dante Studies*, 109, pp. 71–88.

Castagnoli, F., Cozza, L., Fenelli, M., Guaitoli, A., La Regina, M., Mazzolani, E., Paribeni, E., Piccareta, F., Sommella, P. and Torelli, M., 1975. *Lavinium II: le tredici are*. Rome: De Luca Editore.

Castiglione, L., 1967. Tables votives à empreintes de pied dans les temples d'Egypte. *Acta Orientalia Academiae Scientiarium Hungaricae*, 20(2), pp. 239–52.

Castiglione, L., 1968. Inverted footprints: A contribution to the ancient popular religion. *Acta Ethnographica Academiae Scientiarum Hungaricae*, 17, pp. 121–37.

Castiglione, L., 1970. Vestigia. *Acta Archaeologica Academiae Scientiarum Hungaricae*, 22, pp. 95–132.

Cenci, C., 2013. Terrecotte votive. In: A. Capodiferro, ed. *Museo Nazionale Romano: Evan Gorga: la collezione di archeologia*. Milan: Electa, pp. 384–98.

Chaniotis, A., 1995. Illness and cures in the Greek propitiatory inscriptions and dedications of Lydia and Phrygia. In: P.J. van der Eijk, H.F.J. Horstmanschoff and P.H. Schrijvers, eds. *Ancient medicine in its socio-cultural context: Papers read at the congress held at Leiden University, 13–15 April 1992*. Volume Two. Amsterdam: Rodopi, pp. 323–44.

Chaniotis, A., 1997. 'Tempeljustiz' im kaiserzeitlichen Kleinasien: Rechtliche Aspekte der Sühneninschrift Lydiens und Phrygiens. In: G. Thür and J. Vélissaropoulos-Karakostas, eds. *Symposion 1995: Vorträge zur grieschischen und hellenistischen Rechtsgeschichte*. Cologne, Weimar and Vienna: Böhlau, pp. 353–84.

Chaniotis, A., 2004. Under the watchful eyes of the gods: Divine justice in Hellenistic and Roman Asia Minor. In: S. Colvin, ed. *The Greco-Roman East: Politics, culture and society*. Cambridge: Cambridge University Press, pp. 1–43.

Chaniotis, A., 2009. Ritual performances of divine justice: The epigraphy of confession, atonement, and exaltation in Roman Asia Minor. In: H.M. Cotton, R.G. Hoyland, J.J. Price and D.J. Wasserstein, eds. *From Hellenism to Islam: Cultural and linguistic change in the Roman Near East*. Cambridge: Cambridge University Press, pp. 115–53.

Chaplin, S.D.J., 2009. *John Hunter and the 'museum oeconomy', 1750–1800*. Ph.D thesis. University of London, King's College, London.

Chapman, J., 2000. *Fragmentation in archaeology: People, places and broken objects in the prehistory of South-Eastern Europe*. London and New York: Routledge.

Chapman, W.R., 1985. Arranging ethnology: A.H.L.F. Pitt Rivers and the typological tradition. In: G.W. Stocking Jr., ed. *Objects and others: Essays on museums and material culture*. Madison, WI: University of Wisconsin Press, pp. 15–48.

Charcot, J.-M. and Dechambre, A., 1857. De quelques marbres antiques concernant des études anatomiques. *Gazette hebdomadaire de médecine et de chirurgie*, 4, pp. 425–9, pp. 457–61 and pp. 513–18.

Charlier, P., 2000. Nouvelles hypothèses concernant la répresentation de utérus dans les ex-voto étrusco-romains. Anatomie et histoire de l'Art. *Ocnus*, 8, pp. 33–46.

Chaviara-Karahaliou, S., 1990. Eye votives in the Asklepieion of ancient Corinth. *Documenta ophthalmologica*, 74, pp. 135–9.

Cheselden, W., 1733. *Osteographia, or the anatomy of the bones*. London: s.n.

Chidester, D., 2005. The American touch: Tactile imagery in American religion and politics. In: C. Classen, ed. *The book of touch*. Oxford and New York, NY: Berg, pp. 49–65.

Ciaghi, S., 1993. *Le terrecotte figurate da Cales del Museo nazionale di Napoli: sacro, stile, committenza*. Rome: 'L'Erma' di Bretschneider.

Cilliers, L. and Retief, F.P., 2013. Dream healing in Asclepieia in the Mediterranean. In: S.M. Oberhelman, ed. *Dreams, healing and medicine in Greece: From antiquity to the present*. Farnham: Ashgate, pp. 69–92.

Cionci, A., 2004. *Il tenore collezionista. Vita, carriera lirica e collezioni di Evan Gorga*. Florence: Nardini.

Clark, K., 1956. *The nude: A study of ideal art.* London: John Murray.

Clarke, J.R. and Larvey, M., 2003. *Roman sex: 100 B.C. to A.D. 250.* New York, NY and London: Harry N. Abrams.

Clinton, K., 1993. The sanctuary of Demeter and Kore at Eleusis. In: N. Marinatos and R. Hägg, eds. *Greek sanctuaries: New approaches.* London and New York, NY: Routledge, pp. 88–98.

Clinton, K., 2004. Epiphany in the Eleusinian mysteries. *Illinois Classical Studies*, 29, pp. 85–109.

Clinton, K., ed. 2005–8. *Eleusis: The inscriptions on stone. Documents of the two goddesses and public documents of the Deme.* Two volumes. Athens: The Archaeological Society at Athens.

Clinton, K., 2007. The mysteries of Demeter and Kore. In: D. Ogden, ed. *A companion to Greek religion.* Malden, MA and London: Wiley-Blackwell, pp. 342–56.

Coarelli, F. ed. 1986a. *Fregellae 2. Il santuario di Esculapio.* Rome: Quasar.

Coarelli, F., 1986b. Introduzione. In: F. Coarelli, ed. *Fregellae 2. Il santuario di Esculapio.* Rome: Quasar, pp. 7–10.

Coarelli, F. and Rossi, A., 1980. *Templi dell'Italia antica.* Milan: Touring Club Italiano.

Cole, M.W. and Zorach, R. eds. 2009. *The idol in the age of art: Objects, devotions and the early modern world.* Aldershot: Ashgate.

Coltman, V., 2006. *Fabricating the antique: Neoclassicism in Britain, 1760–1800.* Chicago, IL: University of Chicago Press.

Comella, A., 1978. *Il materiale votivo tardo di Gravisca.* Rome: Giorgio Bretschneider Editore.

Comella, A., 1981. Tipologia e diffusione dei complessi votivi in Italia in epoca medio- e tardo-repubblicana. *Mélanges de l'École française de Rome, Antiquité*, 93, pp. 717–803.

Comella, A., 1982. *Il deposito votivo presso l'Ara della Regina.* Materiali del Museo Archeologico Nazionale di Tarquinia IV. Rome: Giorgio Bretschneider Editore.

Comella, A., 1982–83. Riflessi del culto di Asclepio sulla religiosità popolare etrusco-laziale e campana di epoca medio- e tardo-Repubblicana. *Annali della Facoltà di Lettere e Filosofia dell' Università degli studi di Perugia*, 20, pp. 217–44.

Comella, A., 1986. *I materiali votivi di Falerii.* Corpus delle stipi votive in Italia I. Regio VII.1. Rome: Giorgio Bretschneider Editore.

Comella, A., 1996. Sacralità e divinità nei votivi anatomici. In: G. Baggieri and M.L. Rinaldi Veloccia, eds. 1999. *L'antica anatomia nell'arte dei donaria (Ancient anatomy in the art of votive offerings).* Rome: Ministero per i Beni e le Attività Culturali, pp. 10–15.

Comella, A., 2001. *Il santuario di Punta della Vipera: Santa Marinella, Comune di Civitavecchia. 1. I materiali votivi.* Corpus delle stipi votive in Italia XIII. Regio VII.6. Rome: Giorgio Bretschneider Editore.

Comella, A., 2002. *I rilievi votivi greci di periodo arcaico e classico: diffusione, ideologia, committenza.* Bari: Edipuglia.

Comella, A., 2005. Il messagio delle offerte dei santuari Etrusco-italici di periodo medio- e tardo-repubblicano. In: A. Comella and S. Mele, eds. *Depositi votivi e culti dell'Italia antica dall'età arcaica a quella tardo-repubblicana: atti del convegno di studi, Perugia, 1–4 giugno 2000.* Bari: Edipuglia, pp. 47–59.

Comella, A. and Mele, S., eds. 2005. *Depositi votivi e culti dell'Italia antica dall'età arcaica a quella tardo-repubblicana: atti del convegno di studi, Perugia, 1–4 giugno 2000.* Bari: Edipuglia.

Costantini, S., 1995. *Il deposito votivo del santuario Campestre di Tessennano.* Corpus delle stipi votive in Italia VIII. Regio VII.4. Rome: Giorgio Bretschneider Editore.

Coulon, G., 2004. *L'enfant en Gaule romaine.* 2nd ed. Paris: Editions Errance.

Craik, E.M., 1998. *Hippocrates: Places in man.* Oxford: Clarendon Press.

Craik, E.M., 2006. *Two Hippocratic treatises: On sight and on anatomy.* Leiden and Boston: Brill.

Craik, E.M., 2009. Hippocratic bodily 'channels' and oriental parallels. *Medical History*, 53(1), pp. 105–16.

Crawford-Brown, S., 2010. Votive children in Cyprus and Italy. *Etruscan News*, 12, p. 5, p. 31.

Crişan, E., 1970. Ex voto-uri anatomice de la Veii în Muzeul de Istorie Cluj. *Acta Musei Napocensis*, 7, pp. 489–97.

D'Arcy Dicus, K., 2012. *Actors and agents in ritual behavior: The sanctuary at Grasceta dei Cavallari as a case-study of the E-L-C votive tradition in Republican Italy*. Ph.D. thesis. University of Michigan, Michigan.

Dasen, V., 2012. Anatomical votives. In: R.S. Bagnall, K. Brodersen, C.B. Champion, A. Erskine and S.R. Huebner, eds. *The encyclopedia of ancient history*. Malden, MA: Wiley-Blackwell, pp. 402–3.

Dasen, V. ed. 2013. *La petite enfance dans le monde grec et romain*. Dossiers de l'archéologie, 356. Dijon: Faton.

Dasen, V. and Ducaté-Paarmann, S., 2006. Hysteria and metaphors of the uterus in classical antiquity. In: S. Schroer, ed. *Images and gender: Contributions to the hermeneutics of reading ancient art*. Fribourg and Göttingen: Academic Press, pp. 239–61.

Davenport, J., 1869. *Aphrodisiacs and anti-aphrodisiacs: Three essays on the powers of reproduction; with some account of the judicial 'congress' as practised in France during the seventeenth century*. London: privately printed.

Davies, G., 2005. What made the Roman toga virilis? In: L. Cleland, M. Harlow and L. Llewellyn-Jones, eds. *The clothed body in the ancient world*. Oxford: Oxbow, pp. 121–30.

Davis, L.J., 1995. *Enforcing normalcy: Disability, deafness and the body*. London and New York, NY: Verso.

Davis, L.J., 2005. Visualizing the disabled body: The classical nude and the fragmented torso. In: M. Fraser and M. Greco, eds. *The body: A reader*. London and New York, NY: Routledge, pp. 167–81.

Davis, W., 2001. Homoerotic art collection from 1750–1920. *Art History*, 24(2), pp. 247–77.

Davis, W., 2008. Wax tokens of libido: William Hamilton, Richard Payne Knight, and the phalli of Isernia. In: R. Panzanelli, ed. *Ephemeral bodies: Wax sculpture and the human figure*. Los Angeles, CA: Getty Research Institute, pp. 107–29.

Davis, W., 2010. *Queer beauty: Sexuality and aesthetics from Winckelmann to Freud and beyond*. New York, NY and Chichester: Columbia University Press.

Dean-Jones, L., 1994. *Women's bodies in Classical Greek science*. Oxford: Clarendon Press.

de Caro, S. ed. 2000a. *The secret cabinet in the National Archaeological Museum of Naples: Quick guide*. Naples: Electa Napoli and Soprintendenza Archeologica di Napoli e Caserta.

de Caro, S., 2000b. Up and down, in and out: The story of the erotic collection. *The Art Newspaper*, 102, pp. 44–5.

de Cazanove, O., 1991. Ex-voto de l'Italie républicaine: sur quelques aspects de leur mise au rebut. In: J.-L. Brunaux, ed. *Les sanctuaires celtiques et leurs rapports avec le monde méditerranéen*. Paris: Errance, pp. 203–14.

de Cazanove, O., 2000. Some thoughts on the 'religious romanisation' of Italy before the Social War. In: E. Bispham and C. Smith, eds. *Religion in Archaic and Republican Rome and Italy: Evidence and experience*. Edinburgh: Edinburgh University Press, pp. 71–6.

de Cazanove, O., 2008. Enfants en langes: Pour quels voeux? In: G. Greco and B. Ferrara, eds. *Doni agli dei: il sistema dei doni votivi nei santuari*. Naples: Naus, pp. 271–84.

de Cazanove, O., 2009. Oggetti muti? Le iscrizioni degli ex voto anatomici nel mondo romano. In: J. Bodel and M. Kajava, eds. *Dediche sacre nel mondo Greco-Romano: diffusione, funzioni, tipologie. Religious dedications in the Greco-Roman world: Distribution, typology, use. Institutum Romanum Finlandiae, American Academy in Rome 19–20 Aprile 2006*. Rome: Acta Instituti Romani Finlandiae 35, pp. 355–71.

de Cazanove, O., 2012. Le lieu de culte d'Apollon Moritasgus à Alésia. Données anciennes et récentes. *Revue archéologique*, 53(1), pp. 158–69.

de Cazanove, O., 2013. Enfants au maillot en contexte cultuel, en Italie et en Gaule. In: V. Dasen, ed. *La petite enfance dans le monde grec et romain*. Dossiers d'archéologie, 356. Dijon: Faton, pp. 8–13.

de Cazanove, O., 2015a. Per la datazione degli ex voto anatomici d'Italia. In: T.D. Stek and G.-J. Burgers, eds. *The impact of Rome on cult places and religious practices in ancient Italy*. BICS Supplement 132. London: Institute of Classical Studies, pp. 29–66.

de Cazanove, O., 2015b. Water. In: R. Raja and J. Rüpke, eds. *A companion to the archaeology of religion*. Malden, MA: Wiley-Blackwell, pp. 181–93.

de Cazanove, O., Vidal, J., Dabas, M. and Caraire, G., 2012a. Alésia, forme urbaine et topographie religieuse: l'apport des prospections et des fouilles récentes. *Gallia*, 69(2), pp. 127–49.

de Cazanove, O., Barrière, V., Creuzenet, F., Dessales, H., Dobrovitch, L., Féret, S., Leclerc, Y., Popovitch, L., Simon, J. and Vidal, J., 2012b. Le lieu de culte du dieu Apollon Moritasgus à Alésia. Phases chronologiques, parcours de l'eau, distribution des offrandes. In: O. de Cazanove and P. Méniel, eds. *Étudier les lieux de culte de Gaule romaine: actes de la table-ronde de Dijon 18–19 septembre 2009*. Montagnac: Éditions Monique Mergoil, pp. 95–121.

de Cohën, A.-S. and Bailly, L., eds. 1994. *L'œil dans l'antiquité romaine*. Lons-le-Saunier: Centre Jurassien du Patrimoine.

de Coppet, D., 1981. The life-giving death. In: S.C. Humphreys and H. King, eds. *Mortality and immortality: The anthropology and archaeology of death*. London: Academic Press, pp. 175–204.

Decouflé, P., 1960. Sur un mannequin anatomique étrusque (note préliminaire). *Bulletin de la Société médicale française*, 5(2), p. 157.

Decouflé, P., 1961. Introduction à l'étude des mannequins anatomiques: l'incision du corps humain dans la plastique archaïque. *Semaine des hôpitaux de Paris*, 20 décembre 1961, pp. 3608–20.

Decouflé, P., 1964. *La notion d'ex-voto anatomique chez les Étrusco-Romains. Analyse et synthèse*. Bruxelles: Latomus, revue d'études latines.

de Grummond, N.T. and Edlund-Berry, I. eds. 2011. *The archaeology of sanctuaries and ritual in Etruria*. Portsmouth, RI: Journal of Roman Archaeology supplementary series 81.

Delpino, F., 1999. La 'scoperta' di Veio etrusca. In: A. Mandolesi and A. Naso, eds. *Ricerche archeologiche in Etruria meridionale nel XIX secolo (Atti dell'incontro di studio, Tarquinia, 6–7 luglio 1996)*. Florence: All'insegna del giglio, pp. 73–85.

De Lucia Brolli, M.A. and Tabolli, J., 2015. *I tempi del rito: il santuario di Monte Li Santi-Le Rote a Narce*. Rome: Officina edizioni.

Demma, F., 2002. Palestrina, santuari e domus: nuovi dati sulla città bassa. In: S. Gatti and G. Cetorelli Schivo, eds. *Il Lazio regione di Roma (Palestrina, Museo Archeologico Nazionale, 12 luglio – 10 settembre 2002)*. Rome: De Luca, pp. 91–106.

Denajar, L., 2005. *Carte archéologique de la Gaule 10: L'Aube*. Paris: Académie des Inscriptions et Belles-lettres.

de Peyer, R.M. and Johnston, A.W., 1986. Museum supplement: Greek antiquities from the Wellcome Collection: A distribution list. *Journal of Hellenic Studies*, 106, pp. 286–94.

D'Ercole, M.C., 1990. *La stipe votiva del Belvedere a Lucera*. Rome: Giorgio Bretschneider Editore.

Derks, T., 1998. *Gods, temples and ritual practice: The transformation of religious ideas in Roman Gaul*. Amsterdam: Amsterdam University Press.

Derks, T., 2014. Seeking divine protection against untimely death: Infant votives from Roman Gaul and Germany. In: M. Carroll and E.-J. Graham, eds. *Infant health and death in Roman Italy and beyond*. Ann Arbor, MI: Journal of Roman Archaeology supplementary series 96, pp. 47–68.

Deyts, S., 1983. *Les bois sculptés des sources de la Seine.* Gallia Suppléments, 42. Paris: Editions du Centre national de la recherche scientifique.

Deyts, S., 1994. *Un peuple de pèlerins. Offrandes de pierre et de bronze aux sources de la Seine.* Supplement 13. Dijon: Revue archéologique de l'Est et du Centre-Est.

Deyts, S., 2004. La femme et l'enfant au maillot en Gaule: iconographie et épigraphie. In: V. Dasen, ed. *Naissance et petite enfance dans l'Antiquité: actes du colloque de Fribourg, 28 novembre– 1er décembre 2001.* Fribourg and Göttingen: Academic Press, pp. 227–37.

d'Hancarville, P.-F.H., 1771. *Veneres uti observantur in gemmis antiquis.* Two volumes. Naples: Lugduni Batavorum.

d'Hancarville, P.-F.H., 1782. *Monumens de la vie privée des douze Césars: d'après une suite de pierre et médailles gravées sous leur règne.* Capri: Sabellius.

Diakonoff, I., 1979. *Artemidi Anaeiti anestesen.* The Anaeitis dedications in the Rijksmuseum van Oudhehen at Leyden and related material from Eastern Lydia: A reconsideration. *Bulletin Antieke Beschaving,* 54, pp. 139–55.

Didi-Huberman, G., 1998. Revenance d'une forme. In: G. Didi-Huberman, ed. *Phasmes. Essais sur l'apparition 1.* Paris: Éditions de Minuit, pp. 35–46.

di Gennaro, F. and Ceccarelli, L., 2012. Fidenae. Santuari urbani e del territorio. In: E. Marroni, ed. *Sacra Nominis Latini: I santuari del Lazio arcaico e repubblicano: atti del convegno internazionale, Roma, Palazzo Massimo, 19–21 febbraio 2009.* Volume One. Ostraka, volume speciale. Naples: Loffredo, pp. 211–26.

Dillon, M.P.J., 1994. The didactic nature of the Epidaurian *iamata. Zeitschrift für Papyrologie und Epigraphik,* 101, pp. 239–60.

Di Luca, M.T., 1984. Il Lucus Pisaurensis. In: M.R. Valazzi, ed. *Pesaro nell'antichità: storia e monumenti.* Venice: Marsilio, pp. 91–107.

Dolansky, F., 2008. *Togam virilem sumere*: Coming of age in the Roman world. In: J. Edmondson and A. Keith, eds. *Roman dress and the fabrics of Roman culture.* Toronto, Buffalo and London: University of Toronto Press, pp. 47–70.

Dondin-Payre, M. and Cribellier, C., 2011. Un ex-voto oculaire inscrit trouvé au Clos du Détour à Pannes (Loiret), sanctuaire du territoire sénon. *Revue archéologique du centre de la France,* 50, pp. 555–68.

Dondin-Payre, M. and Raepsaet-Charlier, M.-T., 2001. *Noms, identités culturelles et romanisation sous le Haut-Empire.* Brussels: Le livre Timperman.

Dowling, L., 1994. *Hellenism and homosexuality in Victorian Oxford.* Ithaca, NY and London: Cornell University Press.

Draycott, J., 2014. Who is performing what, and for whom? The dedication, construction and maintenance of a healing shrine in Roman Egypt. In: E. Gemi-Iordanou, S. Gordon, R. Matthew, E. McInnes, and R. Pettitt, eds. *Medicine, healing, performance: Interdisciplinary approaches to medicine and material culture.* Oxford: Oxbow, pp. 42–54.

Drew-Bear, T., Thomas, C.M. and Yildizturan, M., 1999. *Phrygian votive steles.* Ankara: Turkish Republic Ministry of Culture.

Ducaté-Paarmann, S., 2007. Voyage à l'intérieur du corps féminin. Embryons, utérus et autres organes internes dans l'art des offrandes anatomiques antiques. In: V. Dasen, ed. *L'embryon humain à travers l'histoire.* Gollion: Infolio editions, pp. 65–82.

Dunbabin, K.M.D., 1990. *Ipsa deae vestigial . . .* Footprints divine and human on Graeco-Roman monuments. *Journal of Roman Archaeology,* 3, pp. 85–109.

Durand, M. ed. 2000. *Le temple gallo-romain de la Forêt d'Halatte (Oise).* Numéro spécial, 18. Amiens: Revue archéologique de Picardie.

Ebenstein, W., 2006. Toward an archetypal psychology of disability based on the Hephaestus myth. *Disability Studies Quarterly,* 26(4). [online] Available at: http://dsq-sds.org/article/view/805/980 [Accessed 5 March 2015].

Edelstein, E. J. and Edelstein, L., 1945 and 1998. *Asclepius: Collection and interpretation of the testimonies*. Two volumes. Baltimore, MD: Johns Hopkins University Press.

Edinburgh Cast Collection, n.d. *Smugglerius unveiled: A visual essay*. [online] Available at: https://sites.eca.ed.ac.uk/casts/activities/smugglerius-unveiled-a-visual-essay/ [Accessed 21 March 2015].

Edlund-Berry, I., 2006. Healing, health, and well-being: Archaeological evidence for issues of health concerns in ancient Italy. *Archiv fur Religionsgeschichte*, 8, pp. 81–8.

Elsner, J., 2007. *Roman eyes: Visuality and subjectivity in art and text*. Princeton, NJ: Princeton University Press.

Elsner, J. and Rutherford, I. eds. 2005. *Pilgrimage in Graeco-Roman and early Christian antiquity: Seeing the gods*. Oxford: Oxford University Press.

Engineer, A., 2000. Wellcome and the 'great past'. *Medical History*, 44(3), pp. 389–404.

Espérandieu, E., 1910. *Recueil général des bas – reliefs, statues et bustes de la Gaule romaine, III, Lyonnaise*, 1. Paris: s.n.

Espérandieu, E., 1911. *Recueil général des bas – reliefs, statues et bustes de la Gaule romaine, IV, Lyonnaise*, 2. Paris: s.n.

Espérandieu, E., 1925. *Recueil général des bas – reliefs, statues et bustes de la Gaule romaine, IX, Gaule Germanique*, 3. Paris: s.n.

Fabbri, F., 2004–05. Votivi anatomici fittili e culti delle acque nell'Etruria di età medio- e tardo-repubblicana. *Rassegna di Archeologia*, 21(B), pp. 103–52.

Fabbri, F., 2010. Votivi anatomici dell'Italia di età medio e tardo-repubblicana e della Grecia di età classica: due manifestazioni cultuali a confronto. *Bollettino di Archeologia Online volume speciale: Roma 2008 – International congress of Classical archaeology: Meetings between cultures in the ancient Mediterranean*, pp. 22–32. [online] Available at: www.archeologia.beniculturali. it/pages/pubblicazioni.html [Accessed 26 March 2015].

Fagan, G.G., 1999. *Bathing in public in the Roman world*. Ann Arbor, MI: University of Michigan Press.

Faraone, C.A., 2011. Magical and medical approaches to the wandering womb in the ancient Greek world. *Classical Antiquity*, 30, pp. 1–32.

Fauduet, I. ed. 2014. *Dieux merci! Sanctuaires, dévots et offrandes en Gaule romaine*. Saint-Marcel: Musée et site archéologiques Argentomagus.

Fauth, W., 1985–86. Aphrodites Pantoffel und die Sandale der Hekate. *Grazer Beiträge*, 12–13, pp. 193–211.

Fend, M., 2005. Bodily and pictorial surfaces: Skin in French art and medicine 1790–1860. *Art History*, 28(3), pp. 311–39.

Fenelli, M., 1975. Contributo per lo studio del votivo anatomico: i votivi anatomici di Lavinio. *Archeologia Classica*, 27, pp. 206–52.

Fenelli, M., 1992. I votivi anatomici in Italia, valore e limite delle testimonianze archeologiche. In: A. Krug, ed. *From Epidaurus to Salerno. Symposium held at the European University Centre for Cultural Heritage, Ravello, April, 1990*. Rixensart: PACT Belgium, pp. 127–37.

Fenelli, M., 1995. Depositi votivi in area etrusco-italica. *Medicina nei secoli: Arte e Scienze*, 7(2), pp. 367–82.

Ferrari, F., ed. 2001. *Omero, Odissea*. Torino: UTET.

Ferrea, L. and Pinna, A., 1986. Il deposito votivo. In: F. Coarelli, ed. *Fregellae 2. Il santuario di Esculapio*. Rome: Quasar, pp. 89–144.

Fiorini, L., 2005. *Gravisca. Scavi nel santuario greco. Topografia generale e storia del santuario. Analisi dei contesti e delle stratigrafie*. Bari: Edipuglia.

Fisher, K. and Langlands, R., 2011. The censorship myth and the secret museum. In: S. Hales and J. Paul, eds. *Pompeii in the public imagination from its rediscovery to today*. Oxford: Oxford University Press, pp. 301–15.

Fisher, K. and Funke, J., 2015. Cross-disciplinary translation: British sexual science, history and anthropology. In: H. Bauer, ed. *Sexology and translation: cultural and scientific encounters across the Modern world*. Philadelphia: Temple University Press, pp. 95–114.

Flemming, R., 2012. Antiochus and Asclepiades: Medical and philosophical sectarianism at the end of the Hellenistic era. In: D. Sedley, ed. *The philosophy of Antiochus*. Cambridge: Cambridge University Press, pp. 55–79.

Flemming, R., 2013. The invention of infertility in the classical Greek world: Medicine, divinity, and gender. *Bulletin of the History of Medicine*, 87(4), pp. 565–90.

Flemming, R., 2016. Anatomical votives: Popular medicine in Republican Italy? In: W.V. Harris, ed. *Popular medicine in the ancient world*. Leiden: Brill, pp. 105–125.

Flemming, R., forthcoming. *Medicine and empire in the Roman world*. Cambridge: Cambridge University Press.

Fletcher, J., 2002. Ancient Egyptian wigs and hairstyles. *Ostracon: Journal of the Egyptian Study Society*, 13(2), pp. 2–8.

Fletcher, J., 2005. The decorated body in ancient Egypt: Hairstyles, cosmetics and tattoos. In: L. Cleland, M. Harlow and L. Llewellyn-Jones, eds. *The clothed body in the ancient world*. Oxford: Oxbow, pp. 3–13.

Forsén, B., 1996. *Griechische Gliederweihungen: eine Untersuchung zu ihrer Typologie und ihrer religions- und sozialgeschichtlichen Bedeutung*. Helsinki: Suomen Ateenan-instituutin säätiö.

Forsén, B., 2004. Model body parts. In: *Thesaurus Cultus et Rituum Antiquorum (ThesCRA)*. Volume One. Los Angeles, CA: J. Paul Getty Museum, pp. 311–13.

Fowler, C., 2001. Personhood and social relations in the British Neolithic, with a study from the Isle of Man. *Journal of Material Culture*, 6(2), pp. 137–63.

Fowler, C., 2004. *The archaeology of personhood: An anthropological approach*. London and New York, NY: Routledge.

Franco, P., Seret, N., Van Hees, J.-N., Scaillet, S., Groswasser, J. and Kahn, A., 2005. Influence of swaddling on sleep and arousal characteristics of healthy infants. *Pediatrics*, 115(5), pp. 1307–11.

Fraser, M. and Greco, M., 2005. Introduction. In: M. Fraser and M. Greco, eds. *The body: A reader*. London and New York, NY: Routledge, pp. 1–42.

Frateantonio, C., 2006. Votive offerings. In: H. Cancik and H. Schneider, eds. *Brill's New Pauly*. [e-book] Leiden: Brill. [Online] Available at: http://referenceworks.brillonline.com/entries/brill-s-new-pauly/votive-offerings-e12209510 [Accessed 26 March 2015].

Fridh-Haneson, B.-M., 1987. Votive terracottas from Italy: Types and problems. In: T. Linders and G. Nordquist, eds. *Gifts to the gods: Proceedings of the Uppsala Symposium. Boreas* 15. Uppsala: Academiae Upsaliensis, pp. 67–75.

Frohmann, C., 1956. Votivgaben in der Antike, insbesondere bei Augenerkrankungen. *Zeitschr ärzliche Fortbildung*, 50, pp. 133–5.

Frost, S., 2007. The Warren Cup: Highlighting hidden histories. *International Journal of Art and Design Education*, 26(1), pp. 63–72.

Frost, S., 2008. Secret museums: Hidden histories of sex and sexuality. *Museums and Social Issues*, 3(1), pp. 29–40.

Frost, S., 2010. The Warren Cup: Secret museums, sexuality and society. In: A.K. Levin, ed. *Gender, sexuality, and museums: A Routledge reader*. London: Routledge, pp. 138–50.

Funke, J., 2015. Navigating the past: Sexuality, race, and the uses of the primitive in Magnus Hirschfeld's *The World Journey of a Sexologist*. In: K. Fisher and R. Langlands, eds. *Sex, knowledge and receptions of the past*. Oxford: Oxford University Press, pp. 111–34.

Funnell, P., 1982. The symbolical language of antiquity. In: M. Clarke and N. Penny, eds. *The arrogant connoisseur: Richard Payne Knight 1751–1824: Essays on Richard Payne Knight together with a catalogue of works exhibited at the Whitworth Art Gallery, 1982*. Oxford: Alden Press, pp. 50–64.

Gabelmann, H., 1985. Römische Kinder in Toga Praetexta. *Jahrbuch des Deutschen Archäologischen Instituts*, 100, pp. 497–541.

Gaimster, D., 2000. Sex and sensibility at the British Museum. *History Today*, 50(9), pp. 10–15.

Garland, R., 2010. *The eye of the beholder: Deformity and disability in the Graeco-Roman world*. 2nd ed. London: Bristol Classical Press.

Gatti, S. and Demma, F., 2012. Praeneste: un luogo di culto suburbano in località Colombella. In: E. Marroni, ed. *Sacra Nominis Latini: I santuari del Lazio arcaico e repubblicano: atti del convegno internazionale, Roma, Palazzo Massimo, 19–21 febbraio 2009*. Volume One. Ostraka, volume speciale. Naples: Loffredo, pp. 341–69.

Gatti, S. and Onorati, M.T., 1996. Dalle argille alle devozioni. In: G. Baggieri and M.L. Rinaldi Veloccia, eds. 1999. *L'antica anatomia nell'arte dei donaria (Ancient anatomy in the art of votive offerings)*. Rome: Ministero per i Beni e le Attività Culturali, pp. 16–18.

Gatti Lo Guzzo, L., 1978. *Il deposito votivo dall'Esquilino detto di Minerva Medica*. Florence: Sansoni.

Gaultier, F., Haumesser, L. and Chatziefremidou, K., 2013. *L'art étrusque. 100 chefs-d'oeuvre du musée du Louvre*. Paris: Musée du Louvre editions.

Gell, A., 1998. *Art and agency: An anthropological theory*. Oxford: Clarendon Press.

Georgoulaki, E., 1997. Votives in the shape of human body parts: Shaping a framework. *Platon*, 49, pp. 188–206.

Ghirardini, G., 1888. Este. Intorno alla antichità scoperte nel fondo Baratella. *Notizie degli scavi di Anchità*, pp. 3–210.

Ginge, B., Becker, M. and Guldager, P., 1989. Of Roman extraction. *Archaeology*, 42(4), pp. 34–7.

Ginzburg, C., 2000. *Miti emblemi spie: morfologia e storia*. 2nd ed. Turin: Einaudi.

Ginzburg, C., 2008. *Storia notturna: una decifrazione del sabba*. 2nd ed. Turin: Einaudi.

Girardon, S., 1993. Ancient medicine and anatomical votives in Italy. *Bulletin of the Institute of Archaeology*, 30, pp. 29–40.

Gleba, M. and Becker, H. eds. 2009. *Votives, places and rituals in Etruscan religion*. Leiden: Brill.

Glinister, F., 2000. Sacred rubbish. In: E. Bispham and C. Smith, eds. *Religion in Archaic and Republican Italy: Evidence and experience*. Edinburgh: Edinburgh University Press, pp. 54–70.

Glinister, F., 2006. Reconsidering 'religious Romanization'. In: C.E. Schultz and P.B. Harvey, eds. *Religion in Republican Italy*. Cambridge: Cambridge University Press, pp. 10–33.

Glinister, F., 2009. Veiled and unveiled: Uncovering Roman influence in Hellenistic Italy. In: M. Gleba and H. Becker, eds. *Votives, places and rituals in Etruscan religion*. Leiden: Brill, pp. 193–215.

Godwin, J., 1994. *The theosophical enlightenment*. Albany, NY: State University of New York Press.

Goette, H.R., 1986. Die Bulla. *Bonner Jahrbücher*, 186, pp. 133–64.

Gordon, R., 2004. Raising a sceptre: Confession narratives from Lydia and Phrygia. *Journal of Roman Archaeology*, 17, pp. 177–96.

Gould, T., ed. 2007. *Cures and curiosities: Inside the Wellcome Library*. London: Profile Books.

Graells, R. and Fabregat, I., 2011. Tres cascos Italo-Calcídicos de la antigua colección Marqués de Salamanca en el Museo Arqueológico Nacional de Madrid. *Oebalus*, 6, pp. 7–49.

Graham, E.-J., 2013. The making of infants in Hellenistic and early Roman Italy: A votive perspective. *World Archaeology*, 45(2), pp. 215–31.

Graham, E.-J., 2014. Infant votives and swaddling in Hellenistic Italy. In: M. Carroll and E.-J. Graham, eds. *Infant health and death in Roman Italy and beyond*. Ann Arbor, MI: Journal of Roman Archaeology supplementary series 96, pp. 23–46.

Graham, E-J., 2016. Mobility impairment in the sanctuaries of early Roman Italy. In: C. Laes, ed. *Disabilities in antiquity*. London and New York, NY: Routledge, pp. 248–66.

Graham, E-J., forthcoming. Holding the baby? Sensory dissonance and the ambiguities of votive objects. In: E. Betts, ed. *Senses of the empire: Multisensory approaches to Roman culture.* London and New York, NY: Routledge.

Greco, E., 1985. Un santuario di età repubblicana presso il Foro di Paestum. *La parola del passato,* 40, pp. 223–32.

Greco, E., 1988. Archeologia della colonia latina di Paestum. *Dialoghi di archeologia,* 3(6), pp. 79–86.

Green, M., 1992. *Dictionary of Celtic mythology and legend.* London: Thames and Hudson.

Grenier, A., 1960. *Manuel d'archéologie gallo-romaine. Volume Four. Les monuments des eaux. Part 2. Villes d'eau et sanctuaires de l'eau.* Paris: Picard.

Grmek, M.D. and Gourevitch, D., 1998. *Les maladies dans l'art antique.* Paris: Fayard.

Guarducci, M., 1942–43. Le impronte del Quo Vadis e monumenti affini, figurati ed epigrafici. *Rendiconti della Pontificia Accademia Romana di Archeologia,* 19, pp. 305–44.

Guarducci, M., 1995. *Epigrafia greca.* Volume Three. 2nd ed. Roma: Istituto Poligrafico e Zecca dello Stato.

Guarnaccia, M., 2001. *Le terrecotte del Museo Nazionale Romano: materiali dai depositi votivi di Palestrina collezioni 'Kircheriana' e 'Palestrina'.* Rome: 'L'Erma' di Bretschneider.

Haack, M.-L., 2007a. Il concetto di 'transferts culturels': un'alternativa soddisfacente a quello di 'romanizzazione'? Il caso etrusco. In: G. Urso, ed. *Patria diversis gentibus una? Unità politica e identità etniche nell'Italia antica.* Pisa: ETS, pp. 135–46.

Haack, M.-L., 2007b. Apollon médecin en Etrurie. *Ancient Society,* 37, pp. 167–90.

Haddow, A., 1936. Historical notes on cancer from the MSS. of Louis Westenra Sambon. *Proceedings of the Royal Society of Medicine, Section on the History of Medicine,* 29(9), pp. 1015–28.

Hahn, F.H., 2012. Vow, Greece and Rome. In: R.S. Bagnall, K. Brodersen, C.B. Champion, A. Erskine and S.R. Huebner, eds. *The encyclopedia of ancient history.* Malden, MA: Wiley-Blackwell, pp. 7031–3.

Halperin, D.M., 1990. *One hundred years of homosexuality: And other essays on Greek love.* New York, NY and Abingdon: Routledge.

Hallpike, C.R., 1969. Social hair. *Man,* 4, pp. 256–64.

Hamilton, W., 1786 [1894]. *An account of the remains of the worship of Priapus.* In: R. Payne Knight and T. Wright, eds. *Two essays on the worship of Priapus.* 2nd ed. (1894), London: s.n. Electronic reprint 2003, Leeds: Celephaïs Press.

Hamilton, W., 1894. An account of the remains of the worship of Priapus. In: R.P. Knight, W. Hamilton and T. Wright, eds. *An account of the remains of the worship of Priapus: A discourse on the worship of Priapus, and its connection with the mystic theology of the ancients . . . A new edition: To which is added an essay (by Thomas Wright and others) on the worship of the generative powers during the middle ages of Western Europe. Reprinted, with a new preface and some corrections.* London: privately published, pp. 3–12.

Handbook, 1913. *Handbook to the Wellcome Historical Medical Museum founded by Henry S. Wellcome.* London: Wellcome Historical Medical Museum.

Handbook, 1920. *Handbook to the Wellcome Historical Medical Museum founded by Henry S. Wellcome.* 2nd ed. London: Wellcome Historical Medical Museum.

Hanson, A.E., 1990. The medical writers' woman. In: D. Halperin, J. Winkler and F. Zeitlin, eds. *Before sexuality: The construction of erotic experience in the ancient Greek world.* Princeton, NJ: Princeton University Press, pp. 309–38.

Harris, J., 2007. *Pompeii awakened: A story of rediscovery.* London: I. B. Tauris.

Haskell, F., 1984. The Baron d'Hancarville: An adventurer and art historian in eighteenth-century Europe. In: E. Chaney, N. Ritchie and H. Acton, eds. *Oxford, China and Italy: Writings in honour of Sir Harold Acton on his eightieth birthday.* London: Thames and Hudson, pp. 177–91.

Haskell, F. and Penny, N., 1981. *Taste and the antique: The lure of classical sculpture 1500–1900.* New Haven, CT and London: Yale University Press.

Haumesser, L., 2013. Archéologie et anatomie: un buste votif étrusque du musée du Louvre. *La revue des musées de France – Revue du Louvre*, décembre, 5, pp. 16–23.

Helbig, W., 1885. Scavi di Civita Lavinia. *Bullettino dell'Istituto di corrispondenza archeologica*, 7 and 8 (July and August), pp. 145–9.

Hermann, P. and Malay, H., 2007. *New documents from Lydia.* Vienna: Verlag der Österreichischen Akademie der Wissenschaften.

Hill, J.M., 2004. *Cultures and networks of collecting: Henry Wellcome's collection.* Ph.D. thesis. University of London, London.

Hirschberg, J., 1982. *The history of ophthalmology, Volume 1, Antiquity.* Bonn: J.P. Wayenborgh.

Hogarth, W., 1753. *The analysis of beauty: Written with a view of fixing the fluctuating ideas of taste.* London: s.n.

Holländer, E., 1912. *Plastik und Medizin.* Stuttgart: F. Enke.

Holmes, M., 2009. *Ex-votos*: Materiality, memory and cult. In: M.W. Cole and R. Zorach, eds. *The idol in the age of art: Objects, devotions and the early modern world.* Aldershot: Ashgate, pp. 159–81.

Hooper-Greenhill, E., 1992. *Museums and the shaping of knowledge.* London and New York, NY: Routledge.

Hughes, J., 2008. Fragmentation as metaphor in the Classical healing sanctuary. *Social History of Medicine*, 21(2), pp. 217–36.

Hughes, J., 2010. Dissecting the classical hybrid. In: K. Rebay-Salisbury, M.L.S. Sørenson and J. Hughes, eds. *Body parts and bodies whole: Changing perspectives and meanings.* Oxford: Oxbow Books, pp. 101–10.

Hughes, J., 2016. The biography of a votive offering from Hellenistic Italy. In: I. Weinryb, ed. *Ex voto: Votive images across cultures.* Ann Arbor, MI: University of Michigan Press, pp. 23–48.

Hughes, J., forthcoming. *Votive body parts in Greek and Roman religion.* Cambridge: Cambridge University Press.

Hume, D., 1758. *Essays and treatises on several subjects.* London: s.n.

Hunter, W., 1774. *The anatomy of the human gravid uterus exhibited in figures.* Birmingham and London: John Baskerville, and S. Baker and G. Leigh.

Ikram, S., 2003. Barbering the beardless: A possible explanation for the tufted hairstyle depicted in the 'Fayum' portrait of a young boy (J. P. Getty 78.AP.262). *Journal of Egyptian Archaeology*, 89, pp. 247–51.

Iozzo, M., 2013. *Iacta stips: il deposito votivo della sorgente di Doccia della Testa a San Casciano dei Bagni (Siena).* Florence: Polistampa.

Isager, J., 1991. *Pliny on art and society: The Elder Pliny's chapters on the history of art.* Odense: Odense University Press.

Jaeger, W., 1988. Eye votives in Greek antiquity. *Documenta ophthalmologica*, 68, pp. 9–17.

James, R.R., 1994. *Henry Wellcome.* London: Hodder and Stoughton.

Jamme, A., 1962. *Sabaean inscriptions from Maḥram Bilqîs (Mârib).* American Foundation for the Study of Man 3. Baltimore, MD: Johns Hopkins University Press.

Janes, D., 2009. *Victorian reformation: The fight over idolatry in the Church of England, 1840–1860.* Oxford and New York, NY: Oxford University Press.

Jayne, W.A., 1925. *The healing gods of ancient civilizations.* New Haven, CT: Yale University Press.

Jenkins, I., 1992. *Archaeologists and aesthetes in the sculpture galleries of the British Museum 1800–1939.* London: British Museum Press.

Jenkins, I. and Sloan, K., 1996. *Vases and volcanoes: Sir William Hamilton and his collection.* London: British Museum Press.

Johannowsky, W., 1963. Relazione preliminare sugli scavi di Teano. *Bollettino d'Arte*, 48(1–2), pp. 131–65.

Johns, C., 1982. *Sex or symbol: Erotic images of Greece and Rome*. London: British Museum Press.

Joly, M. and Lambert, P.-Y., 2004. Un ex-voto dédié à Minerve trouvé sur le sanctuaire de Mirebeau-sur-Bèze (Côte-d'Or). *Revue archéologique de l'Est et du Centre-Est*, 175, pp. 233–7.

Jones, A., 2005. Lives in fragments? Personhood and the European Neolithic. *Journal of Social Archaeology*, 5(2), pp. 193–224.

Jordanova, L., 1989. *Sexual visions*. Madison, WI: University of Wisconsin.

Kamash, Z., Shipley, L., Galakis, Y. and Skaltsa, S., 2013. Iron Age and Roman Italy. In: D. Hicks and A. Stevenson, eds. *World archaeology at the Pitt Rivers Museum: A characterization*. Oxford: Archaeopress, pp. 336–57.

Kästner, V., ed. 2010. *Etrusker in Berlin: Etruskische Kunst in der Berliner Antikensammlung. Eine Einführung*. Berlin and Regensburg: Staatliche Museen zu Berlin, and Schnell and Steiner.

Kemp, M. and Wallace, M., 2000. *Spectacular bodies: The art and science of the human body from Leonardo to now*. London: Haywood Gallery.

Kendrick, W.M., 1987. *The secret museum: Pornography in modern culture*. New York, NY: Viking.

Kiernan, P., 2009. *Miniature votive offerings in the north-west provinces of the Roman empire*. Mainz: Verlag Franz Philipp Rutzen.

King, H., 1998. *Hippocrates' woman: Reading the female body in ancient Greece*. London and New York, NY: Routledge.

King, H., 2002. Chronic pain and the creation of narrative. In: J. Porter, ed. *Constructions of the classical body*. Ann Arbor, MI: University of Michigan Press, pp. 269–86.

King, H. and Dasen, V., 2008. *La médecine dans l'Antiquité grecque et romaine*. Lausanne: Bibliothèque d'Histoire de la Médecine et de la Santé.

Kinnard, J.N., 2000. The polivalent Pādas of Visnu and the Buddha. *History of Religions*, 40(1), pp. 32–57.

Kirk, T., 2006. Materiality, personhood and monumentality in early Neolithic Britain. *Cambridge Archaeological Journal*, 16(3), pp. 333–47.

Kötting, B., 1972. Fuß. In: T. Klauser, ed. *Reallexikon für Antike und Christentum: Sachwörterbuch zur Auseinandersetzung des Christentums mit der antiken Welt. Band 8*. Stuttgart: Anton Hiersemann, pp. 722–43.

Kötting, B., 1983. Fußspuren als Zeichen göttlicher Anwesenheit. *Boreas*, 6, pp. 197–201.

Kron, G., 2013. Fleshing out the demography of Etruria. In: J.M. Turfa, ed. *The Etruscan world*. London and New York, NY: Routledge, pp. 56–75.

LaCroix, P. and Duchesne, A., 1862. *Histoire de la chaussure depuis l'antiquité la plus reculée jusqu'à nos jours: suivie de l'histoire sérieuse et drolatique des cordonniers et des artisans dont la profession se rattaché à la cordonnerie*. Paris: Adolphe Delahays.

Laes, C., Goodey, C. and Rose, M.L., eds. 2013. *Disabilities in Roman antiquity: Disparate bodies 'A capite ad calcem'*. Leiden: Brill.

La Follette, L., 1994. The costume of the Roman bride. In: J.L. Sebesta and L. Bonfante, eds. *The world of Roman costume*. Madison, WI: University of Wisconsin Press, pp. 54–64.

Lanciani, R., 1889. Veio. Scoperte nell'area della città e della necropoli veientana. *Notizie degli scavi di antichità*, pp. 10–2, pp. 29–31, pp. 60–5, pp. 154–8 and pp. 238–9.

Lang, M.L., 1977. *Cult and cure in ancient Corinth: A guide to the Asklepieion*. Princeton, NJ: American School of Classical Studies at Athens.

Lapper, A., 2005. *My life in my hands*. London: Simon and Schuster.

Larson, F., 2009. *An infinity of things: How Sir Henry Wellcome collected the world*. Oxford: Oxford University Press.

Lascaratos, J. and Marketos, S., 1997. Unknown ancient Greek ophthalmological instruments and equipment. *Documenta Ophthalmologica*, 94(1–2), pp. 151–9.

Lawrence, G., 2003. Wellcome's museum for the science of history. In: K. Arnold and D. Olsen, eds. *Medicine man: The forgotten museum of Henry Wellcome.* 2nd ed. London: British Museum Press, pp. 51–71.

Leigh, M., 1995. Wounding and popular rhetoric at Rome. *Bulletin of the Institute of Classical Studies*, 40(1), pp. 195–215.

Leitao, D.D., 2003. Adolescent hair-growing and hair-cutting rituals in ancient Greece: A sociological approach. In: D.B. Dood and C.A. Faraone, eds. *Initiation in ancient Greek rituals and narratives: New critical perspectives.* London: Routledge, pp. 109–29.

Le Roux, P., 2004. La romanisation en question. *Annales. Histoire, Sciences Sociales*, 59(2), pp. 287–311.

Lesk, A.L., 1999. *The anatomical votive terracotta phenomenon: Healing sanctuaries in the Etrusco-Latial-Campanian region during the fourth through first centuries BC.* MA thesis. University of Cincinnati, Cincinnati.

Lesk, A.L., 2002. The anatomical votive terracotta phenomenon in central Italy: Complexities of the Corinthian connection. In: G. Muskett, A. Koltsida and M. Georgiadis, eds. *SOMA 2001 Symposium on Mediterranean Archaeology.* Oxford: Archaeopress, pp. 193–202.

Levine, M.M., 1995. The gendered grammar of ancient Mediterranean hair. In: H. Eilberg-Schwartz and W. Doniger, eds. *Off with her head! The denial of women's identity in myth, religion, and culture.* Berkeley, CA: University of California Press, pp. 76–130.

Licht, H., 1925. *Sittengeschichte Griechenlands: in zwei Bänden und einem. Ergänzungsband.* Bd. 3. Dresden and Zurich: Aretz.

LiDonnici, L.R., 1992. Compositional background of the Epidaurian 'iamata'. *American Journal of Philology*, 113(1), pp. 25–41.

Linders, T. and Nordquist, G., eds. 1987. *Gifts to the gods: Proceedings of the Uppsala symposium. Boreas 15.* Uppsala: Academiae Upsaliensis.

LiPuma, E., 1998. Modernity and forms of personhood in Melanesia. In: M. Lambek and A. Strathern, eds. *Bodies and persons: Comparative perspectives from Africa and Melanesia.* Cambridge: Cambridge University Press, pp. 53–79.

Liverani, M., 1977. Segni arcaici di individuazione personale. A proposito del motivo del riconoscimento nei tragici greci. *Rivista di Filologia e di Istruzione Classica*, 105, pp. 106–18.

Liverani, P., 2004. Excavations in Etruria in the 1880s: The case of Veii. In: I. Bignamini, ed. *Archives and excavations: Essays on the history of archaeological excavations in Rome and southern Italy from the Renaissance to the nineteenth century.* London: British School at Rome, pp. 267–80.

Lloyd, G.E.R., 1983. *Science, folklore and ideology: Studies in the life sciences in ancient Greece.* Cambridge: Cambridge University Press.

Lolos, Y.A., 2005. The sanctuary of Titane and the city of Sikyon. *Annual of the British School at Athens*, 100, pp. 275–98.

London Catalogue, 1918. *Catalogue of old European and Oriental armour, old Oriental and European china, bronzes, etc. sold by order of the trustees of the late William Burges, A.R.A; and J. Ollis Pelton, Esq., 18–19 November 1918.* London: s.n.

LoPresti, R., 2008. *Aisthesis polytropos. Teorie e rappresentazioni della percezione sensoriale e della cognizione negli scritti della Collezione Ippocratica.* Ph.D. thesis. University of Palermo, Palermo.

Lowe, C., 1978. The historical significance of early Latin votive deposits (up to 4th century BC). In: H.M. Blake, T.W. Potter and D.B. Whitehouse, eds. *Papers in Italian archaeology I: The Lancaster seminar. Recent research in prehistoric, classical and medieval archaeology. Part 1.* BAR Supplementary Series 41(1). Oxford: Archaeopress, pp. 141–51.

Lyons, A.P. and Lyons, H.D., 2004. *Irregular connections: A history of anthropology and sexuality.* Lincoln, NE and London: University of Nebraska Press.

Mack, J., 2003. Medicine and anthropology in Wellcome's collection. In: K. Arnold and D. Olsen, eds. *Medicine man: The forgotten museum of Henry Wellcome.* London: British Museum Press, pp. 213–33.

Maetzke, G., 1982–84. Il santuario etrusco italico di Castelsecco (Arezzo). *Rendiconti della Pontificia Accademia di Archeologia*, 55–6, pp. 35–53.

Maioli, M.G. and Mastrocinque, A., 1992. *La stipe di Villa di Villa e i culti degli antichi Veneti.* Corpus delle stipi votive in Italia VI. Regio X, 1. Rome: Giorgio Bretschneider Editore.

Malay, H., 1999. *Researches in Lydia, Mysia and Aiolis.* Vienna: Verlag der Österreichischen Akademie der Wissenschaften.

Malay, H., 2003. A praise on Men Artemidorou Axiottenos. *Epigraphica Anatolica*, 36, pp. 13–8.

Malay, H. and Sayar, M.H., 2004. A new confession to Zeus 'from Twin Oaks'. *Epigraphica Anatolica*, 37, pp. 183–4.

Malul, M., 2001. Foot symbolism in the ancient Near East: Imprinting foundlings' feet in clay in ancient Mesopotamia. *Zeitschrift für Altorientalische und Biblische Rechtgeschichte*, 7, pp. 353–67.

Mansfield, E.C., 2007. *Too beautiful to picture: Zeuxis, myth, and mimesis.* Minneapolis, MN and London: University of Minnesota Press.

Martin, M., 2004. *Sorcières et magiciennes dans le monde gréco-romain.* Paris: Éditions Le Manuscrit.

Matzner, S., 2010. From Uranians to homosexuals: Philhellenism, Greek homoeroticism and gay emancipation in Germany 1835–1915. *Classical Receptions Journal*, 2(1), pp. 60–91.

Mazzei, M. and D'Ercole, M.C., 2003. Le stipi lucerine del Belvedere: nuovi ritrovamenti. Nota preliminare. In: L. Quilici and S. Quilici Gigli, eds. *Santuari e luoghi di culto nell'Italia antica.* 'L'Erma' di Bretschneider. Atlante tematico di topografia antica, 12, pp. 273–8.

Melfi, M., 2007. *I santuari di Asclepio in Grecia.* Rome: 'L'Erma' di Bretschneider.

Melis, F. and Quilici Gigli, S., 1983. Votivi e luoghi di culto nella campagna di Velletri. *Archeologia Classica*, 35, pp. 1–44.

Méniel, P., 1997. Les restes animaux et la définition des lieux de culte en Gaule septentrionale au deuxième âge du fer. *Cahiers du Centre Gustave-Glotz*, 8, pp. 171–80.

Méniel, P., 2006. Religion et sacrifices d'animaux. In: C. Goudineau, ed. *Religion et société en Gaule.* Paris: Errance, pp. 165–75.

Meyer-Steineg, T., 1912. *Darstellungen normaler und krankhaft veränderter Körperteile an antiken Weihgaben.* Volume Two. Jena: Verlag von Gustav Fischer.

Miari, M., 1997. Grotte Maritza, di Ciccio Felice, delle Marmitte. In: M. Pacciarelli, ed. *Acque, grotte e dei 3000 anni di culti preromani in Romagna, Marche e Abruzzo.* Fusignano: Musei Civici di Imola, pp. 103–11.

Middleton, C., 1729. *A letter from Rome, shewing an exact conformity between popery and paganifm: Or, the religion of the prefent Romans derived from that of their heathen ancestors.* London: W. Innys.

Middleton, C., 1733. *A letter from Rome, shewing an exact conformity between popery and paganifm: Or, the religion of the prefent Romans derived from that of their heathen ancestors.* London: s.n. Reprinted 2010. Whitefish, Montana: Kessinger Publishing.

Miller, K.M., 1985. Apollo Lairbenos. *Numen*, 32(1), pp. 46–70.

Millett-Gallant, A., 2000. *The disabled body in contemporary art.* Basingstoke: Palgrave Macmillan.

Mingazzini, P., 1938. Il santuario della Dea Marica alle foci del Garigliano. *Monumenti Antichi*, 37(2), pp. 693–956.

Minto, A., 1925. Saturnia etrusca e romana. Le recenti scoperte archeologiche. *Monumenti Antichi*, 30, pp. 585–705.

Mitchell, S., 1993. *Anatolia: Land, men and gods in Asia Minor*. Oxford: Clarendon Press.

Moltesen, M., ed. 1997. *I Dianas hellige lund: fund fra en helligdom i Nemi (In the sacred grove of Diana: Finds from a sanctuary at Nemi)*. Copenhagen: Ny Carlsberg Glyptotek.

Monson, J., 2000. The new 'Ain Dara temple: Closest Solomonic parallel. *Biblical Archaeology Review*, 26(3), pp. 20–35, p. 66.

Moreau, A.M., 1994. *Le mythe de Jason et Médée: le va-nu-pied et la sorcière*. Paris: Les Belles Lettres.

Moretti, M., 1967. *Il Museo Nazionale di Villa Giulia*. Rome: Tipografia Artistica editrice.

Moretti Sgubini, A.M., ed. 2004. *Scavo nello scavo: gli Etruschi non visti. Ricerche e 'riscoperte' nei depositi dei musei archeologici dell'Etruria meridionale (Catalogo della Mostra, Viterbo, Fortezza Giulioli, 5 marzo–30 giugno 2004)*. Rome: Union Printing.

Moretti Sgubini, M., Ricciardi, L. and Costantini, S., 2005. Testimonianze da Vulci. In: A.M. Comella and S. Mele, eds. *Depositi votivi e culti dell'Italia antica dall'età arcaica a quella tardo-repubblicana*. Bari: Edipuglia, pp. 259–66.

Morgan, D., 2010. Introduction: The matter of belief. In: D. Morgan, ed. *Religion and material culture: The matter of belief*. Abingdon: Routledge, pp. 1–17.

Motte, A., 1963. Le pré sacré de Pan et des nymphes dans le Phèdre de Platon. *L'Antiquité Classique*, 32, pp. 460–76.

Murgia, E., 2013. *Culti e romanizzazione: resistenza, continuità, trasformazioni*. Trieste: Edizioni Università Di Trieste.

Murray, D., 1904. *Museums: Their history and their use, with a bibliography and list of museums in the United Kingdom*. Glasgow: James MacLehose and Sons.

Mylonas, G.E., 1961. *Eleusis and the Eleusinian mysteries*. Princeton, NJ: Princeton University Press.

Mylonopoulos, J., 2006. Greek sanctuaries as places of communication through rituals: An archaeological perspective. In: E. Stavrianopoulou, ed. *Ritual and communication in the Graeco-Roman world*. Kernos Supplement 16. Liège: Centre international d'étude de la religion grecque antique, pp. 69–110.

Myres, J., 1902–03. The sanctuary site of Petsofa. *Annual of the British School at Athens*, 9, pp. 356–87.

Nacht, J., 1923. Der Fuß. Eine folklorische Studie. *Jahrbuch für Judische Volkskunde*, 25, pp. 123–77.

Nagy, H., 2013. Etruscan terracotta figurines. In: J.M. Turfa, ed. *The Etruscan world*. London and New York, NY: Routledge, pp. 2373–407.

Namur, A., 1848. *Rapport sur les inscriptions votives et statuettes trouvée à Géromont près de Girou-ville (Luxembourg belge) et sur les tombes gallo-franques de Wecker découvertes en 1848*. s.l.: s.n.

Naso, A., 2011. La salute della bocca. Protesi dentarie auree in Etruria e nel Lazio. In: S. Rafanelli and P. Spaziani, eds. *Etruschi. Il privilegio della bellezza*. Sansepolcro: Aboca, pp. 146–54.

Nead, L., 1992. *The female nude: Art, obscenity and sexuality*. London and New York, NY: Routledge.

Nicolson, F.W., 1891. Greek and Roman barbers. *Harvard Studies in Classical Philology*, 2, pp. 41–56.

Nochlin, L., 1994. *The body in pieces: The fragment as a metaphor of modernity*. London: Thames and Hudson.

Nuttens, T., Goossens, R., Tytgat, C., De Wulf, A., Van Damme, D., Hennau, M. and Devriendt, D., 2007. The virtual reconstruction of the Titane archaeological site (Greece) by aims of photogrammetry. *International Archives of the Photogrammetry, Remote Sensing and Spatial Information Sciences*, 34(3). [online] Available at: http://cipa.icomos.org/fileadmin/template/doc/ATHENS/FP108.pdf [Accessed 5 March 2015].

Nutton, V., 2013. *Ancient medicine*. 2nd ed. London and New York, NY: Routledge.

Oberhelman, S.M. ed. 2013. *Dreams, healing, and medicine in Greece: From antiquity to the present*. Aldershot: Ashgate.

Oberhelman, S.M., 2014. Anatomical votive reliefs as evidence for specialization at healing sanctuaries in the ancient Mediterranean world. *Athens Journal of Health*, 1, pp. 47–62.

Oliver, M. and Barnes, C., 2012. *The new politics of disablement*. Basingstoke: Palgrave Macmillan.

Olson, K., 2008. *Dress and the Roman woman: Self-presentation and society*. Abingdon and New York, NY: Routledge.

Onians, R.B., 1951. *The origins of European thought: About the body, the mind the soul, the world time, and fate*. Cambridge: Cambridge University Press.

Opper, T., 2003. Ancient glory and modern learning: The sculpture-decorated library. In: K. Sloan and A. Burnett, eds. *Enlightenment: Discovering the world in the eighteenth century*. London: British Museum Press, pp. 58–67.

Orrells, D., 2011. *Classical culture and modern masculinity*. Oxford: Oxford University Press.

Orrells, D., Bhambra, G.K. and Roynon, T., 2011. *African Athena: New agendas*. Oxford: Oxford University Press.

Osborne, R., 2004. Hoards, votives, offerings: The archaeology of the dedicated object. *World Archaeology*, 36(1), pp. 1–10.

Paduano, G., 1970. La scena del 'riconoscimento' nell'Elettra di Euripide e la critica razionalistica alle Coefore. *Rivista di Filologia e di Istruzione Classica*, 98, pp. 385–405.

Paglieri, S., 1960. Una stipe votiva vulcente. *Rivista dell'Istituto Nazionale di Archeologia e Storia dell'Arte*, new series 9, pp. 74–96.

Painter, K., 1971. A Roman gold ex voto from Wroxeter. *Antiquaries Journal*, 51(2), pp. 329–31.

Palmer, R.E.A., 1996. Locket gold, lizard green. In: J.F. Hall, ed. *Etruscan Italy: Etruscan influences on the civilizations of Italy from antiquity to the modern era*. Provo, Utah, UT: Museum of Art, Brigham Young University, pp. 17–27.

Palmer, R.E.A., 1998[1989]. Bullae insignia ingenuitatis. *American Journal of Ancient History* 14(1), pp. 1–69.

Pannella, S. ed. 2013. *Scavi ad Aprilia: condotti nel corso della realizzazione di una centrale elettrica a ciclo combinato: via della Cogna, Campo di Carne: rinvenimento di un impianto rustico, via del Tufetto, Campoleone: rinvenimento di due stipi votive*. Viterbo: Betagamma.

Paris exhibition, 1989. *Fautrier 1898–1964 (catalogue de l'exposition, Paris, Musée d'art moderne de la Ville de Paris, 25 mai-24 septembre 1989)*. Paris: Amis du Musée d'art moderne de la ville de Paris.

Parker, R., 1996. *Miasma: Pollution and purification in early Greek religion*. Oxford: Clarendon Press.

Paulhan, J., 1949. *Fautrier l'enragé*. Paris: s.n.

Pautasso, A., 1994. *Il deposito votivo presso la porta Nord a Vulci*. Corpus delle stipi votive in Italia VII. Regio VII.3. Rome: Giorgio Bretschneider Editore.

Payne Knight, R., 1805. *Analytical inquiry into the principles of taste*. 2nd ed. London: s.n.

Payne Knight, R., 1809. *Specimens of antient sculpture: Egyptian, Etruscan, Greek and Roman: Selected from different collections in Great Britain, by the Society of Dilettanti*. London: T. Payne and J. White and Co.

Payne Knight, R., 1894. A discourse on the worship of Priapus, and its connection with the mystic theology of the ancients. In: R. Payne Knight, W. Hamilton and T. Wright, *An account of the remains of the worship of Priapus: A discourse on the worship of Priapus, and its connection with the mystic theology of the ancients . . . A new edition: To which is added an essay (by Thomas Wright and others) on the worship of the generative powers during the middle ages of western Europe. Reprinted, with a new preface and some corrections*. London: privately published, pp. 13–113.

Payne Knight, R., 1894[1865]. *Discourse on the worship of Priapus*. In: R. Payne Knight and T. Wright, eds. *Two essays on the worship of Priapus*. 2nd ed. (1894), London: s.n. Electronic reprint 2003, Leeds: Celephaïs Press.

Paz de Hoz, M., 2009. The aretalogical character of the Maionian 'confession' inscriptions. In: Á. Martínez Fernández, ed. *Estudios de Epigrafía*. La Laguna, Santa Cruz de Tenerife: Universidad de La Laguna, Servicio de Publicaciones, pp. 357–68.

Pazzini, A., 1935. Il significato degli 'ex voto' ed il concetto della divinità guaratrice. *Rendiconti della Reale Accademia dei Lincei, Classe di scienze morali, storiche e filologiche*, 6(11), pp. 42–79.

Peacock, J., 2005. *Chaussures: un répertoire des modèles de l'Antiquité à nos jours*. Paris: Éditions De la Martinière.

Peatfield, A.A.D. and Morris, C., 2012. Dynamic spirituality on Minoan peak sanctuaries. In: K. Rountree, C. Morris and A.A.D. Peatfield, eds. *Archaeology of spiritualities*. New York, NY: Springer, p. 227–45.

Pensabene, P., 1979. Doni votivi fittili di Roma: contributo per un inquadramento storico. *Archeologia Laziale*, 2, pp. 217–22.

Pensabene, P. ed. 2001. *Le terrecotte del Museo Nazionale Romano II. Materiali dai depositi votivi di Palestrina: collezioni 'Kircheriana' e 'Palestrina'*. Rome: 'L'Erma' di Bretschneider.

Pensabene, P., Rizzo, M.A., Roghi, M. and Talamo, E., 1980. *Terrecotte votive dal Tevere*. Studi Miscellanei 25. Rome: 'L'Erma' di Bretschneider.

Petherbridge, D., 1997. Art and anatomy: The meeting of text and image. In: D. Petherbridge and L. Jordanova, eds. *The quick and the dead: Artists and anatomy*. London: Southbank Centre, pp. 7–99.

Petridou, G., 2009. *Artemidi to ichnos*: Divine feet and hereditary priesthood in Pisidian Pogla. *Anatolian Studies*, 59, pp. 81–93.

Petridou, G., 2013. 'Blessed is he, who has seen . . .' The power of ritual viewing and ritual framing in Eleusis. *Helios*, 40(1–2), pp. 309–41.

Petridou, G., 2014. Asclepius the physician, Asclepius *theos soter*: Epiphanies as diagnostic and therapeutic tools. In: D. Michaelides, ed. *Medicine and healing in the ancient Mediterranean*. Oxford: Oxbow Books, pp. 297–308.

Petridou, G., 2016. Healing shrines. In: G.L. Irby, ed. *A companion to science, technology, and medicine in ancient Greece and Rome*. Malden, MA: Wiley-Blackwell, pp. 434–49.

Petrone, G., 2004. I piedi di Medea. In: G. Petrone and S. D'Onofrio, eds. *Il corpo a pezzi. Orizzonti simbolici a confronto*. Palermo: Flaccovio, pp. 39–51.

Petsalis-Diomidis, A., 2005. The body in space: Visual dynamics in Graeco-Roman healing pilgrimage. In: J. Elsner and I. Rutherford, eds. *Pilgrimage in Graeco-Roman and early Christian antiquity: Seeing the gods*. Oxford: Oxford University Press, pp. 183–218.

Petsalis-Diomidis, A., 2006. Amphiaraos present: Images and healing pilgrimage in classical Greece. In: R. Maniura and R. Shepherd, eds. *Presence: The inherence of the prototype within images and other objects*. Aldershot: Ashgate, pp. 205–29.

Petsalis-Diomidis, A., 2010. *Truly beyond wonders: Aelius Aristides and the cult of Asklepios*. Oxford: Oxford University Press.

Pettazzoni, R., 1936. *La Confessione dei Peccati*. Volume Three. Bologna: Zanichelli.

Petzl, G., 1994. Die Beichtinschriften Westkleinasiens. *Epigraphica Anatolica*, 22, pp. 1–143.

Petzl, G., 1997. Neue Inschriften aus Lydien (II): Addenda und Corrigenda zu 'Die Beichtinschriften Westkleinasiens'. *Epigraphica Anatolica*, 28, pp. 69–79.

Petzl, G., 2006. God and physician: Competitors or colleagues? In: A. Marcone, ed. *Medicina e società nel mondo antico: atti del convegno di Udine 4–5 ottobre 2005*. Florence: Le Monnier Università, pp. 55–62.

Pfuhl, E. and Möbius, H., 1977. *Die ostgriechischen Grabreliefs*. Mainz: Von Zabern.

Phillips, O., 2002. The witches' Thessaly. In: P. Mirecki and M. Meyer, eds. *Magic and ritual in the ancient world*. Leiden: Brill, pp. 378–86.

Pickel, H., Winter, R. and Young, R.H., 2009. History of gynecological pathology XXII. Johann Veit, M.D. *International Journal of Gynecological Pathology*, 28(2), pp. 103–6.

Pistorius, O., 2012. *Blade runner: My story*. London: Virgin.

Platt, V.J., 2011. *Facing the gods: Epiphany and representation in Greco-Roman art, literature, and religion*. Cambridge: Cambridge University Press.

Pointon, M., 1999. Materializing mourning: Hair, jewellery and the body. In: M. Kwint, C. Breward and J. Aynsley, eds. *Material memories*. London and New York, NY: Berg, pp. 39–57.

Postle, M., 2004. Flayed for art: The écorché figure in the English art academy. *British Art Journal*, 5(1), pp. 55–63.

Potter, T.W. and Wells, C., 1985. A Republican healing-sanctuary at Ponte di Nona near Rome and the classical tradition of votive medicine. *Journal of the British Archaeological Association*, 138, pp. 23–47.

Poux, M., 2004. *L'âge du vin: rites de boisson, festins et libations en Gaule indépendante*. Montagnac: M. Mergoil.

Prettejohn, E., 2012. *The modernity of ancient sculpture: Greek sculpture and modern art from Winckelmann to Picasso*. London and New York, NY: I.B. Tauris.

Provost, M. ed. 2009a. *Carte archéologique de la Gaule. La Côte-d'Or. 21/1. Alésia*. Paris: Académie des Inscriptions et Belles-Lettres.

Provost, M. ed. 2009b. *Carte archéologique de la Gaule. La Côte-d'Or. 21/2. d'Allerey à Normier*. Paris: Académie des Inscriptions et Belles-Lettres.

Provost, M. ed. 2009c. *Carte archéologique de la Gaule. La Côte-d'Or. 21/3. De Nuits-Saint-Georges à Voulaines-les-Templiers*. Paris: Académie des Inscriptions et Belles-Lettres.

Quagliotti, A.M., 1998. *Buddhapadas: An essay on the representations of the footprints of the Buddha with a descriptive catalogue of the Indian specimens from the 2nd century BC to the 4th century AD*. Kamakura: Institute of the Silk Road Studies.

Quilici, L., 1983. Palestrina: luoghi di rinvenimento di materiale votivo. *Archeologia Laziale*, 5, pp. 88–103.

Quinn, M., 2006. *Fourth plinth*. Göttingen: Steidl.

Radt, W., 1999. *Pergamon: Geschichte und Bauten einer antiken Metropole*. Darmstadt: Primus.

Rauh, N.K., 1993. *The sacred bonds of commerce: Religion, economy, and trade society at Hellenistic Roman Delos, 166–87 BC*. Amsterdam: J.C. Gieben.

Rawson, E., 1982. The life and death of Asclepiades of Bithynia. *Classical Quarterly*, 32(2), pp. 358–70.

Rebay-Salisbury, K., Sørenson, M.L.S. and Hughes, J. eds. 2010. *Body parts and bodies whole: Changing relations and meanings*. Oxford: Oxbow.

Recke, M., 2013. Science as art: Etruscan anatomical votives. In: J.M. Turfa, ed. *The Etruscan world*. London and New York, NY: Routledge, pp. 1068–85.

Recke, M. and Wamser-Krasznai, W., 2008. *Kultische Anatomie: etruskische Körperteil-Votive aus der Antikensammlung der Justus-Liebig-Universität Giessen*. Ingolstadt: Deutsches Medizinhistorisches Museum.

Reddé, M. ed. 2011. *Aspects de la Romanisation dans l'Est de la Gaule*. Two volumes. Glux-en-Glenne: Centre archéologique européen.

Reggiani Massarini, A.M., 1988. *Santuario degli Equicoli a Corvaro: oggetti votivi del Museo Nazionale Romano*. Rome: De Luca edizioni d'arte.

Regnault, F., 1900. Les terres cuites grecques de Smyrne. *Bulletin et mémoires de la Société d'anthropologie de Paris*, 1(1), pp. 467–77.

Regnault, F., 1909a. Terres cuites pathologiques de Smyrne. *Bulletin et mémoires de la Société d'anthropologie de Paris*, 10(1), pp. 633–5.

Regnault, F., 1909b. Collection d'ex-voto romains du Musée Archéologique de Madrid. *Bulletins et mémoires de la Société d'anthropologie de Paris*, 10(1), pp. 258–64.

Regnault, F., 1926. Les ex-voto polysplanchniques de l'Antiquité. *Bulletin de la Société française d'histoire de la médecine*, 20(3–4), pp. 135–50.

Reilly, J., 1997. Naked and limbless: Learning about the feminine body in ancient Athens. In: A.O. Koloski-Ostrow and C.I. Lyons, eds. *Naked truths: Women, sexuality and gender in classical art and archaeology*. London and New York, NY: Routledge, pp. 154–73.

Rellini, U., 1920. Cavernette e ripari preistorici nell'agro falisco. *Monumenti Antichi*, 26, pp. 5–170.

Renberg, G.H., 2006–7. Public and private places of worship in the cult of Asclepius at Rome. *Memoirs of the American Academy in Rome*, 51–2, pp. 87–172.

Rey-Vodoz, V., 1991. Les offrandes dans les sanctuaires gallo-romains. In: J.-L. Brunaux, ed. *Les sanctuaires celtiques et leurs rapports avec le monde méditerranéen*. Paris: Errance, pp. 215–20.

Rey-Vodoz, V., 1994. La Suisse dans l'Europe des sanctuaires gallo-romains. In: C. Goudineau, G. Coulon and I. Fauduet, eds. *Les sanctuaires de tradition indigène en Gaule romaine. Actes du colloque d'Argentomagus (Argenton-sur-Creuse, Saint-Marcel, Indre) 8, 9, et 10 octobre 1992*. Paris: Errance, pp. 7–16.

Rey-Vodoz, V., 2006. Offrandes et rituels votifs dans les sanctuaires de Gaule romaine. In: M. Dondin-Payre and M.T. Raepsaet-Charlier, eds. *Sanctuaires, pratiques culturelles et territoires civiques dans l'Occident romain*. Brussels: Le livre Timperman, pp. 219–38.

Ricciardi, L., 1988–89. Canino (Viterbo) – Il santuario etrusco di Fontanile di Legnisina a Vulci. Relazione delle campagne di scavo 1985 e 1986: l'altare monumentale e il deposito votivo. *Notizie degli scavi di Anchità*, 42–3, pp. 137–209.

Richardson, R., 2003. Human remains. In: K. Arnold and D. Olsen, eds. *Medicine man: The forgotten museum of Henry Wellcome*. 2nd ed. London: British Museum Press, pp. 319–45.

Ricl, M., 1991. Hosios kai dikaios. Première partie: Catalogue des inscriptions. *Epigraphica Anatolica*, 18, pp. 1–70.

Ricl, M., 1995. The appeal to divine justice in the Lydian confession-inscriptions. In: E. Schwertheim, ed. *Forschungen in Lydien*. Asia Minor Studien 17. Bonn: Habelt, pp. 67–76.

Ricl, M., 1997. CIG 4142 – a forgotten confession inscription from north-west Phrygia. *Epigraphica Anatolica*, 29, pp. 35–43.

Ritti, T., Şimşek, C. and Yıldız, H., 2000. Dediche e καταγραφαί nel santuario frigio di Apollo Lairbenos. *Epigraphica Anatolica*, 32, pp. 1–88.

Rivers, W.H.R., 1924. *Medicine, magic and religion*. London: Kegan Paul, Trench and Trübner.

Rives, J.B., 2007. *Religion in the Roman empire*. Malden, MA and Oxford: Wiley-Blackwell.

Rodriguez Oliva, P., 1987. Representaciones des pies en el arte antiguo de los territorios malacitanos. *Baetica: Estudios de Arte, Geografia e Historia*, 10, pp. 189–209.

Roebuck, C., 1951. *Corinth: Results of excavations conducted by the American School of Classical Studies at Athens. Volume 14: The Asklepieion and Lerna*. Princeton, NJ: American School of Classical Studies at Athens.

Roghi, M., 1999. Le terrecotte votive. In: M. Barbera, ed. *Museo Nazionale Romano: la collezione Gorga*. Milan and Rome: Electa and Ministero per i beni e le attività culturali, Soprintendeza Archeologica di Roma, pp. 137–8.

Roman, J., 1890. Séance du 5 mars 1890. *Bulletin de la Société nationale des antiquaires de France*, pp. 117–18.

Romeuf, A.-M. and Dumontet, L., 2000. *Les ex-voto gallo-romains de Chamalières (Puy-de-Dôme): bois sculptés de la source des Roches*. Documents d'archéologie française, 82. Paris: Editions de la Maison des sciences de l'homme.

Rose, M.L., 2003. *The staff of Oedipus: Transforming disability in ancient Greece.* Ann Arbor, MI: University of Michigan Press.

Rostad, A., 2002. Confession or reconciliation? The narrative structure of the Lydian and Phrygian 'confession inscriptions'. *Symbolae Osloenses*, 77(1), pp. 145–64.

Rostad, A., 2006. The religious context of the Lydian propitiatory inscriptions. *Symbolae Osloenses*, 81(1), pp. 88–108.

Rouquette, P., 1911. Les ex-voto médicaux d'organes internes dans l'Antiquité romaine. *Bulletin de la Société française d'histoire de la médecine*, 10, pp. 504–19.

Rouquette, P., 1912a. Les ex-voto médicaux d'organes internes dans l'Antiquité romaine. *Bulletin de la Société française d'histoire de la médecine*, 11, pp. 270–87.

Rouquette, P., 1912b. Les ex-voto médicaux d'organes internes dans l'Antiquité romaine. *Bulletin de la Société française d'histoire de la médecine*, 11, pp. 370–414.

Rouse, W.H.D., 1902. *Greek votive offerings: An essay in the history of Greek religion.* Cambridge: Cambridge University Press.

Rousseau, G.S., 1988. The sorrow of Priapus: Anticlericalism, homosocial desire and Richard Payne-Knight. In: R. Porter and G.S. Rousseau, eds. *Sexual underworlds of the Enlightenment.* Chapel Hill, NC: University of North Carolina Press, pp. 101–55.

Rubensohn, O., 1895. Demeter als Heilgottheit. *Mitteilungen des Deutschen Archäologischen Instituts, Athenische Abteilung*, 20, pp. 360–7.

Rüpke, J., 2007. *Religion of the Romans.* Cambridge: Polity Press.

Russell, G., 1987. The Wellcome Historical Medical Museum's dispersal of non-medical material, 1936–1983. *Newsletter (Museum Ethnographers Group)*, 20, pp. 21–45.

Russell, N.U., 2014. Aspects of baby wrappings: Swaddling, carrying and wearing. In: S. Harris and L. Douny, eds. *Wrapping and unwrapping material culture: Archaeological and anthropological perspectives.* Walnut Creek, CA: Left Coast Press, pp. 43–58.

Ruta Serafini, A., ed. 2002. *Este preromana. Una città e i suoi santuari.* Treviso: Canova.

Rynearson, N., 2003. Constructing and deconstructing the body in the cult of Asklepios. *Stanford Journal of Archaeology*, 2. Available at: http://www.stanford.edu/dept/archaeology/journal/newdraft/2003_Journal/rynearson/paper.pdf [Accessed 27 March 2015].

Sambon, L., 1895a. Donaria of medical interest in the Oppenheimer collection of Etruscan and Roman antiquities. *British Medical Journal*, 2(1803), pp. 146–50.

Sambon, L., 1895b. Medical antiquities. *The Times*, 2 August, p. 4.

Sannibale, M., 1998. *Le armi della collezione Gorga al Museo Nazionale Romano.* Rome: 'L'Erma' di Bretschneider.

Sawday, J., 1995. *The body emblazoned: Dissection and the human body in Renaissance culture.* London and New York, NY: Routledge.

Scarpellini, M.G., 2001. La collezione Vincenzo Funghini nel Museo Archeologico Nazionale di Arezzo. In: S. Vilucchi, P. Zamarchi Grassi and S. Baldassari, eds. *Etruschi nel tempo: i ritrovamenti di Arezzo dal '500 ad oggi: luglio–dicembre, 2001, Basilica Inferiore di San Francesco, Museo Archeologico Nazionale Gaio Cilnio Mecenate, Arezzo.* Arezzo: Provincia di Arezzo, pp. 177–241.

Scarpellini, M.G., 2013. The bronze votive tradition in Etruria. In: J.M. Turfa, ed. *The Etruscan world.* London and New York, NY: Routledge, pp. 2452–87.

Scheffer, C., 2006. Sinister birds and other unpleasant Etruscan motifs. In: E. Herring, I. Lemnos, F. Lo Schiavo, L. Vagnetti, R. Whitehouse and J. Wilkins, eds. *Across frontiers: Etruscans, Greeks, Phoenicians and Cypriots: Studies in honour of David Ridgway and Francesca Serra Ridgway.* Accordia Specialist Studies on the Mediterranean 6. London: Accordia Research Institute, University of London, pp. 507–15.

Scheid, J., 1991. Sanctuaires et thermes sous l'Empire. In: *Les thermes romains: actes de la table ronde organisée par l'École française de Rome (Rome, 11–12 novembre 1988).* Collection École Française de Rome 142. Rome: École Française de Rome, pp. 205–16.

Scheid, J., 2003. *An introduction to Roman religion.* Translated from French by J. Lloyd. Edinburgh: Edinburgh University Press.

Schultz, C.E., 2006. *Women's religious activity in the Roman Republic.* Chapel Hill, NC and London: University of North Carolina Press and Eurospan.

Sebesta, J.L., 1994. Symbolism in the costume of the Roman woman. In: J.L. Sebesta and L. Bonfante, eds. *The world of Roman costume.* Madison, WI: University of Wisconsin Press, pp. 46–53.

Sima, A., 1999. Kleinasiatische Parallelen zu den altsüdarabischen Buß- und Sühneinschriften. *Altorientalische Forschungen,* 26, pp. 140–53.

Sirano, F., 2007. *Il museo di Teanum Sidicinum.* Naples: Electa.

Skinner, G.M., 1986. Sir Henry Wellcome's museum for the science of history. *Medical History,* 30(4), pp. 383–418.

Smith, J.Z., 1987. *To take place: Toward theory in ritual.* Chicago, IL and London: University of Chicago Press.

Smithers, S., 1993. Images of piety and hope: Select terracotta votives from west-central Italy. *Studia varia from the J. Paul Getty Museum,* 1, pp. 13–32.

Sobchack, V., 2006. A leg to stand on: Prosthetics, metaphor, and materiality. In: M. Smith and J. Morra, eds. *The prosthetic impulse: From a posthuman present to a biocultural future.* Cambridge, MA and London: MIT Press, pp. 17–41.

Söderlind, M., 2002. *Late Etruscan votive heads from Tessennano: Production, distribution, sociohistorical context.* Rome: 'L'Erma' di Bretschneider.

Söderlind, M., 2005. Heads with *velum* and the Etrusco-Latial-Campanian type of votive deposit. In: A. Comella and S. Mele, eds. *Depositi votivi e culti dell'Italia antica dall'età arcaica a quella tardo-repubblicana: atti del convegno di studi, Perugia, 1–4 giugno 2000.* Bari: Edipuglia, pp. 359–65.

Sourvinou-Inwood, C., 2003. Festival and mysteries: Aspects of the Eleusinian cult. In: M. Cosmopoulos, ed. *Greek mysteries: The archaeology and ritual of ancient Greek secret cults.* London and New York, NY: Routledge, pp. 25–49.

Squire, M., 2009. *Image and text in Graeco-Roman antiquity.* Cambridge and New York, NY: Cambridge University Press.

Squire, M., 2011. *The art of the body: Antiquity and its legacy.* London and New York, NY: I.B. Tauris.

Stafford, E., 2005. 'Without you, no one is happy': The cult of health in ancient Greece. In: H. King, ed. *Health in antiquity.* London: Routledge, pp. 120–35.

Stalter, M.-A., 1989. Fautrier, du permanent au fugace: de quelques aspects de son art entre 1920 et 1943. In: S. Pagé, ed. *Fautrier 1898–1964 (catalogue de l'exposition, Paris, Musée d'art moderne de la Ville de Paris, 25 mai–24 septembre 1989).* Paris: Amis du Musée d'art moderne de la ville de Paris, pp. 18–24.

Steingräber, S., 1980. Zum Phänomen der etruskisch-italischen Votivköpfe. *Mitteilungen des Deutschen Archäologischen Instituts: Römisch Abteilung,* 87, pp. 215–53.

Steinhart, M., 1995. *Das Motiv des Auges in der griechischen Bildkunst.* Mainz: P. non Zabern.

Stieda, L., 1899. Über altitalische Weihgeschenke. *Mitteilungen des Deutschen Archäologischen Instituts,* 14, pp. 230–43.

Stieda, L., 1901. Anatomisches über alt-italische Weihgeschenke (Donaria). *Anatomische Hefte,* 16(1), pp. 3–83.

Stocking, G.W., 1987. *Victorian anthropology.* New York, NY: The Free Press.

Storer, S.K. and Skaggs, D.L., 2006. Developmental dysplasia of the hip. *American Family Physician,* 15 October, 74(8), pp. 1310–16.

Strathern, M., 1988. *The gender of the gift: Problems with women and problems with society in Melanesia.* Berkeley, CA: University of California Press.

Tabanelli, M., 1960. Conoscenze anatomiche ed 'ex-voto' poliviscerali, etrusco romani di Tessennano, presso Vulci. *Rivista di Storia della Medicina*, 2, pp. 295–313.

Tabanelli, M., 1962. *Gli 'ex-voto' poliviscerali etruschi e romani: storia, ritrovamenti, interpretazioni*. Florence: Olschki.

Tabanelli, M., 1963. *La medicina nel mondo degli Etruschi*. Florence: Olschki.

Takács, S.A., 2005. Divine and human feet: Records of pilgrims honouring Isis. In: J. Elsner and I. Rutherford, eds. *Pilgrimage in Graeco-Roman and early Christian antiquity: Seeing the gods*. Oxford: Oxford University Press, pp. 353–69.

Tarlow, S., 2011. *Ritual, belief and the dead body in early modern Britain and Ireland*. Cambridge and New York, NY: Cambridge University Press.

Tassie, G.J., 1996. Hair-offerings: An enigmatic Egyptian custom. *Papers from the Institute of Archaeology*, 7, pp. 59–67.

Terra, A., 2014. Santa Quitéria das Frexeiras. *Ideias de fim de semana*, [blog] 24 July 2014. Available at: http://ideiasdefimdesemana.com/santa-quiteria-das-frexeiras/ [Accessed 10 March 2015].

Terrosi Zanco, O., 1966. Stipi votive di epoca Italico-Romana in grotte Abruzzesi. *Atti della Societa Toscana di Scienze Naturali*, 72, pp. 268–90.

Thomas, C.M., 1998. The sanctuary of Demeter at Pergamum: Cultic space for women and its eclipse. In: H. Koester, ed. *Pergamon citadel of the gods: Archaeological record, literary description, and religious development*. Harrisburg, PA: Trinity Press International, pp. 277–98.

Thomas, P.B., 2008. The riddle of Ishtar's shoes: The religious significance of the footprints of 'Ain Dara from a comparative perspective. *Journal of Religious History*, 32(3), pp. 303–19.

Thompson, A., 2005. *Cities of God: The religion of the Italian Comunes 1125–1325*. Pennsylvania, PA: Pennsylvania State University Press.

Thompson, C.J.S., 1922. *Greco-Roman votive offerings for health in the Wellcome Historical Medical Museum*. London: Hazell Watson & Viney.

Tisserand, N. and Nouvel, P., 2013. Sanctuaire de source, sanctuaire des eaux ou simple sanctuaire en milieu humide? Découverte d'un complexe cultuel antique à Magny-Cours (Nièvre). *Revue archéologique de l'Est et du Centre-Est*, 62, pp. 157–85.

Tomasini, G.F., 1639. *De donariis ac tabellis votivis liber singularis*. Padua: P. Frambotti.

Tommasi-Crudeli, C., 1882–84. *Istituzioni di anatomia patologica*. Two volumes. Turin: s.n.

Töpperwein, E., 1976. *Terrakotten von Pergamon*. Berlin: W. De Gruyter.

Torelli, M., 1984. *Lavinio e Roma: riti iniziatrici e matrimonio tra archeologia e storia*. Rome: Quasar.

Torelli, M., 1999. *Tota Italia: Essays in the cultural formation of Roman Italy*. Oxford: Clarendon Press.

Torelli, M., and Pohl, I., 1973. Veio. Scoperta di un piccolo santuario etrusco in località Campetti. *Notizie degli scavi*, 27, pp. 40–258.

Τσουκαλᾶς, Γ., 1851. Ἱστοριογεωγραφικὴ περιγραφὴ τῆς ἐπαρχίας Φιλιππουπόλεως. Vienna: s.n.

Turfa, J.M., 1986. Anatomical votive terracottas from Etruscan and Italic sanctuaries. In: J. Swaddling, ed. *Italian Iron Age artefacts in the British Museum: Papers of the sixth British Museum classical colloquium*. London: British Museum Press, pp. 205–13.

Turfa, J.M., 1994. Anatomical votives and Italian medical traditions. In: R.D. De Puma and J.P. Small, eds. *Murlo and the Etruscans: Art and society in ancient Etruria*. Madison, WI: University of Wisconsin Press, pp. 224–40.

Turfa, J.M., 2004. [Weihgeschenke: Altitalien und Imperium Romanum 1. Italien.] B. anatomical votives. In: *Thesaurus Cultus et Rituum Antiquorum (ThesCRA), vol. 1*. Los Angeles, CA: J. Paul Getty Museum, pp. 359–68.

Turfa, J.M., 2005. *Catalogue of the Etruscan gallery of the University of Pennsylvania Museum of Archaeology and Anthropology*. Philadelphia, PA: University of Pennsylvania Press.

Turfa, J.M., 2006a. Votive offerings in Etruscan religion. In: N.T. de Grummond and E. Simon, eds. *The religion of the Etruscans*. Austin, TX: University of Texas Press, pp. 90–115.

Turfa, J.M., 2006b. Was there room for healing in the healing sanctuaries? *Archiv für Religionsgeschichte*, 8, pp. 63–80.

Turfa, J.M., 2012. *Divining the Etruscan world: The brontoscopic calendar and religious practice*. Cambridge: Cambridge University Press.

Turfa, J.M. and Becker, M.J., 2013. Health and medicine in Etruria. In: J.M. Turfa, ed. *The Etruscan world*. London and New York, NY: Routledge, pp. 855–81.

Turner, F.M., 1981. *The Greek heritage in Victorian Britain*. New Haven, CT and London: Yale University Press.

Turner, H., 1980. *Henry Wellcome: The man, his collection and his legacy*. London: Wellcome Trust and Heinemann.

Unge Sörling, S., 1994. A collection of votive terracottas from Tessennano (Vulci). *Medelhavsmuseet Bulletin*, 29, pp. 47–54.

Vagnetti, L., 1971. *Il deposito votivo di Campetti a Veii (Materiali degli scavi 1937–1938)*. Studi e Materiali di Etruscologia e Antichità Italiche IX. Florence: Sansoni.

van der Horst, P.W., 2014. *Studies in ancient Judaism and early Christianity: Ancient Judaism and early Christianity, 87*. Leiden and Boston: Brill.

van Driel-Murray, C., 1999. And did those feet in ancient time . . . Feet and shoes as a material projection of the self. In: P. Baker, C. Forcey, S. Jundi and R. Witcher, eds. *TRAC 98: Proceedings of the eighth annual Theoretical Roman Archaeology Conference*. Oxford: Oxbow, pp. 131–40.

van Sleuwen, B.E., Engelberts, A.C., Boere-Boonekamp, M.M., Kuis, W., Schulpen, T.W.J. and L'Hoir, M.P., 2007. Swaddling: A systematic review. *Pediatrics*, 120(4), pp. 1097–106.

van Straten, F.T., 1981. Gifts for the gods. In: H.S. Versnel, ed. *Faith, hope and worship: Aspects of religious mentality in the ancient world*. Leiden: Brill, pp. 65–151.

van Straten, F.T., 1990. Votives and votaries in Greek sanctuaries. In: A. Schachter, ed. *Le Sanctuaire grec*. Entretiens sur l'Antiquité classique 37. Geneva: Fondation Hardt, pp. 247–84.

Varbanov, I., 2007. *Greek imperial coins and their values. Volume III: Thrace (from Perinthus to Trajanopolis), Chersonesos Thraciae, Insula Thraciae, Macedonia*. Adicom: Bourgas.

Varone, A., 2001. *Eroticism in Pompeii*. Los Angeles, CA: J. Paul Getty Museum.

Verhoeven, C., 1956. *Symboliek van de voet*. Assen: Van Gorcum.

Verneau, F., 2014. Évolution des espaces et des pratiques dans le sanctuaire de la Fontaine de l'Étuvée à Orléans/Cenabum. *Gallia*, 71(1), pp. 97–108.

Vernou, C. ed. 2011. *Ex-voto, retour aux sources: les bois des sources de la Seine*. Dijon: Musée archéologique de Dijon.

Versnel, H., 1991. Beyond cursing: The appeal to justice in judicial prayers. In: C.A. Faraone and D. Obbink, eds. *Magika hiera: Ancient Greek magic and religion*. Oxford: Oxford University Press, pp. 60–106.

Verstraete, B.C. and Provencal, V. eds. 2005. *Same-sex desire and love in Greco-Roman antiquity and in the classical tradition of the West*. New York, NY: Harrington Park Press.

Vikela, E., 2006. Healer gods and healing sanctuaries in Attica: Similarities and differences. *Archiv für Religionsgeschichte*, 8, pp. 41–62.

Villard, L., 2005. La vision du malade dans la Collection hippocratique. In: L. Villard, ed. *Études sur la vision dans l' antiquité classique*. Mont-Saint-Aignan: Publications des universités de Rouen et du Havre, pp. 109–30.

Vlahogiannis, N., 1998. Disabling bodies. In: D. Monserrat, ed. *Changing bodies, changing meanings: Studies on the human body in antiquity*. London and New York, NY: Routledge, pp. 13–36.

Vlahogiannis, N., 2005. Curing disability. In: H. King, ed. *Health in antiquity.* London and New York, NY: Routledge, pp. 180–91.

von Staden, H., 1989. *Herophilus: The art of medicine in early Alexandria: Edition, translation and essays.* Cambridge: Cambridge University Press.

von Staden, H., 1992. The discovery of the body: Human dissection and its cultural contexts in ancient Greece. *Yale Journal of Biology and Medicine,* 65(3), pp. 223–41.

von Staden, H., 1995. Anatomy as rhetoric: Galen on dissection and persuasion. *Journal of the History of Medicine and Allied Sciences,* 50, pp. 47–66.

Wanning Harries, E., 1994. *The unfinished manner: Essays on the fragment in the later eighteenth century.* Charlottesville, VA and London: University Press of Virginia.

Weinryb, I. ed. 2016. *Ex voto: Votive images across cultures.* Ann Arbor, MI: University of Michigan Press.

Weis, A., 2014. The public face of girlhood at Latin Lavinium in the 4th–3rd centuries BCE. In: S. Moraw and A. Kieburg, eds. *Mädchen im Altertum. Girls in antiquity.* Münster: Waxmann Verlag, pp. 287–307.

Wellcome Collection, n.d. *Medicine Man.* [online] Available at: http://wellcomecollection. org/exhibitions/medicine-man [Accessed 5 March 2015].

Weniger, L., 1923–24. Theophanien, altgriechische Götteradvente. *Archiv für Religionswissenschaft,* 22, pp. 16–57.

WHO, 2011. *World report on disability.* Malta: World Health Organization.

WHMM Handbook, 1927. Wellcome, H.S. and Malcolm, L.W.G., eds. *The Wellcome Historical Medical Museum: Handbook indicating the chief features and objects exhibited in the museum.* London: The Wellcome Foundation Ltd.

Wickkiser. B.L., 2008. *Asklepios, medicine, and the politics of healing in fifth-century Greece: Between craft and cult.* Baltimore, MD: Johns Hopkins University Press.

Wilken, G.A., 1886. Über das Haaropfer und einige andere Trauergebräucher bei den Völkern Indonesiens. *Revue Coloniale Internationale,* 2, pp. 225–69.

Yche-Fontanel, F., 2001. Les boiteux, la boiterie et le pied dans la littérature grecque ancienne. *Kentron,* 17(2), pp. 65–90.

Zamarchi Grassi, P., 1989. Recenti scoperte archeologiche ad Arezzo e nel suo agro. *Atti e Memorie Aacademia Petrarca di Lettere, Arti e Scienze,* 51, pp. 333–56.

Zifferero, A., 2002. The geography of the ritual landscape in complex societies. In: P. Attema, G.-J. Burgers, E. van Joolen, M. van Leusen and B. Mater, eds. *New developments in Italian landscape archaeology.* BAR International Series 1091. Oxford: Archaeopress, pp. 246–65.

Zingerle, J., 1926. Heiliges Recht. *Jahreshefte des Osterreichischen Archdologischen Institutes* 23, pp. 5–72.

Index

Page locators in italics indicate Figures

Printed and bound by CPI Group (UK) Ltd, Croydon, CR0 4YY

24/10/2024

01778283-0006